Treating Health Anxiety

Treating Health Anxiety

A Cognitive-Behavioral Approach

Steven Taylor
Gordon J. G. Asmundson

Foreword by Adrian Wells

THE GUILFORD PRESS
New York   London

© 2004 The Guilford Press
A Division of Guilford Publications, Inc.
72 Spring Street, New York, NY 10012
www.guilford.com

Printed in the United States of America

This book is printed on acid-free paper.

Last digit is print number: 9   8   7   6   5   4   3   2   1

Library of Congress Cataloging-in-Publication Data

Taylor, Steven, 1960–
    Treating health anxiety: a cognitive-behavioral approach / Steven Taylor, Gordon J. G.
Asmundson.
        p. cm.
Includes bibliographical references and index.
    ISBN 1-57230-998-9 (cloth)
    1. Hypochondria.   2. Cognitive therapy.   I. Asmundson, Gordon J. G.   II. Title.
    RC552.H8T39 2004
    616.85′25—dc22

                                                    2003020515

To Amy S. Janeck—S. T.
To Aleiia and Kimberley—G. J. G. A.

About the Authors

Steven Taylor, PhD, is a clinical psychologist and professor in the Department of Psychiatry at the University of British Columbia, Canada. For 10 years he was associate editor of *Behaviour Research and Therapy*, and he is now an associate editor of the *Journal of Cognitive Psychotherapy*. He has published more than 130 journal articles and book chapters and is the author of six books, including the monograph *Understanding and Treating Panic Disorder* (New York: Wiley, 2000) and the edited volume *Health Anxiety* (with Gordon J. G. Asmundson and Brian J. Cox; New York: Wiley, 2001). He served as a consultant on the recent text revision of the *Diagnostic and Statistical Manual of Mental Disorders* (DSM-IV-TR). Dr. Taylor has received early career awards from the Canadian Psychological Association, the Association for Advancement of Behavior Therapy, and the Anxiety Disorders Association of America. He is actively involved in clinical teaching and supervision, and maintains a private practice in Vancouver, British Columbia. His clinical and research interests include cognitive-behavioral treatments and mechanisms of anxiety disorders and related conditions.

Gordon J. G. Asmundson, PhD, is professor and research director in the Faculty of Kinesiology and Health Studies at the University of Regina, Canada, and adjunct professor of psychiatry at the University of Saskatchewan. He is currently the North American editor of *Cognitive Behaviour Therapy* and serves on the editorial boards for the *Journal of Anxiety Disorders*, the *Clinical Journal of Pain*, and the *European Journal of Pain*. He has published more than 110 journal articles and book chapters, as well as several books, including *Clinical Research in Mental Health* (with G. Ron Norton and Murray B. Stein;

Thousand Oaks, CA: Sage, 2001) and the edited volume *Health Anxiety* (with Steven Taylor and Brian J. Cox; New York: Wiley, 2001). He served as a member of the DSM-IV Text Revision Work Group for the Anxiety Disorders. Dr. Asmundson's research contributions have been recognized by early career awards from the Anxiety Disorders Association of America, the Canadian chapter of the International Association for the Study of Pain, and the Canadian Psychological Association. He is actively involved in clinical research and clinical research supervision and has interests in assessment and basic mechanisms of the anxiety disorders, health anxiety, acute and chronic pain, and the association of these with disability and behavior change.

Foreword

A wide range of disorders may be conceptualized at least partially as health anxiety. These include hypochondriasis, illness phobia, some somatic delusional states, panic disorder, and certain somatoform disorders. More generally, medically unexplained symptoms and health anxiety impose significant health care costs and account for a high proportion of primary care visits.

This book focuses on health anxiety disorders such as full-blown and milder (subclinical) forms of hypochondriasis. These disorders fluctuate in severity, can be highly debilitating, and in over 50% of cases persist for years. They provide a challenge to cognitive-behavioral therapists. Patients can be difficult to engage, show signs of resistance, have rigid belief systems, and offer presentations complicated by psychological and organic comorbidity. In the past hypochondriasis was regarded by many mental health professionals as an intractable condition. Notwithstanding this widespread belief, health anxiety disorders have proven to be responsive to cognitive-behavioral and drug treatments. Several controlled and uncontrolled evaluations indicate that cognitive-behavioral treatments are effective. These findings coupled with the development of models of the factors leading to the persistence of the disorder, are reasons for increased optimism.

As its foundation, the cognitive-behavioral approach assumes that health anxiety and hypochondriasis develop and are maintained by a tendency to misinterpret bodily signs and symptoms in a catastrophic fashion as a sign of serious disease or disability. This tendency to misinterpret bodily events may be linked to styles of processing one's own bodyily sensations, and may be captured in individual-difference measures such as the Somatosensory Amplification Scale and the Illness Attitudes Scales. It appears to be influenced by learning factors such as childhood exposures to illness and family death. The cognitive-behavioral approach helps to explain how the person's coping responses such as avoidance, reassurance seeking, and bodily checking feed the cycle of symptom misinterpretation and disease conviction. The mechanisms linking behavior to persistence of negative cognitions are innumerable, and include increased "perceptual pickup" of normal bodily sensations resulting from bodily checking. Traumatization of bodily tissue caused by repeated palpation can lead to "tender points." Repeated reassurance seeking and "doctor shopping" cause unnecessary tests and prescriptions that may have iatrogenic consequences. Reduced activity and use of "guarded movements" contribute to loss of physical fitness and greater symptoms following physical exertion. Cognitive-behavioral therapy is based on a case formulation approach that aims to capture these elements in an idiosyncratic understanding of cognitive and behavioral factors contributing to the problem.

A key to cognitive-behavioral treatment is shifting the patient away from a disease model of his or her problem and toward acceptance of an alternative explanation. This can be achieved by exploring alternative explanations for symptoms, by changing assumptions in a way that allows an acceptance that unexpected symptoms do not always signal serious illness, and by more direct challenges of specific beliefs about disease when possible. A whole armory of cognitive, behavioral, and interpersonal methods have been devised and used for this purpose. Some are explicitly cognitive in nature and aim to remove the factors that contribute to persistence. Others, such as stress management approaches, which also appear to be effective, may have fewer direct effects on beliefs by providing an alternative, nondisease perspective on symptoms. One way to construe effective cognitive-behavioral therapy is to assume that it equips a patient with an alternative, noncatastrophic knowledge base on which to draw in interpreting ambiguous internal events.

Before treatment can proceed, however, the therapist is faced with the task of engaging clients in treatment. Some patients are ambivalent toward psychological treatment, only attending sessions at the behest of another person. For instance, it is not unheard of for a patient to concede that he or she is pursuing psychological treatment to convince the primary care physician that there is *not* a psychological explanation for the problem, so that medical testing may be resumed. In the quest to enhance patient engagement, therapists have devised a variety of socialization experiments and motivational procedures.

All of these issues and more are covered in this timely book by Steven Taylor and Gordon J. G. Asmundson. It promises to be an invaluable source of information and practical guidance for the clinician faced with the assessment and treatment of health anxiety. It charts the interaction between cognitive and behavioral factors involved in the development and persistence of disease conviction, and describes a wide range of useful treatment strategies. Taylor and Asmundson provide an extensive and useful review of the empirical literature on mechanisms and treatment outcomes as a backdrop for their discussion of assessment and cognitive-behavioral intervention. The authors base their approach on case formulations, which represent the predisposing, precipitating, maintaining, and protective factors thought to be involved in individual presentations. Therapists will also find that the authors of this volume directly consider important issues of patient motivation and engagement.

The review of treatments in this book is impressive in its inclusion of a wide range of approaches, some of which will be familiar to seasoned cognitive-behavioral therapists but many of which, such as attention training, are still quite novel. The book is replete with clinical case examples and material that brings added life to the subject and provides an excellent level of clarity. The wealth of experience the authors bring to the topic is evident in their choice of effective strategies from among the plethora of techniques that exist. The book also includes handouts and appendices for therapist use.

Taylor and Asmundson offer both a practical guide to treatment, and, through their unique synthesis of material, contribute to academic debate about the antecedents, maintenance, and treatment of hypochondriasis and other forms of health anxiety.

ADRIAN WELLS
University of Manchester, United Kingdom

Preface

Like death and taxes, health anxiety is a universal experience, which everyone has had at some time or other to a greater or lesser degree. For most of us, health anxiety is a mild and fleeting reaction to minor ailments, or arises as an appropriate response to life-threatening disease. For some people, however, this anxiety is excessive, debilitating, and chronic. That is, the anxiety is disproportionate, given the person's health status. This is a defining feature of the health anxiety disorders.

We consider these disorders to represent a spectrum of severity. At one end lie the relatively mild conditions known as abridged forms of hypochondriasis, such as transient hypochondriasis. We consider disease phobia to be a form of partial or abridged hypochondriasis. Full-blown hypochondriasis, as defined by DSM-IV, occupies the middle of the spectrum. At the severe end lie poor-insight hypochondriasis and the somatic form of delusional disorder. The latter is characterized by somatic delusions, such as delusions of parasitic infestation, without other psychotic features.

Hypochondriasis afflicts up to 5% of the general population, and its abridged form is even more prevalent. Apart from health anxiety disorders, excessive health anxiety can be a feature of other psychiatric disorders, such as anxiety disorders, mood disorders, and adjustment disorders. Excessive health anxiety places a considerable burden on the health care system, leading to needless medical consultations and unnecessary and potentially harmful medical tests. Thus, excessive health anxiety is a common and costly problem.

Over the past decade there have been major advances in understanding and treating health anxiety disorders. Cognitive-behavioral therapies have shown promise in mental health clinics and in general medical settings. There also have been important advances in pharmacological treatment of health anxiety disorders, particularly in treating somatic delusions. Dissemination of these treatments continues to be a problem, partly because of the lack of practical handbooks for clinicians and trainees. Although there have been several excellent books and book chapters on various aspects of health anxiety, there are few comprehensive texts to guide the clinician in treating health anxiety disorders. Our aim in writing this book was to bridge this gap by providing a clear, detailed, empirically based coverage of the nature, assessment, and treatment of health anxiety disorders, with an emphasis on cognitive-behavioral approaches. We also draw on our own clinical experiences and on the important work of many others, including Arthur Barsky, Hillary Warwick, Paul Salkovskis, Adrian Wells, Theo Bouman, John Walker, and Patricia Furer.

We hope this volume will be a useful resource for a range of health care practitioners, including psychologists and various types of medical practitioners, such as psychiatrists, internists, and primary care physicians. This volume should also be a useful tool for trainees in these disciplines, such as psychology interns and psychiatry residents.

Many people have contributed directly or indirectly to this book. Thanks to our patients who have taught us so much about health anxiety. Thanks also to Amy Janeck and Pam Weigartz for sharing their clinical experiences. We are also grateful to Patricia Furer and John Walker for generously sharing their hypochondriasis treatment manual and clinical experiences. We wish to thank Jim Nageotte, Senior Editor at The Guilford Press, for his helpful advice in guiding this project through to fruition. Case examples described in this book have been modified to protect patient privacy and confidentiality. Following the guidelines set out by Clifft (1986), the case illustrations are either disguised to eliminate identifying information, or represent composite descriptions, combining material from several patients.

Contents

Treating Health Anxiety

1

What Is Health Anxiety?

"I've been sickly ever since I was a kid. For the past week I've been feeling out of sorts, but not in a way I can clearly describe. I'm sure something's wrong. I'm scared I might have MS [multiple sclerosis]. Or maybe it's AIDS."

"Every morning in the bathroom I check my body for unusual moles and lesions. Today I found a bump on my skin that I hadn't noticed before. I couldn't stop worrying that it might be cancer. As I prodded and squeezed the bump to check it out, it got bigger, redder, and angrier. That really frightened me, to the point that I had to snip it off with nail clippers."

These people are physically healthy, as their physicians have told them—repeatedly. They are suffering from excessive health anxiety. The purpose of this book is to describe the nature, assessment, and treatment of health anxiety disorders, including hypochondriasis, the various forms of abridged hypochondriasis (among which we include disease phobia), and delusional disorder (somatic type). These are all characterized by excessive anxiety about one's health, stemming from beliefs that one's physical integrity is threatened. Like other forms of anxiety (Lang, 1985), health anxiety is a multifaceted phenomenon, consisting of distressing emotions (e.g., fear, dread), physiological arousal and associated bodily sensations (e.g., palpitations), thoughts and images of danger, and avoidance and other defensive behaviors. Health anxiety ranges from mild and transient to severe and chronic. Our emphasis is on the

1

more debilitating, persistent forms, particularly hypochondriasis. We begin this chapter by defining health anxiety and distinguishing its adaptive and maladaptive forms. We then describe the clinical features of hypochondriasis and related disorders, and explain why health anxiety disorders are important for health care practitioners to understand, detect, and treat.

WHEN IS HEALTH ANXIETY MALADAPTIVE?

Health anxiety varies in the extent to which it is adaptive versus excessive or maladaptive. Virtually all of us have experienced health anxiety at times in our lives. Often the anxiety is adaptive because it motivates us to seek appropriate medical care. Worry about chest pain in a person with a history of cardiac disease, for example, can lead him or her to promptly summon an ambulance when the pain occurs, thereby reducing the risk of mortality.

Health anxiety is maladaptive if it is out of proportion with the objective degree of medical risk. Low anxiety in the face of high risk or high anxiety in the face of low risk can be maladaptive. Lack of worry about the health risks of smoking, for example, can have deadly consequences. Conversely, excessive worry about minor, harmless bodily changes (e.g., spots or rashes) or bodily sensations (e.g., muscle twinges) can cause undue suffering and impairment in social and occupational functioning. The nature and causes of insufficient concern about one's health are not the primary focus of this volume but are discussed in texts on health psychology (e.g., S. E. Taylor, 1999).

HYPOCHONDRIASIS

Diagnostic Criteria

Table 1.1 lists the DSM-IV criteria for hypochondriasis (American Psychiatric Association [APA], 2000). Table 1.2 expands on these criteria by describing the cognitive, emotional, somatic, and behavioral features of hypochondriasis. Table 1.1 is useful for diagnosing hypochondriasis, whereas Table 1.2 better conveys the clinical features of this disorder. These features often, but not always, co-occur.

Cognitive Features

The belief that one is physically ill is known as *disease conviction*. People with hypochondriasis have strong disease convictions, insisting that they have a serious disease that has been undetected by medical investigations. Disease convictions arise from misinterpretations of bodily changes and sensations.

TABLE 1.1. DSM-IV Diagnostic Criteria for Hypochondriasis

A.	Preoccupation with fears of having a serious disease, or the idea that one has such a disease, based in misinterpretation of one's bodily sensations or changes.
B.	Preoccupation persists despite appropriate medical evaluation and reassurance.
C.	The idea that one has a serious disease is not of delusion intensity (as in delusional disorder) and is not restricted to concerns about one's appearance (as in body dysmorphic disorder).
D.	The preoccupation causes significant distress or impairment in social, occupational, or other important areas of functioning.
E.	Duration for at least 6 months.
F.	The preoccupation is not better accounted for by another disorder, such as another somatoform disorder or major depressive disorder.
Poor-insight specifier:	The person is said to have poor insight if, for most of the time during the course of the disorder, he or she does not recognize that his or her concern about having a serious disease is excessive or unreasonable.

Note. Adapted from American Psychiatric Association (2000, p. 507). Copyright 2000 by the American Psychiatric Association. Adapted by permission.

TABLE 1.2. Clinical Features of Hypochondriasis

Cognitive features
• Disease conviction: Belief that one has a serious disease
• Disease preoccupation: Recurrent thoughts and images of disease and death
• Hypervigilance for bodily changes
• Difficulty accepting medical reassurance

Somatic features
• Anxiety-related bodily reactions (e.g., palpitations)
• Benign bodily changes and sensations (e.g., blemishes, mild aches and pains) that are misinterpreted

Hypochondriacal fears
• Fear of currently having a disease
• Fear of contracting a disease in the future
• Fear or anxiety on exposure to disease-related stimuli

Behavioral responses
• Repeatedly checking one's body
• Reassurance seeking (e.g., from physicians or significant others) that one does not have serious symptoms or diseases
• Repeated requests for medical tests
• Checking other sources of medical information (e.g., Internet searches of medical websites)
• Avoiding or escaping disease-related stimuli

Strong disease conviction is associated with *preoccupation* with the possibility of having some dire disease. This is associated with preoccupation with one's bodily appearance and functioning, and hypervigilance for bodily sensations. People suffering from hypochondriasis experience recurrent thoughts and images of disease and death, which intrude, often unbidden, into the stream of consciousness (Warwick & Salkovskis, 1989). One hypochondriasis patient, for example, was bothered by recurrent thoughts that she was about to die from HIV. Her thoughts were accompanied by distressing images of "being pushed into a coffin and buried alive because she is bad" and "husband and son cheerfully visiting her grave with another woman whom he calls mummy" (Wells & Hackmann, 1993, p. 268).

Disease conviction and preoccupation persist even though the person receives reassurance from physicians that there is no evidence of serious disease, and even though the frightening "symptoms" rarely become progressively worse (as might happen in the case of a serious physical condition). People with hypochondriasis typically resist the idea that they are suffering from a mental disorder. Although they may have poor insight into the excessive nature of their health anxiety, by definition they are not delusional. They are able to acknowledge, at least in their calmer moments, that their health concerns are exaggerated.

Somatic Features

People with hypochondriasis tend to misinterpret the seriousness of innocuous, natural bodily fluctuations, and overestimate the seriousness of symptoms of general medical conditions[1] (Côté et al., 1996). They may complain of highly specific symptoms, or report symptoms that are vague, variable, and generalized (e.g., aching "all over"). Common specific symptoms include localized pain, bowel complaints (e.g., changes in bowel habits), and cardiorespiratory sensations (e.g., chest tightness). People with hypochondriasis are more concerned with the meaning of their physical symptoms than with any associated discomfort or pain (Barsky & Klerman, 1983).

Hypochondriacal Fears

People with hypochondriasis have some form of disease fear (Kellner, 1985; Noyes, Stuart, Longley, Longbehn, & Happel, 2002). There are two types: fear that one *currently has* a disease, and fear that one *might contract* a disease in

---

[1]Throughout this text we adopt the term *general medical condition* (APA, 2000) to refer to all medical disorders apart from psychiatric disorders.

the future. A person can simultaneously have both types of fear, perhaps because both are associated with fears of dying and death. When Jane W. noticed mildly painful sensations around her eyes, she was preoccupied with fear of having a brain tumor. Jane also feared that some day she might have another bout of blepharitis (eyelid inflammation). She had had bouts in the past and worried that further episodes might lead to blindness.

Disease conviction is closely associated with fear of currently having a disease, and is also correlated with fear of contracting a disease in the future (Cox, Borger, Asmundson, & Taylor, 2000; Hadjistavropoulos, Frombach, & Amundson, 1999; Stewart & Watt, 2000). Fear of having a disease is more central to full-blown hypochondriasis than fear of acquiring a future disease (Côté et al., 1996). The latter fear is a core feature of one of the other health anxiety disorders we discuss in this book: disease phobia.

People with disease fears become frightened or anxious when exposed to stimuli that they believe to be disease-related, such as bodily sensations or other somatic changes. These people also become anxious when exposed to disease-related information, such as medical TV programs, which can lead them to worry that they might have acquired the disease in question. They also often become anxious if they come into contact with people who appear to be ill.

The two disease fears can be functionally related: fear of having a disease (and associated disease conviction) can lead to fears of contracting other diseases. Bob H. was frightened that his immune system had been dangerously weakened because of exposure to solvents at work. He interpreted various bodily sensations, such as fatigue and nasal congestion, as evidence of immunological impairment. Bob also feared that he might someday come down with Asian flu, which he thought would certainly kill him because of his compromised immune system. Thus, his fear of Asian flu was a result of his fear (and associated belief) that his immune system had been compromised.

A person can shift from fear of contracting a disease to fear of actually having the disease. George K. had had a serious anaphylactic (allergic) reaction during childhood after eating a handful of peanuts. The attack was rapid and extreme; his face puffed up like a balloon, his tongue swelled, and his throat tightened to the point that he could barely breathe. George would have died if his mother had not rushed him to hospital. As an adult, George constantly feared he would have a future, possibly lethal, anaphylactic attack. On several occasions he believed he was actually having an attack. One day while eating a banana he noticed that the back of his throat felt scratchy. He misinterpreted this as a symptom of anaphylaxis. He became so frightened that he called an ambulance. Thus, there was a shift in George's focus of apprehension, from fear of contracting a disease to fear of actually having the disease.

Behavioral Reactions

Behavioral Consequences of Fear of Having a Disease

It is important to distinguish between the two forms of disease fear because they can lead to different behavioral reactions: reassurance seeking and checking versus avoidance and escape (Côté et al., 1996). Fear of having a disease is associated with reassurance seeking (e.g., from primary care physicians), recurrent checking of one's body (e.g., frequent breast self-examinations), seeking out other sources of information on the dreaded disease (e.g., checking medical textbooks), and trying various kinds of remedies (e.g., herbal preparations).

Sufferers may perpetually adopt a "sick role," living as an invalid and avoiding all effortful occupational and home responsibilities (Barsky, 1992). They may persistently complain about their health, discussing their concerns in great detail with anyone who will listen. They frequently seek medical attention even though these consultations rarely confirm their beliefs about having a serious disease. During medical appointments they are often difficult to interrupt in terms of discussion about their health concerns. This is what some frustrated clinicians disparagingly call the "organ recital." It reflects the patient's preoccupation with disease.

Patients with hypochondriasis often have poor relationships with their physicians. Frustration and anger on the part of physician and patient are not uncommon (APA, 2000). Physicians, particularly those working in primary care settings, may have only 15–20 minutes for each consultation, which makes it difficult to thoroughly assess patients with long detailed histories of health anxiety. Physicians also may lack the expertise required to assess and treat health anxiety disorders. These factors can contribute to physician frustration. On the other side of the coin, patients may feel that their physicians are not taking them seriously, and worry that their physicians are not sufficiently competent. People with hypochondriasis commonly complain that their physicians are unable to satisfactorily explain or treat their bodily complaints. This may prompt the person to go "doctor shopping." That is, he or she may visit many different physicians in the hope of finding help (Kasteler, Kane, Olsen, & Thetford, 1976; Sato, Takerchi, Shirahama, Fukui, & Gude, 1995). As a result of doctor shopping, some people with hypochondriasis undergo many different medical and surgical treatments, which can produce troubling side effects or treatment complications, such as scarring and pain from repeated surgeries. Thus, hypochondriasis can be worsened by iatrogenic (physician-induced) factors.

Many people with hypochondriasis repeatedly visit hospital emergency rooms (ERs), believing that *this time* there is something seriously wrong with them. When the patient repeatedly "cries wolf," the physician may grow dismissive of his or her complaints. Such frequent ER attendees are sometimes put on "time-out" by the attending physicians. That is, the patient is made to wait an inordinate amount of time, sometimes for several hours, before being seen by a physician. This strategy is thought to make ER visits unpleasant for the patient, thereby reducing his or her incentive for repeatedly making unnecessary hospital visits.

Unfortunately, a dismissive approach by physicians can fuel patients' concerns that they are not getting proper medical care. In turn, this can strengthen their belief that they have a serious undiagnosed medical condition. Although it is tempting for busy clinicians to dismiss concerns voiced by the "worried well," one should not assume that their fears are always unfounded. People with hypochondriasis—like everyone else—will eventually succumb to some deadly affliction, such as cancer or cardiovascular disease. Periodic medical evaluations are required for people with hypochondriasis, just as they are necessary for everyone else. Routine evaluations are particularly important for older adults with hypochondriasis, where general medical conditions are quite likely to be present.

Behavioral Consequences of Fear of Contracting a Disease

Fear of acquiring a disease is associated with avoidance and escape from stimuli that the person believes to be associated with disease. For example, he or she may avoid hospitals, avoid sickly looking people, and limiting contact with people exposed to sickness such as physicians and nurses. Fear that one might contract a disease can also lead to avoidance of all reminders of the disease. Alan V., for example, had an extremely strong fear of contracting cancer. He avoided all things associated with cancer, including newspapers and magazines that carried stories about people battling cancer, TV programs about stars who had battled cancer, and foods supposedly containing potential carcinogens.

Understanding Behavior by Understanding the Interplay among Disease Fears

The fact that a person can shift from one disease fear to the other, means that health anxious people may shift from avoidance to repetitive checking and reassurance seeking. Understanding the nature of their patients' fears can therefore help clinicians understand why health-anxious people sometimes avoid and sometimes seek out disease-related stimuli. People who are frightened of contracting a disease tend to avoid disease-related stimuli such as hospitals and physicians. But when they believe they have acquired the disease they will seek out these stimuli, sometimes assiduously.

> Becky A. intentionally avoided performing breast self-examinations as part of her fear and avoidance of all things related to breast cancer. The only checking performed was a yearly mammogram by her doctor. When an annual checkup revealed a small benign cyst, Becky feared that she had developed cancer. Removal of the cyst did not assuage her fears. Becky began to compulsively check her breasts to determine whether she had other cysts. At times she palpated her breasts until they were sore, and she visited her doctor weekly for reassurance.

Health Habits

People with hypochondriasis often pursue various forms of self-diagnosis and self-treatment (Barsky, Wyshak, & Klerman, 1986) and some, in fact, may have little contact with the medical system. "A preoccupation with one's body, disease, and health may be found among the impassioned proponents of health foods, rigid diets, and elaborate vitamin regimens and among physical fitness and exercise fanatics" (Barsky & Klerman, 1983, p. 274). These people probably represent only a subgroup of cases of hypochondriasis. The majority have no better health habits than people without the disorder. They are just as likely to smoke, eat fatty foods, drink too much coffee or alcohol, and fail to exercise regularly (APA, 2000).

How can we account for this paradoxical coexistence of excessively high health anxiety and average or even poor health habits? It appears that many people with hypochondriasis are "symptom-driven" in their behavior. Their activities seem to be motivated largely by the presence of bodily changes and sensations. These people appear to be more intent on escaping current disease threats than on promoting their health. In our clinical experience, this is especially true for people who fear that they currently have a disease. A healthy lifestyle seems to be more common in people who are frightened of acquiring a future disease, particularly people who believe that such a lifestyle will help them avoid some dreaded affliction.

Hypochondriasis and General Medical Conditions

Although a person suffering from hypochondriasis may have a coexisting general medical condition, a diagnosis of hypochondriasis is only made when the general medical condition does not fully account for the person's concerns about disease or for his or her bodily changes or sensations (APA, 2000). This is illustrated by the following examples (Schmidt, 1994):

- Hypochondriasis would be diagnosed when the person catastrophically misinterprets medical information about a general medical condition. Bill B. suffered from benign prostate hypertrophy (enlargement). His primary care physician told him that his screening test for prostate cancer was negative. Bill misinterpreted "negative" as meaning "very bad news," and therefore believed he had cancer. When his physician tried to correct this misconception, Bill worried that the doctor was simply trying to soften the bad news because Bill was so clearly distressed.
- When a person has a serious medical condition with a good prognosis, hypochondriasis would be diagnosed when she or he becomes excessively anxious about the prognosis and is unable to accept the physician's reassurance. Joanne T. had a congenital cardiac defect that required an artificial valve. Despite being told by her cardiologist that the prognosis was excellent, Joanne greatly feared she would soon die. She was preoccupied with the clicking sound made by the valve, and kept focusing on the noise in order to check that her heart was beating properly.
- Hypochondriasis would be diagnosed when the disease fear or disease conviction is based on bodily changes and sensations that have nothing to do with the diagnosed disease. Daniel P. was involved in a serious motor accident that left him a paraplegic. Although he felt distressed and vulnerable as a result of the disability, he was more concerned about developing cancer. During his stay in the hospital he met several terminal cancer patients from an adjacent ward who were obviously in a great deal of pain and suffering. This greatly frightened Daniel, and he became preoccupied with getting cancer.
- Hypochondriasis would be diagnosed when there is evidence that it was present before the development of a general medical condition.

Intermittent bouts of medically verified disease might sometimes reinforce hypochondriacal beliefs. However, the opposite can also occur. The diagnosis of serious medical disease—in patients with accurately diagnosed hypochondriasis—sometimes ameliorates hypochondriacal symptoms because the disease legitimizes the patients' complaints, sanctions their assumption of the sick role, affirms their experience of illness, and lessens the skepticism with which they had been previously regarded (Barsky, Fama, Bailey, & Ahern, 1998b). Patients with hypochondriasis sometimes describe a sense of vindication and validation after receiving a diagnosis of a general medical condition, and they note an improvement in their relationships with their physicians: "Now that I know Dr X. is paying attention to me, I can believe him when he says there's nothing wrong" (Barsky et al., 1998b).

Relationship between Hypochondriasis and Other Psychiatric Disorders

Hypochondriasis frequently co-occurs with mood disorders, anxiety disorders, and somatization disorder (Noyes, 2001). To illustrate, among patients with hypochondriasis assessed in primary care settings, 38–43% had concurrent major depression, which was significantly higher than the frequency of major depression in primary care patients without hypochondriasis (16–18%). Similarly, panic disorder was more common in primary care patients with hypochondriasis (16–17%) than in their counterparts without hypochondriasis (3–6%) (Barsky, Barnett, & Cleary, 1994a; Noyes et al., 1994b).

Comorbidity has two important implications. First, it raises questions about how a particular patient should be treated. If someone has hypochondriasis and major depression, should the clinician try to treat both disorders at once, or should one disorder be treated first? A case formulation (see Chapter 6) can help answer this question. Second, comorbidity patterns might shed light on the causes of hypochondriasis. If hypochondriasis commonly co-occurs with other disorders, then this might indicate a common etiology. A further suggestion of shared etiology arises from the fact that hypochondriasis is phenomenologically similar to several of the disorders with which it commonly co-occurs. Like somatization disorder, hypochondriasis is associated with medically unexplained symptoms. Like obsessive–compulsive disorder, hypochondriasis is associated with behaviors that the person feels compelled to perform, such as reassurance seeking and repeatedly checking one's body. Like major depression, hypochondriasis is associated with somatic complaints (e.g., poor sleep, poor appetite, lack of energy) and pessimism about one's future.

These similarities and comorbidity patterns have led some theorists to speculate that hypochondriasis is really a form of some other disorder. Some investigators have suggested that hypochondriasis and somatization disorder are the same thing (Cloninger, Sigvardsson, von Knorring, & Bohman, 1984; Escobar, Swartz, Rubin-Stipec, & Manu, 1991; Vaillant, 1984). Others have suggested that hypochondriasis is an obsessive–compulsive spectrum disorder (Hollander, 1993; Stein, 2000; Yaryura-Tobias & Neziroglu, 1997).

Other writers have speculated that hypochondriasis is a "masked" form of depression (Goodstein, 1985; Lesse, 1980) or a psychodynamic defense against depression (Dorfman, 1968). If hypochondriasis is a defense against depression, then one would expect patients with hypochondriasis to be less depressed than psychiatric patients without hypochondriasis. Research has failed to support this prediction; hypochondriasis patients tend to be just as depressed as psychiatric controls, if not more so (Kellner, Abbott, Winslow, & Pathak, 1989). Moreover, when hypochondriasis is treated (e.g., with cognitive-behavioral therapy), there is little evidence that an underlying ("unmasked") mood disorder arises. Indeed, the evidence suggests the opposite. When treatment reduces hypochondriasis, there is a tendency for depression also to abate (see Chapter 5). Thus, the "masked depression" and psychodynamic defense hypotheses are inconsistent with empirical findings. The issue of whether hypochondriasis has a common etiology with other disorders is examined in Chapter 2.

OTHER CLINICALLY IMPORTANT FORMS OF HEALTH ANXIETY

Abridged Hypochondriasis

Health anxiety, as the primary (most severe) presenting problem, can be clinically important even when the person does not meet the full DSM-IV criteria for hypochondriasis. This form of health anxiety has been called *abridged hypochondriasis* (Gureje, Üstün, & Simon, 1997), which differs from full-blown hypochondriasis in that one or more of the diagnostic features of hypochondriasis are not present (see Table 1.1). For example, the person might be preoccupied with fears of having a serious disease but eventually responds to appropriate medical reassurance (i.e., she or he meets all but criterion B). Alternatively, the person could be preoccupied with fears of disease and be impervious to medical reassurance, but still be able to function reasonably well (i.e., she or he merits all but criterion D).

> Joan F. had experienced many episodes of health anxiety, often in reaction to news stories she encountered. Most recently, she read a news report claiming that cellular phones caused leukemia. Joan began to worry that she too had leukemia. After all, her cell phone became quite hot after a full day of use. Wasn't that a sign of deadly radiation? A thorough medical evaluation yielded no evidence of leukemia. Joan was eventually able to accept this reassurance, although she soon began to worry about other potential health problems, such as viruses borne through the air conditioning. Despite a long-standing history of health anxiety, her distress was never severe or incapacitating. Therefore, she was diagnosed with abridged rather than full-blown hypochondriasis.

Transient Hypochondriasis

Transient hypochondriasis is another common term used to describe health anxiety that does not fully meet the DSM-IV criteria for hypochondriasis. *Transient hypochondriasis* is actually a form of abridged hypochondriasis in which clinically significant health anxiety lasts for no more than 6 months (i.e., it meets all but criterion E). Transient hypochondriasis, like other forms of excessive health anxiety, can be triggered by general medical conditions and by other life stressors (Barsky, Wyshak, & Klerman, 1990b; Ford, 1983; Kellner, 1986).

Various factors may influence whether hypochondriasis is transient or chronic. The disorder is more likely to be chronic when (1) the person receives incentives ("secondary gains") for remaining in the sick role, (2) when life stressors are persistent (causing arousal-related bodily sensations that the person misinterprets), and (3) when the person is socially isolated and therefore has more opportunity to dwell on his or her body (Barsky et al., 1990b). Hypochondriasis is likely to be transient when the life stressors have abated, such as when a medical condition has resolved (Barsky et al., 1990b) or when the person obtains persuasive medical assurance that he or she does not have a serious medical condition.

> John B. was on vacation in Mexico when he noticed a small amount of rectal bleeding after a bowel movement. John reacted with horror because he vividly recalled his father's slow, painful death from colon cancer. John feared that he too had developed a cancerous polyp. During each day of his week-long vacation he thought of nothing but the possibility of cancer. His wife complained that he seemed distant and distracted, and he often excused himself from recreational activities to go to the washroom and check for blood. John's worries were eventually assuaged when, on returning home, his physician told him that there was no sign of cancer: he simply had hemorrhoids. John's health anxiety quickly abated because he trusted his doctor's opinion and found the explanation to be quite plausible. John's doctor pointed out that the tests were negative, that the bleeding was mild and sporadic, and that this pattern was inconsistent with the progressive development of cancer.

Increased knowledge about diseases can lead to transient increases in health anxiety. This is exemplified by *medical student's disease*, which is the short-lived increase in anxiety that occurs when medical students learn about various life-threatening maladies (see Chapter 4). Another potent source of disease-related information is the news media, which can play a prominent role in triggering transient hypochondriasis. Shortly after the terrorist attacks of September 11, 2001, there was a wave of bioterrorism consisting of a small number of actual exposures to anthrax spores mailed in letters, along with a large number of hoaxes and other false alarms. Some people coped with these threats by telling themselves that "it will never happen to me." They reminded themselves that the likelihood of contamination was minuscule compared to the risk of everyday threats, such as the odds of being in a serious motor vehicle accident. This coping strategy prevented most people from feeling anxious and allowed them to carry on with the important tasks in their lives. But other people reacted by becoming highly anxious and hypervigilant for threat. They became alarmed when they experienced minor ailments, such as sore throats or chest congestion, worrying that their symptoms could be due to anthrax exposure. These people adopted a "better safe than sorry" approach by engaging in various sorts of protective behaviors. Some donned gas masks and protective gloves before opening their mail, while others stockpiled antibiotics. Most episodes of excessive health anxiety appeared to be short-lived, typically lasting for no more than a few weeks and abating once the threat of bioterrorism receded. Nevertheless, these transient hypochondriacal reactions significantly impaired the functioning of many people.

Disease Phobia

Specific phobia of acquiring or being exposed to a disease is a DSM-IV anxiety disorder. It is associated with distress, apprehension, and avoidance of situations that may, in the mind of the person, lead to contracting the dreaded disease (APA, 2000). Disease phobia is commonly a feature of full-blown hypochondriasis (Kellner, 1985; Marks, 1987; Pilowsky, 1967), although it can exist on its own, without the other features of hypochondriasis. The person with disease phobia is fearful of contracting a disease, but does not believe that he or she has already contracted it, and may respond to medical reassurance. Thus, we share Marks's (1987) view that disease phobia is an abridged form of hypochondriasis.

Unlike people with full-blown hypochondriasis, people with disease phobia do not typically possess the symptoms of the disease they fear contracting, although they may present with somatic symptoms of anxiety (Côté et al., 1996). Someone phobic of developing skin cancer, for example, would not typically complain of skin lesions, but might complain of nervousness, muscle tension, sweating, and palpitations.

Disease phobia can take a variety of forms, with the most common being fear of developing cancer or acquiring a communicable disease. Paul S. presented with a severe phobia of contracting HIV, associated with fear and avoidance of public washrooms. Although he acknowledged that it was unlikely that he could get HIV from public washrooms, he believed that infection was still possible. He worried that if he had to use a public washroom, the virus might make its way into his body through the pores of his skin.

Somatic Delusions

We include delusional disorder (somatic type) among the health anxiety disorders because of the increasing recognition that delusions are on a continuum with other beliefs, differing quantitatively rather than qualitatively (Chadwick, Birchwood, & Trower, 1996). People with extremely strong, unshakable, and unfounded beliefs that they have a serious disease are suffering from somatic delusions. The most common forms of somatic delusions are (1) that one is emitting a foul odor from the skin or a body orifice; (2) that one is infested with insects or parasites; (3) that certain parts of the body are misshapen or ugly, contrary to objective evidence; and (4) that parts of one's body (e.g., the circulatory system) are not functioning properly (APA, 2000).

Some people with somatic delusions vociferously complain to public health departments that their dwellings are infested with vermin, and they frequently call on the services of pest control agencies. It is also not uncommon for people with delusions of vermin infestation to consult university zoology departments in the hope of identifying the offending vermin and discovering some method of eradication. This can be seen from a recent account from our zoologist colleague Dr. Karen Needham:

> Ten years ago, when I first began taking care of the Spencer Entomological Museum in the Department of Zoology at UBC [University of British Columbia], I would occasionally (once or twice a year) receive a call from a member of the general public complaining about a serious insect invasion in their home. The insects were described as living in clothing, bedding, furniture, and on or under the skin. They were characterized as tiny and fast moving, with their bite accompanied by a sudden, sharp pain; the feeling of them burrowing under the skin was unbearable. So small were they that their victims could barely see them with the naked eye, so fast moving that capturing a specimen for identification was impossible. The few times that people complaining of such an infestation did manage to send something in for identification, the sample invariably consisted of lint, kitchen crumbs, and sometimes human skin. . . . Sadly, in recent years, the number of these calls that I receive has increased dramatically. . . . One elderly woman had become so distraught that she had rid her home of all of its furnishings and was sleeping each night on her freshly scrubbed, bare kitchen floor. Another elderly gentleman could only get relief from the sensation of "little, black insects" burrowing into his skin by dousing himself daily with undiluted kerosene. (2000, p. 16)

If the delusional person does not meet criteria for schizophrenia or a mood disorder, and if the delusions are not due to substance intoxication, or a cognitive disorder (e.g., delirium), or a general medical condition, then the person would be diagnosed with delusional disorder (somatic type) (APA, 2000). It can be difficult to distinguish this disorder from the poor-insight subtype of hypochondriasis. The difference is a matter of degree; compared to delusional disorder, the disease beliefs in poor-insight hypochondriasis are not as strongly held and are more likely to wax and wane over time and circumstance.

It is unclear whether delusional disorder (somatic type) is best regarded as a psychotic spectrum disorder (related to schizophrenia) or whether it should be considered an extreme form of hypochondriasis (akin to poor-insight hypochondriasis). Certain forms of treatment, such as some pharmaco-therapies and cognitive-behavioral interventions, may be effective for poor-insight hypochondriasis and delusional disorder.

Other Disorders

Excessive health anxiety can also be a feature of other disorders, such as panic disorder and major depressive disorder. For example, worry about dying commonly occurs during panic attacks in people with panic disorder. In these cases, a diagnosis of hypochondriasis would not be given if excessive health anxiety appeared to be part of, or "due to," another disorder (APA, 2000). That is, these presentations would not be considered to be primarily health anxiety disorders. However, if a person with panic disorder also had a broader pattern of disease convictions and disease fears that were unrelated to panic attacks, then a diagnosis of hypochondriasis or other health anxiety disorder would be considered.

PERSONAL AND ECONOMIC COSTS OF HEALTH ANXIETY DISORDERS

The severity of health anxiety is often unrelated to objective measures of physical health (Barsky et al., 1986). Even so, excessive health anxiety—whether in the form of hypochondriasis or related disorders—can seriously impair a person's social and occupational functioning. People with excessive health anxiety, compared to others, are less likely to be employed outside the home, have more days of bed rest, have greater physical limitations, and are more likely to be living on disability benefits (Barsky et al., 1990b, 1998b; Escobar et al., 1998; Noyes et al., 1993). They also pay more visits to primary care physicians and specialists, have more medical laboratory tests and surgical procedures, and impose a greater economic burden on the health care system (Barsky, Ettner, Horsky, & Bates, 2001; Barsky et al., 1986; Hollifield, Paine, Tuttle, & Kellner, 1999). In fact, medically unexplained "symptoms" account for 25–50% of all primary care visits (Barsky, 2000).

PREVALENCE, ONSET, AND COURSE

Despite some inconsistencies, most studies have found that excessive health anxiety is equally common among women and men (Asmundson, Taylor, & Cox, 2001). Estimates suggest that full hypochondriasis has a lifetime prevalence in the general population of 1–5%, and is found in 2–7% of primary care outpatients (APA, 2000). Thus, hypochondriasis is as common as many major psychiatric disorders, such as panic disorder and schizophrenia. Abridged hypochondriasis is more common than the full-blown disorder (Kirmayer & Robbins, 1991; Looper & Kirmayer, 2001; Noyes et al., 1993), suggesting that excessive health anxiety is a widespread clinical problem. The lifetime prevalence of each form of abridged hypochondriasis is unknown. The point prevalence of disease phobia is 3–4% (Agras, Sylvester, & Oliveau, 1969; Malis, Hartz, Doebbeling, & Noyes, 2002). Little is known about the prevalence of delusional disorder (somatic type). Available evidence suggests it is the least common of the health anxiety disorders (APA, 2000), although some investigators believe that its prevalence has been underestimated (Koblenzer, 1997).

Excessive health anxiety can arise at any age although it most commonly develops in early adulthood (APA, 2000). It typically arises when the person is under stress, seriously ill or recovering from a serious illness, or has suffered the loss of a family member (Barsky & Klerman, 1983). Excessive health anxiety also can occur when the person is exposed to disease-related media information, as mentioned earlier.

The course of full-blown hypochondriasis is often chronic (APA, 2000), persisting for years in over 50% of cases (Barsky, Wyshak, Klerman, & Latham, 1990c; Barsky et al., 1998b; Robbins & Kirmayer, 1996). It is most likely to become chronic in people who (1) experience many unpleasant bodily sensations, (2) believe they have a serious medical condition, and (3) have a comorbid psychiatric disorder such as major depression (Barsky, Cleary, Sarnie, & Klerman, 1993a; Noyes et al., 1994a, 1994b). Little is known about the course of other health anxiety disorders. Although the course of transient hypochondriasis is, by definition, less than 6 months, people with this disorder are likely to experience future episodes of excessive health anxiety (Barsky et al., 1993a).

It is unclear whether health anxiety changes with age. The research so far has been based largely on cross-sectional (cohort) studies, which have yielded conflicting findings. Some studies suggest that health anxiety is greater in older than in younger people (Altamura, Carta, Tacchini, Musazzi, & Pioli, 1998; Gureje et al., 1997), while other research has found no difference between age groups (Barsky, Frank, Cleary, Wyshak, & Klerman, 1991). Longitudinal studies are needed to further examine this issue. Such research should attempt to disentangle the effects of declining health and social isolation to assess their relative importance in health anxiety. These variables are often confounded because elderly adults tend to be less healthy and more isolated than younger adults. Recall that social isolation provides a person with more opportunity to dwell on her or his body.

CROSS-CULTURAL CONSIDERATIONS

Cultural factors, such as societally transmitted values, beliefs, and expectations, can influence how a person interprets bodily changes and sensations, and whether treatment seeking is initiated. The tendency to present to primary care physicians with bodily concerns varies across cultures. Clinical and epidemiological studies show that Chinese, African American, Puerto Rican, and other Latin American people tend to present higher levels of medically unexplained "symptoms" than other groups (Escobar, Allen, Hoyas Nervi, & Gara, 2001).

There also appear to be cross-cultural differences in which bodily changes and sensations tend to be feared the most (Escobar, 1995). Some cultures appear to be more concerned about gastrointestinal sensations (e.g., excessive concern about constipation in the United Kingdom), while other cultures appear to be more concerned about cardiopulmonary symptoms (e.g., excessive concern about poor blood circulation and low blood pressure in Germany compared to other countries). Other countries appear to be associated with particularly high concerns about immunologically based symptoms (viruses, "sick building syndrome," "multiple chemical sensitivity" in the United States and Canada) (Escobar et al., 2001).

Whether a person's health concerns are unreasonable must be judged in light of his or her cultural background. One should be cautious about diagnosing hypochondriasis or related disorders in people whose beliefs about disease have been reinforced by traditional healers who disagree with the reassurances provided by physicians (APA, 2000). Even with this caveat, a number of *culture-bound syndromes* in which excessive health anxiety is a prominent feature have been identified. A culture-bound syndrome is a recurrent, locality-specific pattern of aberrant behavior and troubling experience that may or may not be linked to a particular DSM-IV diagnostic category (APA, 2000). Although cultural factors appear to shape culture-bound syndromes, these syndromes are considered to be mental disorders because they are associated with distress and functional impairment, and only a subgroup of the culture develop the disorder (i.e., cultural factors appear to be contributory factors, but fail to fully explain the disorder).

To illustrate a culture-bound health anxiety disorder, consider the dhat syndrome found in India. Dhat is characterized by severe anxiety and hypochondriacal concerns about the discharge of semen, along with complaints of whitish discoloration of the urine and feelings of weakness and mental exhaustion (Chadda & Ahuja, 1990; Malhotra & Wig, 1975). Other somatic complaints, such as aches and pains, are often present. The sufferer attributes his problems to the loss of semen in urine. Urological examination fails to reveal any discoloration or sperm.

Dhat is sometimes a feature of full-blown hypochondriasis, although it also can be a culturally specific from of abridged hypochondriasis. Dhat is reportedly common in India (Chadda & Ahuja, 1990), although its precise prevalence remains unknown. Some patients attribute dhat to early masturbation habits, to pre- or extramarital heterosexual contacts, or to homosexual contacts (Chadda & Ahuja, 1990). The disorder appears to arise from widely held cultural beliefs in India. However, cultural factors are not sufficient to explain the disorder because only a subgroup of Indian men develops dhat. Nevertheless, cultural beliefs can help us to partially understand how the disorder arises. In India, semen is widely regarded as an extremely precious fluid—the elixir of life—formed by a long process of distillation. It is believed that 40 meals give rise to 1 drop of blood; 40 drops of blood give rise to 1 drop of bone marrow; and 40 drops of bone marrow give rise to 1 drop of semen. A single ejaculation is thought to be sufficient to deplete one's mental and physical energy (Malhotra & Wig, 1975).

Dhat is sometimes resolved when the physician assures the patient that there is no semen loss, and that health would not suffer even if semen loss occurred (Chadda & Ahuja, 1990; Malhotra & Wig, 1975). If the patient does not respond to medical reassurance, then dhat is likely a feature of full-blown hypochondriasis or possibly a delusional disorder (somatic type).

SUMMARY AND CONCLUSIONS

There are several components of health anxiety, including disease conviction, disease fears, disease preoccupation, bodily checking and reassurance seeking, and disease-related avoidance and escape behaviors. Health anxiety is excessive when it is out of proportion with the objective evidence of disease. Health anxiety disorders include full and abridged hypochondriasis and delusional disorder (somatic type). Excessive health anxiety is common, costly, and often debilitating. Cultural factors, such as culturally based beliefs, can influence the sorts of symptoms and diseases that are feared. Hypochondriasis commonly co-occurs with, and is phenomenologically similar to, various disorders, particularly panic disorder, major depression, obsessive–compulsive disorder, and somatization disorder.

2

Body and Mind
Biological and Cognitive Factors

THEORETICAL ORIENTATION

Several theories of health anxiety have been proposed over the years, including biological, psychodynamic, behavioral, and cognitive-behavioral models. Rather than review each approach, we will concentrate mainly on the empirical literature to guide our efforts in understanding excessive health anxiety. As the reader will see, the research indicates that a cognitive-behavioral approach is particularly useful for understanding health anxiety. Biological factors also play a role, especially in producing bodily sensations. Perhaps later research will reveal that biological factors play a more important role, although the current research literature suggests that these factors are not major players in causing health anxiety disorders.

CAUSAL ELEMENTS

Ideally, a comprehensive model of health anxiety disorders would explain the four Ps of clinical causation: *predisposing, precipitating, perpetuating,* and *protective* factors. *Predisposing factors* are diatheses, or vulnerability factors. They could include formative learning experiences or a biological propensity to have a "noisy" body; that is, a body that produces a great many intense but benign bodily sensations. *Precipitating factors* are those stimuli or circumstances that trigger health anxiety. Stressful life events, for example, may trigger an episode of severe health anxiety in a person who believes stress–related sensations, such as chest pain, diarrhea, or polyuria (excessive urination), portend some dangerous disease. *Perpetuating factors* are those that maintain the problems. *Protective factors* prevent problems from developing, persisting, or getting worse. They may not be present in every case. Very little is known about the factors that protect people from developing health anxiety disorders, apart from the obvious fact that these disorders are unlikely to occur or persist in the absence of predisposing, perpetuating, and precipitating factors.

The four Ps of clinical causation are the topics of this and the following two chapters, with each chapter dealing with a particular group of variables thought to be involved in health anxiety disorders. The present chapter covers the biological and cognitive factors that appear to play a role in predisposing, precipitating, and perpetuating episodes of excessive health anxiety. Our emphasis in this chapter is on precipitating and perpetuating factors. Chapter 3 discusses the behavioral factors and their consequences. Chapter 4 considers the predisposing factors, particularly learning experiences, that lead to the development of maladaptive health–related beliefs and behaviors. Given that there has been little research on protective factors, our discussion of the latter is limited to case examples discussed later in this volume.

OVERVIEW OF THE PRESENT CHAPTER

In the present chapter we review some of the biological factors that commonly contribute to bodily sensations. If people with excessive health anxiety tend to misinterpret these sensations, then factors that increase the frequency or intensity of bodily sensations should increase the likelihood of mistakenly believing that one's health is in jeopardy. Understanding the common causes of bodily sensations may therefore further our knowledge of the causes of excessive health anxiety, and also should help patients develop realistic (non-catastrophic) interpretations of their feared sensations. We also review the research on the role of biological factors in producing anxiety about one's health, including neurotransmitters implicated in hypochondriasis, and central processing (cortical) structures thought to be involved. We then examine the cognitive factors in health anxiety. The empirical research has been mainly focused on hypochondriasis, although we also attempt to draw inferences about the causes of other forms of health anxiety.

To provide readers with a guide for conceptualizing the material to be reviewed in this chapter, Figure 2.1 provides a general framework for understanding the cognitive and biological factors that appear to be involved in excessive health anxiety.

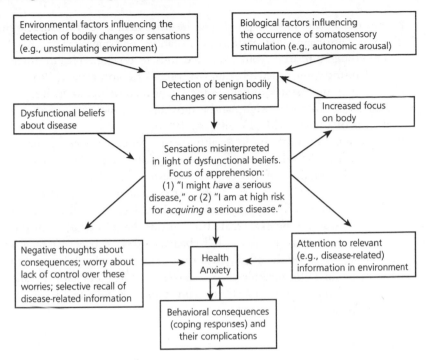

FIGURE 2.1. Factors involved in precipitating and perpetuating episodes of excessive health anxiety.

COMMON CAUSES OF BENIGN BODILY SENSATIONS

Benign bodily sensations arise from any number of sources, including benign bodily perturbations, minor diseases, and autonomic arousal. Regardless of the source, it seems that almost any somatic sensation can be misinterpreted as an indication of disease.

Benign Bodily Perturbations

Health-related worries can be triggered by a variety of things, including external stimuli such as newspaper articles about viral outbreaks, and internal stimuli such as bodily sensations. The human body is "noisy"; bodily sensations are daily or weekly occurrences even for healthy people (Pennebaker, 1982; White, Williams, & Greenberg, 1961). Many of these sensations are mild or transient, and are not associated with disease.

For example, dieting in physically healthy people can induce mild hypoglycemia, associated with faintness, sweating, and tachycardia (Airola, 1977). Trembling can arise from excessive muscle tension. Health-anxious people may misinterpret proctalgia fugax as a sign of colon cancer. Proctalgia fugax is a sudden, brief attack of pain in the lower rectum and anus. It is a benign condition of unknown origin, and is most likely to occur when the person is anxious or under stress (Thompson, 1989).

It is not unusual for physically healthy people to experience momentary dizziness when they stand up (mild postural hypotension). Transient functional alternations in the control of blood pressure are the most common causes (Schatz, 1986). This can arise from factors that inhibit the functioning of mechanisms involved in the regulation of blood pressure (baroreflexes). Postural hypotension can be exacerbated by various things, including heat exposure and alcohol or marijuana use (Chobanian, 1982; Schatz, 1986). Poor physical fitness, as a result of physical inactivity, can result in postural hypotension, along with breathlessness, muscle wasting, and fatigue, all of which can promote further inactivity and reinforce beliefs that one is physically ill (Sharpe & Bass, 1992).

Howard V. worked as a security guard in a large office building. His job required him to sit for most of the day at a reception desk. As a result of prolonged physical inactivity he experienced low back pain (due to muscle wasting) and dizziness on standing. He misinterpreted these sensations as signs that he had some lethal wasting disease that was sapping his strength. He believed that the best way to cope was to get plenty of rest. As a result of inactivity, his physical fitness became very poor and the unwanted sensations persisted.

Symptoms of Minor Disease

Symptoms of minor ailments can lead to disproportionate health anxiety if the person overestimates the seriousness of the sensations. Benign tissue lumps may be fatty deposits or sebaceous cysts. Chest pain can arise from gastrointestinal upset and chest wall syndromes (de Leon & Cheng, 1986). It is quite common for health-anxious people to misinterpret these sensations as indicators of heart disease.

Health-anxious people commonly misinterpret symptoms of dyspepsia (chest pain, burning sensations in the epigastrium, nausea, and vomiting) as indications of heart disease or cancer. A common form of this disorder is nonulcer dyspepsia, which occurs in the absence of identifiable physical disease. A number of factors have been implicated in this condition, including gastric acid reflux, abnormal esophageal motility, and bacterial infection (Kellner, 1991). Dyspepsia can be induced by lying in a recumbent position, by eating large meals, by consuming spicy foods or tomato products, and by consuming caffeinated drinks and foodstuffs.

Gastrointestinal distress may be part of irritable bowel syndrome (IBS), which is characterized by abdominal pain, bowel cramps, diarrhea, constipation, bloating, and flatulence (Thompson, 1984). These symptoms may be exacerbated by stress, and can be worsened by substances that increase bowel motility, such as caffeine or tomato products, and foods that are difficult to digest, such as red meat or fatty foods. IBS appears to be a dysfunction of the bowel smooth muscle or its innervation, causing disruption of normal peristaltic bowel contractions (Gershon, 1998). Health-anxious people may misinterpret IBS symptoms as signs of a more serious disorder, such as bowel cancer. Similarly, bloody stools, which may be misinterpreted as a sign of colon cancer, can arise from hemorrhoids.

The famous French writer Marcel Proust provides a good example of exaggerated responses to medical ailments. Like many of us, Proust suffered from asthma and allergies. Unlike most people, however, Proust's health anxiety was disproportionate to the seriousness of his medical condition, to the point that he spent most of his days in bed, inside a room that was lined with cork to block out noise and dust. On those few occasions when he went out, he wore multiple layers of clothing (e.g., three overcoats and numerous scarves) to prevent himself from catching cold. Once while attending a wedding his clothing was so bulky that he could not fit in the pews and had to stand in the aisle during the service (Fabricant, 1960; Pickering, 1974).

Autonomic Arousal

Autonomic arousal is a concomitant of emotions such as anxiety, anger, grief, and excitement. Arousal-related reactions—even in physically healthy people—include palpitations, muscle tension, shortness of breath, gastrointestinal distress, and increased urinary frequency. Palpitations include rapid heartbeat (tachycardia) and intermittent arrhythmia, which can occur in healthy people during periods of anxiety or stress (Amsterdam, 1990; Shear et al., 1987).

Arousal-related gastrointestinal sensations include nausea, stomach cramps, and diarrhea. Prolonged, stress-related muscle tension can lead to muscle twitches, chest tightness or pain (due to contractions in the intercostal muscles), headache, and pain in the neck, shoulders, or back. Stress-related hyperventilation can result in dizziness, dry throat, and paresthesias (tingling or prickling sensations in the extremities). Hyperventilation produces many of these effects because of decreased carbon dioxide (i.e., hypocapnia and associated alkalosis), which can lead to benign constriction of the cerebral arteries (hence producing dizziness), and paresthesias (Taylor, 2000).

People with excessive health anxiety often fail to recognize that their upsetting bodily sensations may be simply the concomitants of anxiety or other forms of emotional arousal. It is not uncommon for such people to believe that "anxiety and stress can't cause intense bodily reactions," and thereby overestimate the seriousness of harmless arousal-related sensations.

> Karla H. had a history of stomach cramps, which typically occurred during stressful periods at work. At times she thought the cramps were a result of drinking too much coffee. But when cramping persisted for days after she stopped drinking coffee, Karla began to worry that she might have stomach cancer. At times she would become so distressed by this possibility that her gastrointestinal upset would escalate to the point that she had diarrhea. Karla took this as "proof" that she had stomach cancer, which further intensified her fears.

> David P. also experienced an increase in unwanted bodily sensations during hectic times at work, such as headaches and muscle twitches around his eyes. Despite reassurance from a neurologist that he was physically healthy, David worried that he had a degenerative neurological disease such as Lou Gehrig's disease (amyotrophic lateral sclerosis). During his lunch breaks, when David was not occupied with the demands of work, he focused on his body and worried about his "symptoms." At times David's anxiety escalated to the point that he trembled, his heart raced, and he broke into a cold sweat. He regarded these reactions as further evidence of a neurological disorder. At other times, David also misinterpreted stress-related increases in urinary frequency as a sign of kidney disease.

BIOLOGICAL ASPECTS OF HEALTH ANXIETY

Advances in understanding of the biology of health anxiety disorders may be gained by studying the neuroanatomical structures and neurotransmitter systems that may be involved, possibly as predisposing or perpetuating factors.

Neurotransmitters

Findings from pharmacological studies have been used to speculate about the neurotransmitter dysregulations that might be involved in health anxiety disorders. Drug studies of hypochondriasis, although few in number, indicate that medications acting on the serotonergic system (e.g., paroxetine, fluoxetine, clomipramine) are effective in reducing this disorder (see Chapter 5). Unfortunately, these studies have consisted largely of case studies and uncontrolled trials. To our knowledge, there has been only one controlled trial (Fallon et al., 1996), which found that fluoxetine was marginally superior to placebo. Stronger support for the role of serotonergic dysregulation would be garnered if additional studies show that other drugs acting on the serotonergic system (agonists or antagonists) influence health anxiety.

The neurotransmitter systems involved in nondelusional health anxiety disorders might be different from those involved in delusional disorder (somatic type). Most of the research on the latter has focused on delusions of parasitic infestation, which responds to antipsychotic medications, particularly pimozide (see Chapter 5). These medications act on the dopamine system. Although this might suggest that dopaminergic dysregulation is involved in delusional disorder (somatic type), it is noteworthy that pimozide has an antipruritic (anti-itching) effect. This raises the possibility that the drug might work simply by reducing skin sensations in people who suffer from delusions of parasitic infestation. With the reduction of sensations, these people may come to believe that they are no longer infested with vermin.

Neural Structures

Miller (1984) proposed that the second somatosensory area (SII) of the cerebral cortex plays an important role in hypochondriasis and other somatoform disorders. The SII, which lies on the upper bank of the Sylvian fissure, adjacent to the insula, is involved in the abstraction, analysis, and evaluation of complex, meaningful patterns of somesthetic input. The SII may play a special role in the perception of pain (Carpenter, 1976), which is a symptom commonly reported by people with hypochondriasis. Some groups of SII cells have large receptive fields, suggesting that they integrate diffuse input from large areas of the body (Brodal, 1969; Mountcastle, 1974). Similarly, people with hypochondriasis often complain of vague, ambiguous physical sensations. Most cells in the SII react to stimulation of the body surface and visceral structures (Brodal, 1969; Mountcastle, 1974). Electrical stimulation of the SII gives rise to sensations of tingling, numbness, and warmth, and also to abdominal and gastric sensations (Penfield & Faulk, 1955; Penfield & Jasper, 1954). These are sensations commonly reported by people with hypochondriasis.

Although Miller's hypothesis is consistent with observations that people with hypochondriasis report experiencing a lot of different bodily sensations, it is noteworthy that these people generally do not show abnormalities in sensory acuity, as we explain in the following section.

PERCEPTUAL AND COGNITIVE FACTORS

Perceptual Acuity

People with severe health anxiety consider themselves to be especially sensitive to bodily sensations; compared to control groups they more frequently report experiencing pain and other unpleasant bodily sensations (Barsky, Brener, Coeytaux, & Cleary, 1995a; Bond, 1971; Haenen, Schmidt, Kroeze, & van den Hout, 1996). This raises the question of whether health anxiety disorders are associated with greater ability to detect bodily sensations. Two related approaches have addressed this issue: studies of perceptual acuity (e.g., sensory detection thresholds) and studies of perceptual accuracy (e.g., heart rate estimation).

Hanback and Revelle (1978) measured absolute auditory threshold and visual two-flash fusion threshold in college students with either high or low scores on a measure of hypochondriasis. Auditory sensitivity was assessed by asking participants to detect tones of varying intensity. Two-flash fusion threshold was measured by the minimum interval between two flashes of light required for the person to perceive them as two rather than one flash. Students with high scores on the hypochondriasis measure, compared to low scorers, had significantly lower visual thresholds (i.e., they were more sensitive). The two groups did not differ in auditory threshold. The authors suggested that hypochondriasis is associated with greater perceptual acuity. However, two-flash fusion sensitivity increases with arousal. This raises the question of whether the results simply reflect the fact that people with hypochondriacal features are often more anxiously aroused than controls without hypochondriasis. In other words, the results may be due to differences in anxiety rather than differences in perceptual sensitivity per se. Indeed, intensity of bodily sensations is more closely correlated with the person's degree of anxiety or distress than with his or her objective physiological state (Fahrenberg, Frank, Bass, & Jost, 1995; Steptoe & Noll, 1997).

Subsequent research does not provide convincing evidence for heightened somatosensory acuity in people with excessive health anxiety. Pauli, Schwenzer, Brody, Rau, and Birbaumer (1993) found that the threshold for thermal pain in college students was unrelated to the severity of health anxiety, but was negatively correlated with the person's degree of concern about pain—that is, greater concern was associated with greater pain sensitivity. A problem with this study is that a signal detection paradigm was not used, so it is not possible to disentangle pain sensitivity from the person's criterion for reporting that pain is present.

Subsequent research found that excessive health anxiety is not associated with heightened pain sensitivity (Lautenbacher, Pauli, Zaudig, & Burbaumer, 1998) or with greater tactile sensitivity to nonpainful stimuli, as measured by the two-point discrimination threshold (Haenen, Schmidt, Schoenmakers, &

van den Hout, 1997b). The latter is measured by touching the skin with two objects (e.g., two pencil tips) and identifying the smallest distance between the two for which the person can detect two rather than one stimulus.

Gramling, Clawson, and McDonald (1996) compared responses of people with hypochondriasis and controls on a cold pressor task. In this task the person immerses his or her hand into cold water, which induces pain. People with hypochondriasis, compared to controls, terminated the task earlier, rated the task as more unpleasant, and were more physiologically reactive (e.g., their heart rates were higher during the task). The two groups did not differ in their ratings of pain intensity. Although these findings could be taken as evidence that hypochondriasis is associated with greater "physiological reactivity" to pain, an alternative interpretation is that the findings reflect differences in people's beliefs about pain. People with excessive health anxiety commonly believe that pain is a sign of danger (i.e., the belief that "hurt equals harm"). People with these beliefs are most likely to become distressed about pain (with concomitant autonomic arousal) and terminate the task earlier.

Tyrer, Lee, and Alexander (1980) asked patients to estimate their pulse rates before and after viewing a mildly stressful film. Patients with hypochondriasis, compared to psychiatric controls, were more accurate in estimating their heart rates. But when Barsky et al. (1995a, 1998a) corrected for guessing and other artifacts that were not controlled in the Tyrer et al. study, they found that hypochondriasis was not associated with greater accuracy of heart rate estimation.

To summarize, there is little evidence that excessive health anxiety is associated with heightened acuity for detecting bodily sensations. It is possible, however, that people with health anxiety disorders have especially noisy bodies, so that they more often experience bodily sensations than other people. "Noisiness" could be biologically determined, although there is evidence that psychological factors play an important role, as described later in this chapter. Note that a person might have an especially noisy body (compared to other people) without necessarily having heightened somatosensory acuity. In other words, the person may tend to experience a great many bodily sensations (e.g., aches, pains, gastrointestinal upsets, palpitations) without necessarily having greater acuity for detecting those sensations.

Attention

Disease-Related Hypervigilance

Health-anxious people tend to be vigilant for bodily changes and sensations (Miller, Brody, & Summerton, 1988). When attention is directed to one's body, the intensity of perceived sensations increases (Mechanic, 1983;

Pennebaker, 1980; Pennebaker & Skelton, 1978). Some sensations, such as itching, coughing, and yawning, have an infectious quality, spread by observing others with these reactions. Someone's cough in a theater, for example, draws our attention to our own throats and we soon note a mild sensation of dryness or scratchiness that we had previously ignored (Barsky, 1992).

People with excessive health anxiety may spend a great deal of time attending to their bodies, thereby increasing the chances of noticing bodily sensations (Kellner, Abbott, Winslow, & Pathak, 1987). Consistent with this idea, when attention is experimentally manipulated, more bodily sensations are typically reported when people are instructed to deliberately focus on their bodies (Haenen et al., 1996; Schmidt, Wolfs-Takens, Oosterlaan, & van den Hout, 1994; Vervaeke, Bouman, & Valmaggia, 1999). The tendency to focus on one's body is not simply a consequence of aversive somatic sensations because this tendency can be identified even in people who are not currently experiencing such sensations (Ferguson & Ahles, 1998). Attentional focus may be a consequence of beliefs about bodily sensations: people tend to search for, and focus on, these sensations if they believe the sensations are signals of bodily dysfunction.

> James S. was in class when his teacher announced that there was an outbreak of head lice, for which students would be screened by the school nurse. James worried that he might have somehow contracted lice. He focused his attention on his scalp and noticed, to his dismay, that he occasionally had itching sensations, which he hadn't really noticed before. When the wind blew through his hair, James became aware of "crawling" sensations on his scalp. The more James noticed the sensations, the more he worried that he had lice.

Factors Influencing Attentional Focus

Attention to one's body is influenced by environmental factors. Our attentional capacities are limited, and so internal and external stimuli compete for attention (Pennebaker, 1982). Therefore, the detection of bodily changes and sensations depends, in part, on the person's focus of attention. Attention to stimuli outside the body decreases the likelihood of detecting internal body sensations. This is seen in athletes who sustain injuries during sporting competitions. If the competition is intense and demands concentration, then the injury may go unnoticed until later on. Conversely, the probability of detecting sensations increases when attention is directed inward.

Research by Pennebaker and others shows that if the person's external environment is lacking in attention-grabbing stimuli, then body sensations are more likely to be detected, particularly when the person has just experienced an aversive or stressful event (Pennebaker, 2000). People report higher levels of fatigue, increased palpitations, and even more frequent coughs when they are in boring or unstimulating situations (e.g., living at home alone, working at a monotonous job) compared to when they are in stimulating situations. Patients in drab, boring hospital wards are therefore more likely to notice bodily sensations, compared to patients in wards containing diverting activities such as games, books, or TV programs (Pennebaker, 1982, 2000).

Memory

Selective recall of threatening health-related information could contribute to somatic preoccupation and to beliefs that one's health is fragile. To investigate this possibility, Durso, Reardon, Shore, and Delys (1991) administered a memory test to students with either high or low scores on the MMPI Hs (Hypochondriasis) scale. The two groups did not differ in their recollection of health-related information, although high-scoring participants were poorer at recalling the source of the information (i.e., confusion between recall of health-related events concerning oneself vs. health-related events of others). A limitation of this study is its reliance on the MMPI Hs scale, which has questionable validity as a measure of hypochondriasis. Another study found that health anxiety, as assessed in a college student sample, was unrelated to recognition memory for illness-related words (Owens, Asmundson, Hadjistavropoulous, & Owens, 2001).

Studies using patient samples have revealed stronger evidence that health anxiety is related to memory bias, at least when recognition memory is assessed. In a task requiring people to identify and recall difficult-to-read health-related and non–health-related words, people with hypochondriasis had better recall for health-related than non–health-related words (Brown, Kosslyn, Delamater, Fama, & Barsky, 1999). Controls did not show this bias. People with hypochondriasis and control participants did not differ in the detection (perception) of words. Brown et al. conjectured that people with hypochondriasis elaborately process information related to health, perhaps by frequently ruminating about their health. Similar findings were reported by Pauli and Alpers (2002), who found that patients with hypochondriasis, compared to those without this disorder, were better able to recall pain-related words (e.g., *burning, stinging*).

Suggestibility

Health hazards—real or exaggerated—are frequently reported in the media. When health-anxious people learn of these hazards, they often come to fear or believe that they have succumbed to the dreaded threat (Kellner, 1985). After the widely reported outbreak of bovine spongiform encephalopathy ("mad cow disease") in Great Britain, many people avoided eating beef for fear that they would acquire the human counterpart, Creutzfeldt–Jakob disease. Some people misinterpreted fleeting dizziness and other benign sensations as indications that they had fallen prey to the disease. Thus, the perceived threat of serious disease can heighten health anxiety. In many cases the concerns are transient. However, some people might be particularly suggestible, being easily influenced by alarming health-related information, and thereby developing hypochondriasis.

To examine this issue, Haenen, Schmidt, Schoenmakers, and van den Hout (1997a) examined the suggestibility to bodily sensations in people with hypochondriasis and healthy controls. Both groups participated in an experiment in which they were told to expect a weak electric current delivered through a finger electrode over five consecutive trials, with the intensity being initially below detection threshold and gradually increasing. In fact, a shock was never delivered. Participants were asked to report whenever they experienced the shock. This report was used as an index of suggestibility. Contrary to expectation, more shocks were reported by the control group. A limitation of this research is that it assessed only one aspect of suggestibility, suggestibility for the *presence* of sensations (electric shocks). The research would have been more informative if it had tested suggestibility for *interpretations* of sensations.

Media reports of disease outbreaks may influence how people interpret everyday bodily sensations. A dry cough could be interpreted as a mild dust allergy. However, given the recent media reports of bioterrorism, a health-anxious person might interpret such a cough as a sign of anthrax infection. The clinical experience of the authors and others (e.g., Kellner, 1985) indicates that health-anxious people are highly suggestible regarding the interpretation of sensations, especially if media reports suggest that particular bodily reactions (e.g., fever) are harbingers of lethal maladies (e.g., the mosquito-borne West Nile virus). Research is needed to further test this clinical impression. If health-anxious people are especially suggestible in this way, then why is this so? Examining people's beliefs offers some important clues.

Beliefs and Interpretations

There is ample room for misinterpreting bodily sensations, especially when sensations are mild, vague, or diffuse. There is less room for differing interpretations of symptoms that are severe, disabling, very unusual, or obviously externally induced. "This could explain why symptoms such as weakness, fatigue, nausea, or diffuse pain are so common in people with hypochondriasis; non-hypochondriasis individuals would be more likely to attribute them to a non-pathological cause such as aging, overwork, or 'tension'" (Barsky &

Klerman, 1983, p. 277). Thus, hypochondriasis and other forms of excessive health anxiety could be largely cognitive disorders, arising from misinterpretations of benign bodily changes or sensations. In turn, the tendency to misinterpret sensations may be a result of one's beliefs about sickness and health (Barsky & Klerman, 1983; Mechanic, 1972; Salkovskis & Warwick, 2000).

Consistent with this cognitive formulation, health anxiety is more strongly correlated with appraisals of one's health than with objective indices of health (Frazier & Waid, 1999; Hollifield et al., 1999). Cognitive studies have also shown that health-anxious people, compared to non-health-anxious controls:

- Are more likely to interpret bodily sensations as indicators of poor health or serious disease (Barsky & Wyshak, 1989; Barsky, Coeytaux, Sarnie, & Cleary, 1993b; Haenen et al., 1997a; Haenen, Schmidt, Shoenmakers, & van den Hout, 1998; Hitchcock & Mathews, 1992; MacLeod, Haynes, & Sensky, 1998; Marcus, 1999; Rief, Hiller, & Margraf, 1998).
- Are more likely to believe that good health is associated with few or no bodily sensations (Barsky et al., 1993b).
- Are more likely to believe that they are weak and unable to tolerate stress (Rief et al., 1998).
- Show a greater tendency to overestimate the likelihood of contracting diseases and to overestimate the dangerousness of diseases (Ditto, Jemmott, & Darley, 1988; Easterling & Leventhal, 1989).
- Are more likely to regard themselves as being at greater risk for developing various diseases, but do not view themselves as being at greater risk for being the victim of an accident or criminal assault (Barsky et al., 2001; Haenen, de Jong, Schmidt, Stevens, & Visser, 2000). This suggests that severe health anxiety is characterized by a specific tendency to overestimate health risk rather than a general tendency to overestimate danger.
- May have greater knowledge about diseases, according to some studies (Ferguson, 1996; Katz, Meyers, & Walls, 1995; Woods, Natterson, & Silverman, 1966) but not another (Haenen et al., 1998). Disease knowledge could be a result of health anxiety (e.g., checking medical texts for information on bodily concerns). In turn, greater knowledge about deadly diseases could fuel health anxiety by providing the person with more reasons for worrying about his or her health (e.g., learning to become frightened of small cuts in the skin after learning that they can lead to necrotizing fasciitis or "flesh-eating disease").

Table 2.1 gives examples of dysfunctional beliefs associated with excessive health anxiety. These examples are derived from various sources, includ-

TABLE 2.1. Dysfunctional Beliefs Associated with Excessive
Health Anxiety

Theme	Examples
Meaning of bodily changes and sensations	• "I'm healthy only when I don't have any bodily sensations." • "Bodily complaints are always a sign of disease." • "Red blotches are signs of skin cancer." • "Joint pain means that my bones are degenerating." • "Real symptoms aren't caused by anxiety."
Meaning and consequences of diseases	• "If I get sick I'll be in great pain and suffering." • "People will avoid or reject me if I get really ill." • "Serious diseases are everywhere." • "People don't recover from serious diseases."
View of self as weak, vulnerable, or inadequate	• "My circulatory system is very sensitive." • "I need to avoid exertion because I'm physically frail." • "Illness is a sign of failure and inadequacy." • "If I'm ill people will abandon me."
Physicians and medical tests	• "It is possible to be absolutely certain about my health." • "Doctors should be able to explain all bodily complaints." • "Doctors can't be trusted because they often make mistakes." • "If a doctor refers me for further medical tests, then he or she must believe that there's something seriously wrong with me." • "Medical evaluations are unreliable if you don't have symptoms at the time of the test." • "Medical evaluations are unreliable if you don't give your doctor a complete and detailed description of your symptoms." • "If the doctor simply listens to you and says 'Your health is fine,' then the assessment can't be trusted; a reliable evaluation requires a detailed interview and lab tests."
Adaptiveness of worry and bodily vigilance	• "Worrying about my health will keep me safe." • "I need to frequently check my body in order to catch the first signs of illness." • "I need to carefully watch my health, otherwise something terrible will happen."
Death, the afterlife, and superstitious beliefs	• "I'll be trapped and alone forever when I'm dead." • "Death means I'll be eternally aware of what I've lost." • "God makes bad people die early." • "If I tell myself I'm healthy then I'll be tempting fate."

ing our clinical experience and research by other investigators (Barsky et al., 1993b; Rief et al., 1998; Salkovskis, 1989; Wells & Hackmann, 1993). The beliefs are dysfunctional because they contribute to excessive preoccupation and worry about one's health. The strength of these beliefs is correlated with the severity of health anxiety (James & Wells, 2002), and reductions in belief strength coincide with treatment-related reductions in health anxiety (Avia et al., 1996; Clark et al., 1998; Speckens, Spinhoven, van Hemert, Bolk, & Hawton, 1997; Visser & Bouman, 2001).

Health-anxious people typically hold several dysfunctional beliefs, including beliefs about specific bodily sensations (e.g., "Abdominal pain is a sign of malignancy") and more general beliefs (e.g., "I have a weak constitution"). The latter beliefs appear to explain why people with severe health anxiety commonly complain that they always find something health-related to worry about.

> One day Cathy C. worried that her headache might be a symptom of a brain tumor. The following day she worried that her pollen allergies might result in her throat constricting to the point of suffocation. The next week she was alarmed about a rash on her chest; she didn't know what it was, but worried that it was caused by something bad. The following week she worried about the effects of air pollution on her immune system. These numerous, changing concerns appeared to arise from Cathy's beliefs about diseases (e.g., "Viruses are everywhere") and her beliefs about herself ("I've inherited a sickly disposition from my mother").

When health-anxious people are exposed to disease-related information (e.g., bodily changes or sensations, or media information), their dysfunctional beliefs appear to give rise to intrusive thoughts, worries, and images about disease (Easterling & Leventhal, 1989; Wells & Hackmann, 1993). The images are often catastrophic in nature. For instance, lower back pain may give rise to horrific images of being on dialysis for the rest of one's life, or images of killing oneself because the pain and suffering of kidney disease is too great to endure. The distress experienced by health-anxious people is fueled further by their tendency to worry about their lack of control over their illness worries (Bouman & Meijer, 1999).

Cognitive Specificity and Health Anxiety

The cognitive content-specificity hypothesis (Beck, 1976) suggests that hypochondriasis and other forms of excessive health anxiety can be distinguished from other disorders by the content of dysfunctional beliefs. Depression, for example, is said to be associated with beliefs about loss, failure, or self-denigration (Beck, Rush, Shaw, & Emery, 1979). Social phobia is thought to be associated with beliefs about rejection or ridicule by others (Beck & Emery, 1985). Panic disorder is associated with beliefs that arousal-related bodily sensations (e.g., palpitations) will have immediate calamitous consequences, such as death, insanity, or loss of control (Clark, 1986). Hypochondriasis is associated with beliefs that bodily changes and sensations—arousal-related and otherwise—will have calamitous consequences in the more distant future (Warwick & Salkovskis, 1990). Recent research supports this distinction between hypochondriasis and panic disorder (Salkovskis & Warwick, 2001).

Persistence of Dysfunctional Beliefs

Why do dysfunctional beliefs often persist in health-anxious people? These individuals have typically experienced many health-related "false alarms," where their frightening bodily sensations turned out to be innocuous. These experiences sometimes disconfirm beliefs that one's health was at risk. However, often the opposite occurs. The fact that a bodily sensation turned out to be benign today does not preclude the possibility that at some point in the future the same sensation could be due to a serious disease. Mild dyspnea today while climbing the stairs could simply indicate poor physical fitness. But in 15 years time the same symptom could indicate congestive heart failure. Uncertainties like these may prevent hypochondriacal beliefs from being disconfirmed ("I was lucky this time, next time it could be serious"). Beliefs that one is at risk for serious disease can persist even in people who have learned that many of their feared sensations are due to anxiety.

> Hugh L. went through an extensive battery of cardiology tests because of recurrent chest pain. No physical disease was identified and his cardiologist told him that his symptoms were due to "stress and anxiety." Initially Hugh was relieved, but after an Internet search he obtained information that "anxiety can damage your heart." This lead to further worry about the future consequences of recurrent palpitations.

People may become health-anxious partly because they lack the "positive illusions" that characterize many normal people. Many emotionally well-adjusted people hold positive, distorted beliefs about themselves and their environment (Taylor & Brown, 1988). Examples include, "I'm too fit to get sick," "There is no need to worry about my health," and "My doctor is always right."

Why Are Some Beliefs Overvalued or Delusional?

The strength of beliefs about disease varies along a continuum. A person with mild health anxiety might have a nagging doubt that he or she has a disease (e.g., "Sometimes I wonder if my tiredness is due to something serious, like leukemia"). People with hypochondriasis sometimes have strongly held (overvalued) beliefs about disease. Most of the time these people fail to recognize that their concerns about having a serious disease are excessive or unreasonable ("I'm usually quite certain that I have leukemia, although sometimes I wonder if my tiredness is simply due to lack of sleep"). Disease beliefs can, in a minority of cases, be so strong that they are delusional, as in delusional disorder (somatic type) ("I'm absolutely certain I have leukemia—death is just around the corner").

Delusions can arise from various medical conditions, such as vitamin B12 deficiency, pellagra, renal disease, cocaine or amphetamine dependence, steroid psychosis, and cerebral arteriosclerosis and other brain syndromes (Koblenzer, 1997; Lishman, 1987; Matas & Robinson, 1988; Sheppard, O'Loughlin, & Malone, 1986). By definition, delusional disorder (somatic type) is ruled out as a diagnosis, because the delusions are attributable to a general medical condition (APA, 2000). Delusional disorder (somatic type) is not due to an identifiable medical condition, and is found in people with good physical health (Koblenzer, 1997).

What influences the strength of disease beliefs in physically healthy people? Why do some people retain somatic delusions in the face of abundant disconfirmatory evidence? Little is known about these issues. Belief strength can vary over time and circumstance, with beliefs becoming stronger when the person experiences worrisome bodily sensations and weaker in the absence of such sensations. When people encounter potentially risky situations, they tend to selectively look for evidence confirming danger and evidence refuting safety (de Jong, Haenen, Schmidt, & Mayer, 1998; Smeets, de Jong, & Mayer, 2000). This is a "better be prepared" strategy. For people who believe they might have a serious disease, this selective search is biased toward the confirmation of their beliefs. With the selective accrual of supporting evidence, disease beliefs may eventually become overvalued or even delusional.

Bodily sensations themselves may also contribute to delusion disorder (somatic type). Prominent, persistent bodily changes or sensations could provide constant reminders that one's body is "not functioning as it should be." Delusions of parasitic infestation may arise from a combination of bodily changes (e.g., persistent dry, flaking skin, or a minor skin irritation) and particular environmental circumstances (e.g., social isolation, which allows the person more time and opportunity to dwell on his or her "symptoms")

(Koblenzer, 1997). Similarly, delusions of halitosis (and associated delusions about bodily decay) can arise from persistent sensations of bad taste, associated with a history of rhinitis (an inflammation of the lining of the nose, with typical symptoms being nasal obstruction and discharge). Distortions in taste physiology may contribute to the delusion of halitosis (Goldberg, Buongiorno, & Henkin, 1985). Sometimes the delusional person's significant other colludes in the delusion, agreeing that halitosis or parasitic infestation is present. This folie à deux can reinforce and perpetuate delusional beliefs.

Amplifying Somatic Style

In preceding sections we have seen that people with severe health anxiety (1) tend to fear bodily sensations, (2) hold catastrophic beliefs about the implications of these sensations, and (3) tend to be hypervigilant for, and to focus on, bodily sensations (even weak sensations) and on disease-related information. This constellation of features is called an *amplifying somatic style* (Barsky, 1992; Barsky et al., 1999). An *amplifier* is a person who reports a wide range of bodily discomfort and is troubled by uncomfortable sensations that are not generally symptomatic of disease, such as insect bites, loud noises, and normal physiology (Barsky, Ahern, Bailey, & Delamater, 1996). Amplifying somatic style is seen as a predisposing factor rather than simply a correlate of health anxiety (Barsky, 1992).

The concept of amplifying somatic style is useful because it underscores the close links among selective attention, dysfunctional beliefs, and anxiety. A measure that assesses all of these facets would be useful because it captures many of the factors thought to be important in the health anxiety disorders. Accordingly, to measure the person's trait-like degree of somatosensory amplification, Barsky, Goodson, Lane, and Cleary (1988b) developed a 10-item questionnaire called the Somatosensory Amplification Scale (SSAS). Sample items include "I am often aware of various things happening within my body" and "Even something minor, like an insect bite or a splinter, really bothers me." The entire scale appears in Appendix 6.

Scores on the SSAS tend to be stable over months, if not years (Barsky et al., 1988b, 1995b; Weinstein, Berwick, Goldman, Murphy, & Barsky, 1989), and are unrelated to medical morbidity (Barsky, Wyshak, & Klerman, 1990a). The SSAS is positively correlated with the severity of health anxiety (Barsky et al., 1988b, 1990a; Barsky & Wyshak, 1990), and predicts the persistence of health anxiety (Barsky et al., 1993a). Persistent bodily sensations, such as recurrent palpitations, appear to be best predicted by the interaction between amplifying somatic style and the occurrence of minor daily stressors (Barsky et al., 1996). These two factors work in concert to increase the frequency and perceived intensity of bodily sensations.

Somatosensory amplification could be learned in childhood by upbringing and other formative experiences, or could be "hard-wired" into the nervous system from birth (Barsky, 1992). The behavioral-genetic research, as reviewed in Chapter 4, suggests that learning experiences may be particularly important.

Alexithymia

Sifneos and colleagues suggested that hypochondriasis arises from alexithymia (Nemiah & Sifneos, 1970; Sifneos, 1972). People with high levels of alexithymia have difficulty identifying, describing, and distinguishing among their emotions. They tend to express psychological distress in somatic rather than emotional form, and have difficulty distinguishing between feelings and bodily sensations of emotional arousal. People with high levels of alexithymia also have an impoverished fantasy life, and tend to be preoccupied with the details of objects and events in their external environment (Nemiah, 1996). High levels of alexithymia are thought to reflect deficits in the cognitive processing and regulation of emotions: deficits in both the cognitive–experiential component of emotion response systems and deficits in the interpersonal regulation of emotion (G. J. Taylor, 2000).

> Unable to identify accurately their own subjective feelings, not only are individuals with high degrees of alexithymia limited in their ability to reflect on and regulate their emotions, but they also verbally communicate emotional distress to other people very poorly, thereby failing to enlist others for aid and comfort. In turn, the lack of emotion-sharing may contribute to the difficulty in identifying emotions. The constricted imaginal capacities of high-alexithymia individuals limit the extent to which they can modulate emotions by fantasy, dreams, interests, and play. (G. J. Taylor, 2000, p. 135)

Consistent with the hypothesized role of alexithymia in hypochondriasis, scores on measures of alexithymia are correlated with measures of hypochondriasis (Bagby, Taylor, & Ryan, 1986; Wise, Mann, Hryvniak, Mitchell, & Hill, 1990). However, elevated alexithymia is also associated with a range of other disorders, including schizophrenia, mood disorders, anxiety disorders, eating disorders, borderline personality disorder, antisocial personality disorder, somatization disorder, and some sexual disorders (Bankier, Aigner, & Bach, 2001; Cedro, Kokoszka, Popiel, & Narkiewicz, 2001; Fukunishi, Kikuchi, Wogan, & Takabo, 1997; Honkalampi, Hintikka, Tanskanen, Lehtonen, & Viinamacki, 2000; Madioni & Mammana, 2001; Mazzeo & Espelage, 2002; Sayar, Ebrine, & Ak, 2001; Sureda, Valdes, Jodar, & de Pablo, 1999; Yehuda et al., 1997; Zlotnick, Mattia, & Zimmerman, 2001). Research so far has produced no convincing evidence that alexithymia is more strongly associated with somatic complaints than with emotional complaints, and some research suggests that alexithymia is uncorrelated with somatic complaints once anxiety and depression are statistically controlled (Lundh & Simonsson, 2001). It has also yet to be shown that alexithymia is causally related to hypochondriasis. Experimental research is required to address this issue (e.g., by experimentally reducing alexithymia and observing the effects on hypochondriasis).

A recent study by Kooiman, Bolk, Brand, Trijsburg, and Rooijmans (2000) found that people with medically unexplained symptoms attending an outpatient clinic did not have elevated alexithymia, even though many had a mental disorder such as hypochondriasis. Alexithymia was unrelated to subjective health experience and with the use of medical services. This suggests that among the majority of people with medically unexplained physical symptoms, alexithymia does not play a clinically significant role.

To summarize, if alexithymia does play a role in hypochondriasis, it is a nonspecific one, and therefore insufficient to explain hypochondriasis (or other forms of health anxiety). Alexithymia might be important in shaping the manner of presentation of hypochondriasis and other health anxiety disorders. People with high alexithymia might present mainly with disease conviction without expressing anxious feelings about their health problems.

SUMMARY AND CONCLUSIONS

Despite a rapidly growing corpus of research, much remains to be learned about the biological and psychological factors in hypochondriasis and other health anxiety disorders. As mentioned at the outset of this chapter, the biological and cognitive factors that seem to be involved in precipitating and perpetuating episodes of undue health anxiety are illustrated in Figure 2.1.

People with hypochondriasis report that they frequently experience all sorts of bodily sensations. Yet there is no persuasive evidence that they possess a heightened sensitivity for detecting sensations. It could be that these people have especially "noisy" bodies, yielding a high frequency of intense, benign sensations, which may be catastrophically misinterpreted. Abnormalities in somatosensory processing may be particularly important in delusional disorder (somatic type), because these people often complain of unusual sensations (e.g., abnormal cutaneous or taste sensations).

The detection of disturbing sensations is enhanced by selective attention toward disease-related information. This information can originate from the body (bodily sensations or changes) or from the environment. There is also evidence of memory bias in hypochondriasis, favoring the selective recall of threatening health-related information. This bias could be the result of rumination about one's health, thereby enhancing the encoding and retrieval of health threat information. In turn, selective recall of such information may heighten the person's perceived vulnerability to health threats.

Hypochondriasis, and possibly other health anxiety disorders, is associated with a range of dysfunctional beliefs about one's health and its medical care. This includes specific beliefs about particular sensations (e.g., "Lumps mean cancer") and general beliefs (e.g., "I'm vulnerable to disease"). These beliefs appear to contribute to the catastrophic misinterpretation of benign bodily changes and sensations. These beliefs also may promote selective attention to one's body, and may lead to rumination about possible health threats. Further adding to their anxiety, health-anxious people not only worry about illnesses, but also worry about their inability to control their disease-related worries. This "worry about worry" may induce some people to seek out mental health professionals for treatment of health anxiety.

3

Behavioral Factors and Their Consequences

Behavioral factors, particularly maladaptive coping strategies, play an important role in excessive health anxiety. These strategies arise largely from beliefs that one has a serious disease or that one is at high risk for acquiring such a disease. Maladaptive coping strategies can reinforce dysfunctional disease-related beliefs, thereby perpetuating health anxiety. In this chapter we consider four common maladaptive coping strategies: (1) persistent reassurance seeking, (2) other forms of repetitive checking (e.g., bodily checking), (3) reliance on safety signals, and (4) avoidance. We also consider some of the complications that arise from these coping strategies, such as iatrogenic (physician-induced) worsening of health anxiety.

REASSURANCE SEEKING

Reassurance Can Perpetuate Health Anxiety

Reassurance about one's health, provided by physicians or significant others, is an age-old remedy for many sorts of health-related worry. Balint (1964) was among the first to voice concerns about "overprescription" of reassurance by physicians:

> In spite of our almost pathetic lack of knowledge about the dynamisms and possible consequences of "reassurance" and "advice," these two are perhaps the most often used forms of medical treatment. (p. 116)

> Reassurance is not in itself necessarily wrong. It may even be a powerful drug which, if correctly prescribed, can be highly beneficial. The trouble with it is that it is prescribed wholesale, without proper diagnosis. . . . Reassurance is much too often administered for the benefit of the doctor, who cannot bear the burden of either not knowing enough or of being unable to help. (p. 231)

Reassurance may allay excessive health anxiety, although its effectiveness depends on what one considers to be "reassurance." Some therapists define reassurance broadly (e.g., Starcevic & Lipsitt, 2001), to the point that it seems little different from cognitive restructuring, involving the provision of new health-related information. *Reassurance* is more commonly defined as the repeated presentation of the simple message that there is nothing wrong with the person's health. Reassurance may be based on a review of bodily concerns, a physical examination, and/or medical tests (Warwick & Salkovskis, 1985). This sort of reassurance is what health-anxious people typically receive from their physicians. Studies have shown that for people with hypochondriasis, reassurance has an initial calming effect, but health anxiety subsequently returns, often within 24 hours (Haenen et al., 2000; Salkovskis & Warwick, 1986).

Repeated reassurance seeking is not only ineffective in producing lasting reductions in health anxiety disorders, it may also perpetuate these disorders (Warwick, 1992; Warwick & Salkovskis, 1990; Wells, 1997). Repeatedly seeking and receiving reassurance can have the following adverse effects:

- It can prolong the person's preoccupation with illness by extending the amount of time he or she spends discussing his or her health, and by exposing him or her to alarming information about rare but lethal medical conditions.
- It can infantilize the person. By repeatedly turning to others for help, health-anxious people can "train" their significant others to repeatedly inquire about their health and offer assurance. This fosters helplessness and reinforces the view that the person is weak and vulnerable
- It can have other iatrogenic effects. Repeated medical tests or physician–patient miscommunication can perpetuate health anxiety (as described later in this chapter).

Why Do Health-Anxious People Persistently Seek Reassurance?

If reassurance seeking is not beneficial in the long term, then why do health-anxious people persistently seek it out? Reassurance seeking and other checking behaviors appear to be maintained because they are negatively reinforced.

That is, the person engages in these behaviors because they are reinforced, usually temporarily, by a reduction in anxiety (Lucock, Marley, White, & Peake, 1997). The next time a bodily change or sensation is detected, the health-anxious person therefore feels compelled to check or seek reassurance again in order to attain immediate (but temporary) relief. Doubts about the accuracy of the reassuring information often arise, which can lead the health-anxious person to repeatedly check or persistently seek reassurance in order to be 100% certain that serious disease has been ruled out.

Why Does Reassurance Have Transient Effects?

Why are the effects of reassurance short-lived in people with severe health anxiety? Why do their health concerns return? Although there has been little research on these important questions, there are several plausible explanations. One is that the calming effects of reassurance persist until the person notices more bodily changes or sensations. This can lead the health-anxious person to wonder, "Why would I be experiencing more symptoms if I my doctor said I'm healthy?" As the person ponders this question a myriad of doubts may arise about the accuracy of the physician's assessment, resulting in a resumption of health-related preoccupation. Such doubts may be especially likely to arise if the physician does not give the patient a good explanation of what *is* causing the sensations (Lucock, White, Peake, & Morley, 1998): "My doctor told me that my stomach cramps aren't due to cancer, but she hasn't told me why I keep having them."

A second likely reason for the transience of reassurance concerns the lack of complete certainty associated with medical tests and evaluations. Medical tests are rarely, if ever, 100% accurate, and physicians sometimes make mistakes. Successful, routine medical procedures are rarely deemed newsworthy, but disastrous medical errors are regularly reported in the media. One newspaper article described "horror stories of people having the wrong leg amputated or being diagnosed with a drug overdose when they were actually having a heart attack." The article went on to report that medical errors occur in 16% of people admitted to the hospital (*Vancouver Sun*, May 8, 2002, p. A5). Thus, media reports can lead health-anxious people to be highly aware of the fallibility of medical evaluations.

"Reassuring" messages from physicians provide fertile grounds for doubt and rumination in the health-anxious person. A diagnosis of a "clean bill of health" is a probabilistic determination; a heart murmur may be judged as "probably benign," or a biopsy specimen may be deemed to be "likely normal." Thus, the person receives a *diagnosis of uncertain wellness* (Cioffi, 1991). For people who are very worried about their health, this lack of certainty can be troubling. It can lead to persistent doubting (Fallon, 1999). This is seen in patients who ask the same question over and over, in slightly different ways, or repeatedly request additional tests to reduce their uncertainty:

"But doctor, how can you be certain that I don't have MS [multiple sclerosis]? . . . Are these tests completely accurate? . . . Is there another test we could do, just to make sure? . . . And what about the tingling in my hands? Are you sure it's not MS? . . . "

Reassurance also may be short-lived if the health-anxious person later wonders whether the physician received "all" the relevant information at the time of the medical consultation.

"I forgot to tell the doctor that I sometimes feel dizzy. Maybe he failed to make the right diagnosis because he didn't have all the information. And my heart wasn't pounding during the examination, the way it usually is. That could mean that the doctor mightn't have been able to detect an arrhythmia."

People who are unable or unwilling to tolerate the uncertainty inherent in medical diagnoses are quite likely to persist in seeking medical reassurance in the hope that if they obtain enough diagnostic tests and medical opinions, then they will eventually be able to be 100% certain that they are healthy. Of course, the greater the number of medical tests, the greater the odds of obtaining a false-positive result.

McDonald, Daly, Jelinek, Panetta, and Gutman (1996) observed that chance circumstances, called *wild card effects*, can also make patients resistant to reassurance:

A woman, initially successfully reassured [about her health], became mistrustful of the normal result after she learnt that her sister had developed metastatic cancer despite earlier negative ultrasound and computed tomography scans; this belief was reinforced by her conviction that computers were often prone to error. . . . As occurrences such as these could not readily be predicted by doctor or patient we refer to them as "wild card effects." (p. 331)

Another example is the person who was experiencing severe headaches and then learned of a neighbor's death from a brain tumor (Fitzpatrick, 1996). The combination of these circumstances can contribute to health anxiety and may make people persist in seeking medical reassurance. The person's social circle may also contribute to the persistent seeking of reassurance. Family members may express doubt and surprise that one's headaches are "simply due to stress." Significant others may encourage the health-anxious person to seek a second (or third) opinion, and may remind the health-anxious person that medical errors can occur: "Remember what happened to your uncle Rick; the doctors said his heart was fine, and the next week he died of a heart attack."

OTHER FORMS OF REPETITIVE CHECKING

Bodily Checking

Checking one's body is a common "coping" response for health-anxious people. Although some degree of checking is healthy and adaptive (e.g., monthly breast or testicular self-examinations), people with health anxiety disorders often engage in excessive checking, which can perpetuate or intensify their health concerns. Repeatedly checking one's skin for bumps or blemishes increases the chances of noticing minor, harmless irregularities. This can lead the person to become alarmed and then to seek out medical attention. The experience of noticing "suspicious" moles or freckles that one hadn't previously noticed can also reinforce the belief that one's body needs to be constantly monitored in order to be vigilant for suddenly emerging diseases.

Palpating body regions also can worsen the person's health worries and bodily preoccupation. Repeated self-palpation of the lower abdomen to check for liver enlargement can lead to a soreness or tenderness, which the person may misinterpret as evidence of liver disease. Repeated use of a tongue depressant to check the back of one's throat for inflammation can induce soreness, which may be misinterpreted as an indication of infection. Repeatedly swallowing, to check for "throat cancer," can induce the sensation that there is a lump in one's throat, thereby strengthening the person's fear of cancer.

Repeated bodily checking also makes the health-anxious person aware of bodily changes and sensations that other people don't usually notice. Thus, checking, combined with discussing and comparing one's health with that of one's friends and family members, can reinforce the health-anxious person's belief that she or he is particularly weak or sickly.

Another form of bodily checking involves the purchase of home diagnostic tests. Some people with excessive fears of colorectal cancer purchase a Home Fecal Occult Blood Test, which is available at pharmacies without a prescription. This test screens for occult (hidden) blood in the stool, which may be due to cancerous tissue or precancerous polyps. A common version of this test involves placing a small stool sample on a chemically treated card; then another chemical is added. If the card turns blue, then there is blood in the stool. The American Gastroenterological Association recommends that this test be performed yearly for people over age 40 or 50 years. But some health-anxious people excessively perform this test (e.g., weekly), thereby increasing the chances of false-positive results. The latter would occur if, say, blood was present as a result of hemorrhoids or a recent meal of red meat. False positives are not only alarming but also strengthen the person's preoccupation with health threats (e.g., "I was lucky this time. Next time it could be the real thing"). False positives also may strengthen the person's belief in the need to repeatedly check ("The test is not perfectly reliable; a negative result could be a false negative. Therefore, I need to frequently recheck"). With repeated false positives, the health-anxious person may insist on more extensive testing, such as a barium enema or colonoscopy.

The rise of readily available, user-pays methods of diagnostic assessment provides ample opportunity for health-anxious people to engage in excessive checking, and thereby perpetuate their health anxiety. Full-body computerized tomography (CT) or MRI scans and other imaging procedures are now widely available. Newspaper advertisements and promotional materials widely tout the value of these approaches, as illustrated by one recent press release for full-body scanning:

> The old adage that "Knowledge is Power" has never been more relevant than it is today. What you don't know truly *can* hurt you. Having the knowledge of a high risk of heart attack or discovering a cancer early while it can be successfully treated will allow the patient to take preventative and/or treatment measures to put them in charge of their health. The knowledge that he or she is at low risk of heart attack and cancer will certainly give peace of mind. (*www.ldcmir.com/html/ news.html*, extracted June 18, 2002; emphasis in original)

The frequency of using these scans for bodily checking is limited only by one's financial resources. But the value of these scans is dubious. The scans are ineffectual screening methods according to many medical associations, including the Radiological Society of North America, the American College of Radiology, the American Cancer Society, and the U.S. Food and Drug Administration (*UC Berkeley Wellness Letter*, December 2002, p. 2).

Repeated scanning carries risks of radiation exposure. A CT scan of the abdomen, for example, gives the equivalent of about 50 times the radiation from a normal chest x-ray. Thus, repeated scanning with body scans buys, at best, "peace of mind" for the short term. For the health-anxious person, doubts and worries are likely to return.

Checking Health-Related Publications

Health-anxious people check health-related publications for a variety of reasons. Some check in order to reassure themselves that some bodily change or sensation is harmless. Others check in order to learn ways of warding off dreaded diseases, such as foods to eat, activities to do, or medications to take to reduce the risk of cancer. It is not uncommon for such checking to expose the health-anxious person to alarming information. The following quotation, which appeared in a widely published health newsletter, is likely to alarm many a health-anxious person:

> Germs that can make you sick are everywhere. According to an unpublished University of Arizona study, playground equipment, handrails and armrests, surfaces in public bathrooms, and shopping cart handles are among the *surfaces* that are likely to have traces of saliva or other bodily fluids that could contain germs. The *places* where you've got to be especially careful: daycare centres, gyms, doctors' offices, and restaurants. . . . And cold bugs can survive on your skin for several hours. So if you rub your eyes or scratch your nose—the main routes of entry—after touching a contaminated surface, the germs can hitch a ride right into your body. (*Nutrition Action Healthletter*, March, 2002, p. 7; emphases in original)

Some health-anxious people repeatedly phone hotlines, such as AIDS hotlines, to obtain reassurance. Reassurance seeking may be especially frequent in these cases because of the anonymous nature of the hotlines. Health-anxious people may also repeatedly check newspaper obituaries as a way of obtaining reassurance.

> Joel C. was terrified of developing cancer. He checked obituaries to reassure himself that men of his age were "too young" to get cancer. He was reassured when he found obituary listings of men who either died in old age, or men his age who "passed away suddenly," suggesting death by accident or heart attack, rather than cancer. Joel was made anxious by obituary listings of men who "died young after a brave fight" (suggesting cancer). Most times when he checked, Joel found reassuring rather than alarming obituaries. Thus, his checking was usually reinforced by reassuring information.

Cyberchondria

The Internet is a vast source of health-related information—and misinformation. With the widespread availability of the Internet, health-anxious people have been increasingly searching medical websites to learn about feared symptoms and diseases, such as on-line medical reference sites, medical school research sites, health-related websites set up by laypeople or private companies, and bulletin boards devoted to the discussion of symptoms and diseases. Some websites enable users to select particular symptoms from a menu; these symptoms are then matched to a list of corresponding diseases. When "sore throat" was selected at one website, the following possible causes were listed: viral pharyngitis, influenza, strep throat, and infectious mononucleosis. Hyperlinks were provided for each of these diseases, providing information about them.

The Internet provides health-anxious people with a virtually inexhaustible supply of terrifying medical information. For instance, the website for the National Association for Rare Disorders provides information on over 1,100 rare (and often fatal) diseases. People who worry that they may have a deadly disease often seek out this information in an effort to obtain reassurance. Often web searches make the person's health anxiety much worse. Thus, Internet checking can induce or perpetuate what the media has dubbed "cyberchondria."

> Alan M. was a bright young graduate student. Although his coursework and research was intellectually exciting, he also found the workload to be highly taxing. Gradually, he developed increasingly frequent episodes of chest pain, particularly during long evenings of study. He had been to the hospital emergency department on several occasions, and had been evaluated by a cardiologist. Despite reassurance that his pain was due to stress-related tension in his chest muscles, Alan continued to worry that he might have heart disease. Whenever he experienced chest pain he would perform Internet searches for information on chest pain, including searches of the Medline database. He hoped the searches would provide him with reassuring information about how stress could cause chest pain. All too often, however, Alan came across information about rare and deadly heart conditions. This information increased his health anxiety, to the point that he insisted that his cardiologist perform a potentially risky cardiac catheterization to rule out heart disease.

Some websites contain bulletin boards devoted primarily to health anxiety. These boards and their associated websites are intended for people who realize that their health anxiety is excessive, or who have significant others with this problem. The goal of these Internet resources is to provide support and helpful information to health-anxious people. However, a review of the postings on these boards reveals that people are all too often using them for the purpose of reassurance seeking. Some people place weekly postings, with concerns about a different "symptom" each week. They receive temporary reassurance from other people, until the next troubling "symptom" arises. Thus, these bulletin boards may inadvertently perpetuate health anxiety.

Internet searches can create other problems for health-anxious people. On-line pharmacies are available at some websites, dispensing prescription medications (often without requiring a doctor's prescription). This can lead to needless and potentially dangerous self-medication regimens for people who mistakenly believe they have, or might contract, a deadly malady. In the wake of the anthrax scares shortly after September 11, 2001, some health-anxious people began purchasing, via the Internet, large quantities of the antibiotic ciprofloxacin, and taking the drug "prophylactically." Such overuse of antibiotics has been linked to the rise of drug-resistant strains of bacteria.

RELIANCE ON SAFETY SIGNALS

Safety signals are stimuli that the person believes will be associated with the absence of feared outcomes. People with health anxiety disorders often seek out safety signals in order to protect themselves from feared diseases. The list of safety signals is limitless, and health-anxious people are often idiosyncratic in the sorts of safety signals that alleviate their health anxiety. Safety signals include precautionary items—such as a Medic Alert bracelet, cellular telephone, medication, or doctor's business card—that would prove valuable in the event of a medical emergency. Some safety signals are elaborate and expensive. Some health-anxious people have purchased portable medical equipment, such as cardiac defibrillators, after learning of the unpredictability of sudden cardiac death.

> Every year, more than 200,000 people in Canada and the US collapse and die of cardiac arrest. This is not a heart attack, it's worse: Without warning, the electrical signals that pump the heart go haywire and heartbeat stops. . . . Only a defibrillator can restart the heart. . . . [One person bought two of these devices:] "I have one in my home and my car, as a personal safety thing." (*Vancouver Sun*, February 2, 2002, p. A7)

There are two major problems with the unnecessary acquisition of, and reliance on, safety signals. First, they are persistent reminders of disease, and thereby contribute to the person's preoccupation with ill health. Second, the reliance on safety signals fosters helplessness and increases one's sense of vulnerability, because the person comes to believe that these "safeguards" are vital to one's health.

AVOIDANCE

Avoidance of disease-related stimuli is a characteristic of people who are frightened of acquiring a disease. Some forms of avoidance are also seen in people who believe they actually have a disease. In both cases avoidance can be passive or active, and plays a role in perpetuating health anxiety by preventing the person from acquiring information that would disconfirm his or her fears.

Passive Avoidance

Passive avoidance includes the deliberate failure to engage in some normal activity. This might involve avoiding annual medical checkups in order to limit one's exposure to sick people (other patients) and to people who come in contact with the sick (medical staff). People who view themselves as sickly or physically fragile avoid all forms of physical exertion, including physical exercise. This form of passive avoidance leads to physical deconditioning. As discussed in Chapter 2, poor physical fitness can result in postural hypotension, breathlessness, muscle wasting, and fatigue, which can promote further inactivity and reinforce beliefs that one is ill. Conversely, exercise programs that improve fitness can reduce bodily sensations such as musculoskeletal aches and pains (Gerdle et al., 1995), and so can play an important role in treating health anxiety disorders.

Active Avoidance

Active avoidance involves the deliberate performance of some action in order to limit one's exposure to disease. Some health-anxious people engage in drastic forms of active avoidance. To illustrate, some women are so frightened of the prospect of breast cancer that they undergo a prophylactic mastectomy (Easterling & Leventhal, 1989). This is a controversial procedure that is currently being investigated as a preventive intervention for women who have a strong family history of breast cancer and carry the BRCA1/2 genetic mutations (Stefanek, Hartmann, & Nelson, 2001). Some health-anxious women contemplate undergoing this procedure even when there is no evidence that they are in the high-risk population.

> Jane L. frequently worried about breast cancer, even though there was no indication that she was especially at risk. She frequently palpated her breasts in search of lumps, to the point that they became tender and swollen. Her life was so ruled by the fear of breast cancer that she believed she would be better off if she had a mastectomy. Jane consulted several doctors in the hope of eventually obtaining this procedure.

Avoidance versus Vigilance

The tendency to monitor versus distract depends on the person's beliefs about her or his health. People who believe that they could have a serious disease are likely to monitor their "symptoms." These people are likely to become increasingly anxious if they are unable to check their bodies. Conversely, people who believe that they are at risk for some future disease are likely to avoid sources of disease exposure. These differences have important treatment implications. People who tend to monitor their bodies may benefit from a reduction in body checking in order to learn that they do not need to monitor bodily sensations in order to stay healthy. People who avoid may benefit from exposure to "disease-related" stimuli, including exposure to bodily changes and sensations induced by physical exercise, so as to learn that these stimuli have no harmful consequences.

COMPLICATIONS ARISING
FROM MALADAPTIVE COPING STRATEGIES

Iatrogenic (Physician-Induced) Health Anxiety

An unfortunate consequence of repeated reassurance seeking and other forms of medical checking is that it increases the chance of iatrogenic worsening of health anxiety. Performing unnecessary medical tests to placate the patient may strengthen the latter's belief that he or she really has a serious medical condition: "If my doctor was certain my symptoms were due to stress, then why would he order more tests?" Some physicians provide repeated, unnecessary reassurance to their health-anxious patients, which may perpetuate the disorder (as discussed earlier in this chapter).

The tendency to seek opinions from multiple medical specialists ("doctor shopping") in a desperate attempt to seek the causes of one's "symptoms" can be iatrogenic because it increases the risk of unnecessary and possibly harmful medical tests (e.g., repeated exploratory surgeries). Doctor shopping also increases the odds that the patient will receive conflicting medical advice. This can fuel the patient's anxiety and confusion, resulting in more doctor shopping in an effort to obtain a consensus of opinion.

Maladaptive coping strategies on the part of health-anxious people are not the only sources of iatrogenesis. Health anxiety can be increased inadvertently by the physician. One source is poor doctor–patient communication, leading to patient misconceptions—for example, by misinterpreting "degenerative disk" to mean that one's bones are rapidly deteriorating. Health anxiety can also be iatrogenically induced by the overzealous diagnostician in search of a disease to explain the patient's physical complaints:

> Physicians repeatedly fail to recognize somatization . . . and instead, tend to pursue organic possibilities and compulsively evaluate and treat all symptoms. Over time, the result may be that patients undergo multiple hospital admissions, tests,

invasive procedures, operations, and medications without any benefit. . . . Be-
sides being costly, this odyssey through the health care system also has an enor-
mous risk of iatrogenic harm. (Fink, 1993, p. 211)

Medical misdiagnosis can also be iatrogenic. In experimental studies,
people who were incorrectly told that they had a particular illness tended
to report symptoms that they believed were congruent with the illness
(Baumann, Cameron, Zimmerman, & Leventhal, 1989; Croyle & Sande,
1998). The symptoms were often common ambiguous bodily sensations
(e.g., due to normal physiology). Ann M., for example, was told by a neurologist that her muscle weakness could be the beginning of MS. In the
weeks after that she recalled being highly anxious and experienced "all the
MS symptoms under the sun." Later she learned that the diagnosis was
mistaken.

Medications and the Nocebo Effect

Medications are potent sources of bodily sensations that can frighten health-
anxious people. Antihypertensive medications can produce postural hypotension and associated feelings of faintness (Chobanian, 1982; Schatz, 1986).
Cold and allergy preparations, such as those containing caffeine or ephedrine,
can produce arousal-related sensations. Tricyclic antidepressants and selective
serotonin reuptake inhibitors—which are increasingly used to treat health
anxiety—can produce a range of side effects, including agitation, nausea,
sweating, and palpitations (Canadian Pharmacists Association, 2002). Clinically, it is common to encounter health-anxious people who worry about the
possible adverse effects of their medications. Thus, medications can sometimes
perpetuate health anxiety through their side effects.

Side effects are also associated with a phenomenon known as the
"nocebo effect," which is the opposite of the well-known "placebo effect."
The nocebo effect refers to expectation-induced negative side effects (Hahn,
1999). Commonly, these are generalized and diffuse symptoms such as drowsiness, nausea, fatigue, and insomnia (Barsky, Saintforth, Rogers, & Borus,
2002). Nocebo effects may arise from selective attention to, and misinterpretation of, ordinary bodily sensations (e.g., sensations due to anxiety or to normal physiology). People with high levels of health anxiety are especially likely
to show nocebo effects (Barsky et al., 2002). This means that attempts to placate health-anxious patients by unnecessarily prescribing medications can
backfire. A physician might prescribe an antibiotic with the intention of ad-
ministering a placebo, but instead the health-anxious person returns with a
host of nocebo effects. As a result, the patient's health preoccupation persists,
and possibly worsens.

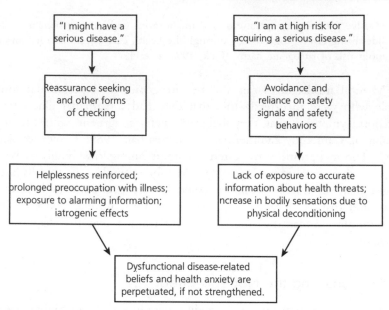

FIGURE 3.1. Maladaptive coping strategies can perpetuate or worsen health anxiety.

SUMMARY AND CONCLUSIONS

This chapter considered four common maladaptive coping strategies associated with excessive health anxiety: persistent reassurance seeking, other forms of repetitive checking, reliance on safety signals, and avoidance. We also considered some of the complications arising from these coping strategies. These strategies appear to be driven primarily by the person's beliefs about having or acquiring a disease. Figure 3.1 illustrates these links.

4

Learning Experiences and the Development of Health Anxiety

What role does learning play in predisposing and precipitating health anxiety disorders? We will examine these issues by first reviewing the literature on the environmental and genetic factors. This will permit some tentative conclusions about the relative importance of environmental factors (e.g., learning experiences) and genes. Then we will consider in more detail the role of particular life experiences, such as stressful life events and experiences with one's parents. As with most of the research on health anxiety, the relevant research has been mainly on hypochondriasis.

ENVIRONMENTAL AND GENETIC FACTORS

Studies of monozygotic (MZ) and dizygotic (DZ) twins have examined the heritability of hypochondriasis using the MMPI Hs (Hypochondriasis) scale. Results suggested that hypochondriasis is moderately heritable, with genetic factors accounting for up to 35% of the variance in Hs scores (DiLalla, Carey, Gottesman, & Bouchard, 1996; Gottesman, 1962). According to the Wiggins content scales, which can be extracted from the MMPI, self-reported poor health is also moderately heritable (26% of variance), as is the tendency to experience somatic symptoms (42%) (DiLalla et al., 1996). A problem with these studies is that the MMPI is a poor measure of hypochondriasis because it assesses awareness of bodily sensations rather than hypochondriasis per se. At best, these studies indicate that one correlate of health anxiety—the tendency to experience recurrent bodily sensations—is moderately heritable.

Torgersen (1986) used a structured interview to assess the lifetime history of somatoform disorders in MZ and DZ twins. The concordance for hypochondriasis was not significantly higher in MZ than in DZ twins, suggesting that hypochondriasis is not heritable. Results also suggested that hypochondriasis is not genetically linked to other somatoform disorders. A caveat in interpreting these results is the very small sample size ($n = 35$ twin pairs), which may make any estimates of concordance unreliable.

To summarize, the research tentatively suggests that the risk for developing hypochondriasis is not strongly influenced by genetic factors. Environmental factors seem to be more important. The heritabilities of other health anxiety disorders are unknown.

Multivariate twin studies by Kendler et al. (1995) indicate that anxiety disorders and mood disorders arise from a combination of specific and nonspecific factors:

- Environmental factors specific to the development of a given disorder.
- Environmental factors common to a number of different disorders.
- Genetic factors specific to a given disorder.
- Genetic factors shared by a number of disorders.

Kendler and colleagues did not study health anxiety disorders, although it is possible that they too are a product of patterns of specific and nonspecific factors. Nonspecific factors may be those that are common to health anxiety disorders and other emotional disorders. Such factors, whether they be genetic or environmental, may explain why health anxiety disorders are commonly comorbid with other disorders. Hypochondriasis, for example, is often comorbid with mood disorders and anxiety disorders (see Chapter 1).

STRESSFUL LIFE EXPERIENCES
AND THE ACQUISITION OF HEALTH ANXIETY

Experiences with Disease and Death

Health anxiety in adulthood is associated with a childhood history of severe diseases in oneself and in one's family members (APA, 2000; Fritz & Williams, 1989; Robbins & Kirmayer, 1996). Childhood diseases—particularly those involving severe pain or discomfort—can induce fear of future disease. Hospitalization and separation from nurturant caregivers can add to the distress, particularly when the child is strongly attached to her or his caregiver.

The death of someone close to the person appears to sometimes precipitate hypochondriasis (APA, 2000). For example, the loss of a loved one in a traffic accident may lead one to believe that life is fragile and that dangers are ever present. In turn, this can lead to bodily preoccupation and worry about one's own health.

According to retrospective reports from patients, a range of factors may be involved in the development of disease phobia, including the personal experience of disease or exposure to environmental toxins, or observations of family members grappling with illness (Malis et al., 2002; Marks, 1987). To illustrate, exposure to air pollution may fuel one's fear of eventually succumbing to emphysema, especially if the person believes that his or her lungs have been damaged by pollution.

In summary, various types of experiences with disease (in oneself or others) and experiences with the death of loved ones have been associated with health anxiety disorders. A limitation of the research is that most studies have been based on retrospective reports, and so it is possible that health-anxious people are engaging in some sort of "effort after meaning" to make sense of their health anxiety. If experiences with disease and death do play a role in health anxiety disorders, then it would be important to determine whether the various classes of experience are specific or nonspecific in the development of health anxiety. Loss of a loved one, for instance, may be a nonspecific factor, linked to hypochondriasis and other disorders (e.g., mood disorders). Childhood experiences with severe painful diseases might be more specific to health anxiety disorders.

Physical and Sexual Abuse

Barsky et al. (1994b) compared adult patients with hypochondriasis with outpatients without hypochondriasis from the same general medical clinic. Hypochondriasis was associated with a higher frequency of sexual abuse (29% vs. 7%), childhood physical violence (32% vs. 7%), and major parental upheaval (29% vs. 9%) before age 17. Stressors such as physical or sexual abuse may lead the young child to believe that he or she is weak, helpless, and generally vulnerable, thereby contributing to anxiety about one's health.

Various psychiatric populations, compared to normal controls, are associated with increased prevalence of sexual abuse, physical abuse, and other sorts of stressful life events. Examples include patients with panic disorder, bulimia nervosa, and borderline personality disorder (Paris, 1998; Taylor, 2000). This suggests that physical and sexual abuse plays, at most, a nonspecific role, possibly influencing health anxiety disorders and many other disorders.

Other Stressors

The occurrence of stressful life events unrelated to disease or death (e.g., financial stressors) are also correlated with increased somatic complaints, health anxiety, and physician visits. These increases are disproportionate to actual medical morbidity (Hankin & Oktay, 1979; Kellner, Pothek, Romanik, & Winslow, 1983; Mechanic, 1978; Rahe & Arthur, 1978). Stressors can produce arousal-related bodily sensations, which some people misinterpret as indications of serious disease. People with hypochondriasis who spend large amounts of money on unnecessary medical tests may encounter financial problems as a result. Therefore, repeated testing can create stressors that give rise to anxiety-related bodily sensations, which, if misinterpreted as evidence of disease, will exacerbate health anxiety.

Stressful life events are insufficient on their own to lead to health anxiety disorders because most people who experience these events don't develop severe health anxiety. A number of factors are probably involved. Various factors might have additive (incremental) or interactive effects on the risk for health anxiety disorders. Particular disease-related beliefs may interact with particular (critical) events to give rise to, or exacerbate, health anxiety. This is illustrated in the following case:

> Warren T. had experienced mild health anxiety for much of his life. He didn't develop full-blown hypochondriasis until he turned 40. At that age he began to worry excessively about having a heart attack. He checked his pulse several times a day and avoided all forms of physical exertion. He carried his cellular telephone wherever he went, "just in case" he developed chest pains. His father and uncle had unexpectedly died of heart attacks in their 40s. Warren believed that he had now reached the age at which he was imminently at risk. Hence, he experienced a worsening of his health anxiety.

PARENT–CHILD INTERACTIONS

Early learning experiences arising from particular patterns of parent–child interaction might predispose a person to develop excessive health anxiety as a child or later in life. Learning experiences may exert their effects by shaping health-related beliefs and coping behaviors. Several sorts of parent–child patterns have been studied:

- *Parental modeling* experiences where the child observes that his or her parents are excused from home or work responsibilities or receive special attention when they are ill.
- *Parental overprotection*, in which parents treat the child as frail and vulnerable, thereby leading the child to believe that he or she is at risk for succumbing to illness.
- *Parental reinforcement* of illness behaviors, which occurs when a child often receives toys, food treats, attention, sympathy, or special care, or is excused from school or home chores, when ill.

Most retrospective studies suggest that severe health anxiety in adulthood is associated with childhood exposure to these parental patterns (Baker & Merskey, 1982; Bianchi, 1971; Parker & Lipscombe, 1980; Schwartz, Gramling, & Mancini, 1994; Watt & Stewart, 2000; Whitehead, Winget, Fedoravicius, Wooley, & Blackwell, 1981; Whitehead, Busch, Heller, & Costa, 1986; Whitehead et al., 1994; but cf. Barsky et al., 1994b; Mabe, Alex, Hobson, Jones, & Jarvis, 1988). Consistent with importance of parental modeling, prospective (longitudinal) studies have found that parental ill health is correlated with medically unexplained symptoms in offspring during childhood and adulthood (Craig, Boardman, Mills, Daly-Jones, & Drake, 1993; Hotopf, Mayou, Wadsworth, & Wessely, 1999; Mechanic, 1980).

The three parent–child interaction patterns may contribute to different aspects of health anxiety. Parental modeling may contribute to beliefs that disease is important and not to be ignored, thereby leading to bodily preoccupation in the child. Parental modeling may also lead the child to vicariously acquire health worries. Parental overprotection may lead the child to fear that he or she is vulnerable, and that diseases are highly dangerous.

Parental reinforcement impresses upon the child the importance of symptoms by adding a desirable (rewarding) component to being sick, such as exemption from chores and other responsibilities (Parsons, 1951). A further reward is that illness provides a ready excuse for poor performance or failure (e.g., poor performance in an exam). Health-anxious people may use this face-saving strategy if they believe that disease is a legitimate excuse (Smith, Snyder, & Perkins, 1983). Thus, learning experiences that teach the child that being sick is "rewarding" can perpetuate excessive health anxiety because the child gains rewards by remaining health anxious, and loses rewards if he or she attempts to overcome the anxiety. This does not mean that health-anxious people are feigning or malingering. The incentives may simply encourage somatic preoccupation in people who are already genuinely worried that they have some serious disease. The incentives probably don't play a major role in health anxiety, because reinforcement of the sick role is not always correlated with the severity of health anxiety (Ferguson, 1998; Stone & Neale, 1981).

Although the available research suggests that parent–child interactions may be important in the development of health anxiety disorders, we are not advocating a "blame your parents" model of health anxiety. It is unhelpful for health-anxious people to blame others (or themselves) for their problems. Parents learn their parenting styles from a variety of sources, including their own experiences during childhood. Parental overprotection and reinforcement may arise because these patterns are reinforcing to both the parent and the child: parents feel they are providing good care, and children feel cared for. It can be difficult for parents to foresee the long-term consequences of well-intentioned actions. Moreover, not all children become health-anxious as a result of parental overprotection, reinforcement, or modeling. Parent–child patterns are but one element in the matrix of factors involved in the etiology of health anxiety disorders.

EXPOSURE TO OTHER FORMS OF DISEASE-RELATED INFORMATION

Media Influences

People draw on environmental information to help decide whether bodily sensations are due to disease (Baumann et al., 1989). The media is a potent source of information. Each day the mass media bombards us with reports—especially sensational reports—about health-related threats. Learning about the "disease du jour" not only increases people's awareness of health threats, but also can teach them to become worried about bodily changes and sensations that had previously, prompted no concerns. Popular magazine articles about actor Michael J. Fox's battle with Parkinson's disease can cause people to become hypervigilant for, and to misinterpret, benign motor reactions (e.g., eyelid twitches). Similarly, media reports concerning sudden acute respiratory syndrome (SARS) have caused many people to misinterpret mild coughs as indications of the dreaded disease. Thus, media reports can cause bodily changes and sensations to acquire new, alarming meanings. The role of disease-related information in the acquisition of health anxiety disorders is vividly illustrated in two phenomena: medical students' disease and mass psychogenic illness. Both are typically transient forms of hypochondriasis.

Medical Students' Disease

As mentioned in Chapter 1, medical students' disease (MSD) is a form of abridged hypochondriasis in which medical students fear they have the diseases they are studying and misinterpret bodily changes and sensations as "symptoms" of these diseases (Woods et al., 1966). MSD has long been recognized by medical instructors, and may be as old as medicine itself. In his classic 1651 treatise *The Anatomy of Melancholy*, Robert Burton (1927) reported the following observation made by one of his medical colleagues: "As Felix Planter notes of some young Physicians, that studying to cure diseases catch them themselves, will be sick, and appropriate all symptoms they find related of others to their own persons" (p. 330).

The first empirical studies of MSD suggested that many medical students—particularly first-year and, to a lesser degree, second-year students—exhibit anxiety about the diseases they are studying (Hunter, Lohrenz, & Schwartzman 1964; Woods et al., 1966). Results from later research have been mixed, with one study finding that medical students have higher health anxiety than nonmedical students (Moss-Morris & Petrie, 2001), whereas others studies failed to find this effect (Howes & Salkovskis, 1998; Kellner, Wiggins, & Pathak, 1986b). The inconsistencies are probably due to sample differences. Studies finding evidence of MSD have focused on first-year students.

MSD includes fears of all kinds of diseases, including cancer, tuberculosis, cardiac disease, and renal disease. The severity of health anxiety ranges from mild or moderate through to severe and disruptive. Woods et al. (1966) observed that 15% of students experienced major impairments, including phobic avoidance of things related to the disease:

> One student who experienced MSD regarding lung cancer at the beginning of his second year then phobically avoided all reading and study about this condition. This persisted into the clinical years as a deliberate avoidance of patients with lung cancer. (Woods et al., 1966, p. 788)

In most cases the episodes of health anxiety abate within weeks, but they may reoccur when the student studies other diseases: "More often it disappeared through the reassurance provided by intensive study of the disease or by direct or covert consultation with an instructor or physician" (Woods et al., 1966, p. 787).

How does this phenomenon arise? MSD is the process of matching one's bodily changes or sensations to known disease labels (Moss-Morris & Petrie, 2001). As students read about the signs and symptoms of various diseases, or observe patients with diseases, the students' bodily events take on new meaning. When students learn about diseases such as diabetes, they may become self-aware of sensations such as thirst or increased urinary frequency, which they may misinterpret as indications of diabetes (Moss-Morris & Petrie, 2001).

Medical school is a stressful experience for many students, especially in their early years. Medical school is therefore a source of stress-related bodily sensations, the most common of which are headache and fatigue. Students who have problems in their personal and academic lives are especially prone to these sensations, and are particularly likely to develop MSD (Pennebaker, 2000; Woods et al., 1966). As the students learn about various kinds of deadly diseases, they may misinterpret stress-related (and other) bodily changes and sensations as indications of severe disease. A student learning about brain diseases may misinterpret a tension headache as a sign of a chronic subdural hematoma (bleeding between the outer membranes that cover the brain). A student learning about kidney disease may misinterpret stress-related polyuria (increased urination) as a symptom of kidney failure.

Mass Psychogenic Illness

Mass psychogenic illness (MPI) provides an instructive illustration of how intense health anxiety can be rapidly acquired in a group of people through exposure to disease-related information. MPI refers to the occurrence, in a group of people, of bodily changes or sensations that the sufferers mistakenly attribute to disease. The most common complaints are headache, dizziness, light-headedness, nausea, abdominal pain, cough, fatigue, drowsiness, and weakness (Jones, 2000). The "symptoms" typically have rapid onset, quickly spread to others, and have a rapid remission.

> In November 1998, a teacher at a Tennessee high school noticed a "gasoline-like" smell in her classroom. Shortly afterward she developed headache, nausea, shortness of breath, and dizziness. The school was evacuated and dozens of students and staff went to a nearby hospital emergency department. The most frequent symptoms were headache, dizziness, nausea, shortness of breath, and drowsiness. The occurrence of symptoms was correlated with seeing another ill person, knowing that a classmate was ill, and reporting an unusual odor at the school. Sixty-five percent of people reported detecting an odor, although there was no consistency in the reported quality or location of the smell. Sixty-eight percent of afflicted people thought their symptoms were caused by exposure to fumes or other toxic substances. Most symptoms resolved quickly after exiting the school. An extensive investigation was performed by several government agencies, along with medical evaluations of the sufferers. No medical or environmental explanation was found (Jones et al., 2000).

This case bears all the hallmarks of MPI. Formerly known as "mass hysteria," MPI is "increasingly recognized as a significant health and social problem that is more common than is presently reported" (Bartholomew & Wessely, 2002, p. 300). Outbreaks typically occur after an environmental event or trigger—such as an innocuous odor, an "unusual" taste in the drinking water, or particularly heavy smog—which is misinterpreted as a sign of danger. Misinterpretations are especially likely if the sufferers have learned of related health threats. White powder, for example, may be misinterpreted as anthrax spores after one learns that there have been cases of anthrax bioterrorism in which spores (in the form of white power) were mailed to people.

The "index person" in MPI—the first person to report the symptoms—may be suffering from a genuine medical condition such as influenza, but misinterprets the significance of the symptoms. People nearby learn of this concern, become anxious, and scan their bodies for indications of the dreaded affliction. Symptoms in these people are probably normal bodily reactions or anxiety-related bodily sensations (Jones, 2000; Wessely, 2000). For some people, anxiety-related hyperventilation occurs, which produces a range of intense bodily sensations, such as faintness, sweating, and tingling in the extremities. Other people notice that their skin is itchy, which they attribute to disease. They scratch themselves and thereby induce skin irritation. Others observe these sufferers and they too become concerned. They scan their bodies and notice bodily sensations, which they take as signs of infection. Thus, MPI rapidly spreads. Studies of MPI outbreaks (Bartholomew & Wessely, 2002; Jones et al., 2000; Wessely, 2000) suggest that its likelihood increases when the following conditions are met:

- Widely held preexisting health concerns (e.g., concerns about bioterrorism or exposure to toxic waste).
- The group of people is closely congregated in an enclosed settings (e.g., people in a school, office building, military unit, or factory).
- Occurrence of some environmental event or trigger.
- People observe or hear that others have symptoms (e.g., "line of sight" transmission).
- In schools, the spread occurs down the age-scale, beginning in older or higher status students.
- The perceived threatening agent is seen as credible.
- A prominent response by emergency services, such as by the arrival of ambulances and fire engines, with sirens blaring.

Uncertainty and fear after disasters commonly generate psychogenic symptoms such as hyperventilation, headache, and nausea, which may be difficult to distinguish from the early stages of a chemical, biological, or toxic insult (Bartholomew & Wessely, 2002). Thus, MPI can be difficult to distinguish from disease caused by general medical conditions (Jones et al., 2000). The uncertainty means that some sort of medical and environmental tests are often warranted. But persistent medical investigations increase the likelihood of false-positive results, which must then be explained to the apprehensive sufferers (Jones et al., 2000).

MPI can persist when sufferers refuse to believe that their symptoms were simply due to anxiety. Some sufferers conclude that medical and environmental investigations had failed to find the real source of their "symptoms," or that some sort of cover-up occurred. In a conjecture that is likely to provoke controversy, Bartholomew and Wessely (2002) suggested that a number of the people involved in the September 11 terrorist attacks were suffering from MPI.

> About 4,000 of a total 10,000 New York firefighters who have visited the site of the World Trade Center attacks have reported respiratory difficulties, dubbed "World Trade Center syndrome." Many others who live and work near ground zero in lower Manhattan are reporting similar symptoms (shortness of breath, chest pressure and pain, coughing, and general anxiety), despite the New York Health Department's continuous monitoring of airborne contaminants by city, state and federal agencies, which continue to indicate contaminant levels below that which poses a public health threat. (p. 303)

The research literature, although limited to a small number of reports, suggests that any of us may succumb to MPI under the right conditions. "No one is immune . . . because humans continually construct reality and the perceived danger needs only to be plausible in order to gain acceptance within a particular group and generate anxiety" (Bartholomew & Wessely, 2002, p. 304).

SUMMARY AND CONCLUSIONS

Research on the acquisition of excessive health anxiety is still in its infancy. There is suggestive evidence that particular life experiences are important, such as stressful life events (e.g., severe painful diseases), particular forms of parent–child interactions, and exposure to disease-related information. These experiences may shape the development of dysfunctional disease-related beliefs, thereby leading to excessive health anxiety. Some experiences, such as a history of serious childhood disease, may specifically lead to health anxiety disorders. Other sorts of experiences, such as childhood physical or sexual abuse, may be nonspecific, predisposing the person to develop any of a number of disorders, depending on the presence or absence of other etiological factors. It is important for the clinician treating health anxiety disorders to understand the patient's disease-related learning experiences because they enable one to understand why the patient holds a particular set of disease-related beliefs. Armed with this knowledge, the clinician may be in a better position to devise corrective learning experiences to modify the patient's dysfunctional beliefs.

5

Treatments
A Review of the Research

When health anxiety is a secondary feature of some other disorder, such as a mood or anxiety disorder, treatment of the latter (with either drugs or cognitive-behavioral therapy) can lead to reductions in health anxiety (Fava, Kellner, Zielezny, & Grandi, 1988; Kellner, Fava, Lisansky, Perini, & Zielezny, 1986a; Noyes, Reich, Clancy, & O'Gorman, 1986; Taylor, 2000). The treatment of health anxiety, as the patient's primary (most severe) problem has, however, been a source of controversy. Until recently there has been a lack of sound empirical work on treatments for health anxiety disorders.

Based largely on clinical experience with early treatment techniques, the prognosis for primary hypochondriasis was widely considered to be poor, and treatments were thought to be of limited value (Kenyon, 1964; Ladee, 1966). As a result, health-anxious patients were often seen as "the despair of their physicians, who soon learn to dread the sound of their voices or their approaching footsteps" (Goldstein & Birnbom, 1976, p. 150). Extreme interventions were often contemplated, and in some cases clinicians performed prefrontal lobotomies in the hope of reducing this disorder (Bernstein, Callahan, & Jaranson, 1975; Greenblatt, 1959).

During the 1980s and 1990s there were several important advances in treatments for health anxiety, particularly in the development of behavioral, cognitive-behavioral, and pharmacological interventions. Yet many textbooks and articles continued to make pessimistic pronouncements about the value of treatments for hypochondriasis and related disorders.

Hypochondriasis as a primary condition does not seem to be responsive to known psychopharmacological drugs. (Martin & Yutzy, 1994, p. 614)

Drugs are of no value unless the patient is depressed. . . . No behaviour therapy is reliably effective. (Gelder, Gath, & Mayou, 1983, pp. 184–185)

Unless hypochondriasis is part of an overt affective disturbance, medications . . . are without effect. (Nemiah, 1985, p. 941)

Neither the benzodiazepines nor behaviour therapy appear to be of use. . . . Drug therapy . . . is not indicated for primary hypochondriasis. (Quality Assurance Project, 1985, pp. 397, 404)

Each of these conclusions turned out to be wrong. This will become apparent throughout this chapter, as we review the research on the treatments for hypochondriasis and other health anxiety disorders. Most of the research has focused on hypochondriasis, in either its full or abridged forms, although there have been several studies on delusional disorder (somatic type).

In the following sections we review the psychosocial and drug treatments for full and abridged nondelusional hypochondriasis, where this is the patient's primary problem. The available research also permits us to perform a meta-analysis of many of these treatments. This will allow us to obtain a preliminary indication of their comparative efficacy. Treatments that are only supported by uncontrolled case studies, such as psychodynamic psychotherapy and hypnotherapy, are not included in the meta-analysis.

This chapter also reviews the treatments for delusional disorder (somatic type). Finally, we consider a number of important treatment-related issues, including prognostic factors and special populations.

PSYCHOSOCIAL TREATMENTS
FOR NONDELUSIONAL HEALTH ANXIETY

Psychotherapies

Psychodynamic Treatments

The pessimism about the treatment of hypochondriasis and other health anxiety disorders arose, in part, from the fact that psychodynamic psychotherapy proved to be of little value in treating these problems. Summarizing the early findings of dynamic psychotherapy, Knight (1941) found that of the eight published case reports of patients with hypochondriasis, only one patient appeared to benefit. Ladee (1966) assessed 23 patients with hypochondriasis who were thought to be good candidates for dynamic therapy. Only four (17%)

achieved a "satisfactory-to-good result" (p. 376). For patients treated predominantly with supportive psychotherapy, Kenyon (1964) reported that only 21% were judged to be recovered or much improved.

Why is psychodynamic psychotherapy of such limited value? The famous German psychiatrist Karl Leonhard offered an explanation in 1961 that still rings true today:

> Hypochondriac neuroses are often thought to be difficult to influence. As a matter of fact they do respond rather badly to analytical psychotherapy in most cases. If patients of this type of neurosis are asked by the therapist to give a complete report of their life history and to go back to childhood as far as possible, it often induces them to devote still more attention to their body and state of health than hitherto. As a result their state of health gets worse because their neurosis developed exactly from this excessive attention to themselves. (p. 123)

Strategic Therapy

Wetchler (1994) reported a case study in which methods from strategic therapy were used to treat hypochondriasis. The patient, Ron, was frightened of having contracted HIV after "deep kissing" and touching the vulva of a prostitute. He had failed to benefit from medical reassurance, including negative HIV tests. Strategic therapy was based on the assumption that the patient's health anxiety was part of an interactional sequence among family members (consisting of his estranged wife and their child), and that his health preoccupations kept the family from dealing with other issues (i.e., the marital breakdown). The focus of treatment was on changing behaviors that maintained Ron's health anxiety. The therapist offered both straightforward and paradoxical suggestions. *Straightforward suggestions* direct the patient to perform a specific behavior that breaks an existing sequence of events. *Paradoxical suggestions* direct the patient to do more of his or her symptom-maintaining behaviors in the hope that the patient will do the opposite.

The therapist noted that Ron's HIV concerns arose on those occasions in which he was separated from his wife: "in his loneliness [Ron] developed HIV hypochondria" (Wetchler, 1994, p. 5). (No explanation was offered as to why loneliness would induce hypochondriasis.) The therapist further noted that Ron's HIV concerns appeared to be maintained by his persistent reassurance seeking from medical professionals and others. Two interventions were used in the first therapy session to disrupt these anxiety-inducing factors: (1) a straightforward intervention, advising Ron to attempt a reconciliation with his wife (which Ron had wanted to do, but had not done because he was anxious about rejection), and (2) a paradoxical intervention, informing Ron that there was indeed a chance that he could have contracted HIV from the prostitute:

> The therapist stated that Ron *should be concerned* about having contracted HIV. As
> studies to date had not totally refuted the theory that HIV could be contracted
> through deep kissing, he may have caught the virus. . . . Ron responded to the
> paradoxical intervention with shock and confusion. He stated that the therapist's
> job was to talk him out of his fears, not enhance them. The therapist maintained
> the paradoxical stance by responding that since Ron's fears were somewhat ap-
> propriate it was unwise to challenge them at this time. . . . Prior to the end of the
> session, Ron again stated that he wanted the therapist to convince him that he
> should not be afraid of having contracted HIV. The therapist again responded
> that Ron should be afraid as there was justifiable cause for his concern.
> (Wetchler, 1994, pp. 5–6, emphasis in original)

Not surprisingly, "prior to the second appointment, Ron called the therapist
to announce that he no longer needed therapy" (p. 6).

As part of the paradoxical intervention the therapist told Ron that in order to overcome his fears he would have to follow the path suggested by a
"sign." As it turned out, Ron found his sign after consulting a priest, who said
it was up to God to decide whether to take him from this world. Apparently,
this advice combined with the reconciliation with his wife was sufficient to allay Ron's health concerns. However, Ron admitted that he planned to have
another HIV test.

Wetchler (1994) claimed that Ron's hypochondriasis had been successfully treated as result of the single session of strategic therapy. This is dubious.
There is no evidence that Ron's hypochondriasis had been reduced. His concerns were allayed by the priest, although this may have simply been a temporary effect. Ron was persisting in seeking reassurance (via another HIV test),
and presumably was still vulnerable to a resurgence of health anxiety if he
again became estranged or separated from his wife. Even if his hypochondriasis had been reduced, there was no evidence that this was due to strategic therapy. The benefits could have been entirely due to his consultation
with the priest. A further concern with the strategic treatment is that the paradoxical intervention involved deception and provided Ron with erroneous
information about the risk of contracting HIV (McCollum, 1994).

Hypnotherapy

Deiker and Counts (1980) described a case study in which hypochondriasis
was successfully treated with three sessions of hypnosis followed by seven sessions of dynamic psychotherapy. Hypnosis was used to facilitate cognitive
change. The patient was hypnotized and given instructions that her daily
problems (e.g., household hassles) would take on more importance than her

health concerns, and that she would overcome her problems if she continued to work on them. The intervention was based on the assumption that complaining about her health and adopting the sick role (i.e., avoidance of responsibilities because of illness) was used to avoid more pressing problems in her life. Treatment was associated with a decrease in physical complaints and an increase in activity level. This occurred over the course of the hypnosis sessions. Strangely, however, the authors did not assess the central features of hypochondriasis—disease fears and beliefs—and so it is not clear whether treatment was sufficient to treat hypochondriasis.

Cognitive-Behavioral Therapy and Related Interventions

There are several treatment packages that are similar to one another in that they incorporate one or more cognitive-behavioral interventions:

- Psychoeducation.
- Explanatory therapy.
- Cognitive therapy.
- Exposure and response prevention.
- Cognitive-behavioral therapy.
- Behavioral stress management.

Table 5.1 summarizes the components of these packages; more detailed discussions appear in Chapters 7–12. All the interventions listed in Table 5.1 are based on the assumption that a thorough medical and psychiatric evaluation has been conducted beforehand. All include nonspecific treatment factors (e.g., therapist warmth and empathy) along with some form of psychoeducation. Nonspecific treatment factors are likely to be very important. Health-anxious people often complain about lack of understanding from others, including their health care providers. An open and accepting attitude by the therapist may enhance the patient's sense of being understood (Bouman & Visser, 1998; Kellner, 1986).

The treatments differ in that some packages contain more components than others, and only explanatory therapy uses reassurance as an intervention. The other treatment packages explicitly avoid giving reassurance because of the concern that reassurance perpetuates health anxiety. Our treatment approach similarly eschews the repeated provision of reassurance. Behavioral exercises in cognitive-behavioral therapy are, in many ways, similar to those used in exposure and response prevention. The main difference is that a broader range of behavioral exercises are used in cognitive-behavioral therapy.

TABLE 5.1. Cognitive-Behavioral and Related Treatments for Health Anxiety

Components	Psycho-education	Explanatory therapy	Cognitive therapy	Exposure and response prevention	Cognitive-behavioral therapy	Behavioral stress management
Thorough medical and psychiatric evaluation	+	+	+	+	+	+
Nonspecific treatment factors (e.g., therapist attention, warmth, and empathy)	+	+	+	+	+	+
Detailed education about the causes of bodily sensations and health anxiety	+	+	+	+	+	+
Monitoring of bodily sensations, emotions, and thoughts	+	+	+	+	+	+
Extensive use of cognitive restructuring exercises	–	–	+	–	+	+
Systematic exposure exercises	–	–	–	+	+	+
Relaxation training	+	–	–	–	+/–	+
Assertiveness training	–	–	–	–	–	+
Stimulus control exercises for reducing worry	–	–	–	–	–	+
Time management training	–	–	–	–	–	+
Provision of repeated assurance that patient does not have a serious disease	–	+	–	–	–	–

Note. +, intervention used; +/–, sometimes used; –, not used.

These exercises are often framed as behavioral experiments that test health-related beliefs. In the following sections we describe each treatment package and review the outcome findings.

Psychoeducation

The provision of information about the patient's disorder and its treatment, presented clearly in verbal, written, or video formats, has long been known to be useful in treating general medical conditions (e.g., Devine, 1992). Psychoeducation can similarly be useful in treating health anxiety disorders. The advantages of psychoeducation are that it is simple to administer, and it can be delivered in groups (e.g., five to eight participants per group).

Bouman (2002) provides an excellent example of a psychoeducational program, which was presented as a course titled "Coping with Illness Anxiety." The program was based in the community (rather than in a mental health clinic) and designed for people who were not considering a referral to a mental health practitioner. This approach may enhance the acceptability of treatment for people with health anxiety disorders, many of whom reject the idea that they are suffering from a mental disorder. The program consisted of a mix of minilectures, demonstrations, video illustrations, focused group discussions, and brief exercises. Homework assignments were brief and optional (e.g., monitoring and challenging thoughts, identifying avoidance behaviors, monitoring daily hassles). The session contents were as follows:

- *Session 1.* Overview of the program.
- *Session 2.* Role of thoughts in producing health anxiety, and how to challenge them.
- *Session 3.* Information on the role of selective attention in health anxiety.
- *Session 4.* Education on the role of checking, reassurance seeking, avoidance, and other maladaptive behaviors in perpetuating health anxiety.
- *Session 5.* Information on the role of stress in producing bodily sensations.
- *Session 6.* Exercises in which participants devise interventions to overcome their health anxiety (e.g., cognitive restructuring exercises) based on their individualized cognitive-behavioral formulation of their health anxiety.

Psychoeducation differs from the provision of reassurance in that the patient is presented with new information. By comparison, the provision of reassurance involves the repeated presentation of old information (e.g., reminding the patient each week that he or she is healthy, or repeatedly performing medical tests to placate the patient). Coping strategies (e.g., relaxation training) are also often used in psychoeducation, but systematic exposure exercises are usually not included.

Three studies have examined the merits of group psychoeducation as the main component of treatment (Avia et al., 1996; Bouman, 2002; Lidbeck, 1997). Using a mixed sample of participants with full and abridged hypochondriasis, Avia et al. (1996) found that psychoeducation (administered in a university setting) was associated with significant reductions in illness fears and attitudes, somatic symptoms, and dysfunctional beliefs. Gains were maintained at 1-year follow-up. There was little change in a comparison wait-list control group.

Lidbeck's (1997) group psychoeducation program was administered to patients with medically unexplained symptoms, most of whom had hypochondriacal features (full or abridged hypochondriasis). Patients were treated in an outpatient clinic at a preventive medicine unit. Psychoeducation emphasized the role of stress in producing bodily sensations, and included relaxation training. Twenty-five percent of referred patients refused treatment, possibly because they did not regard stress management as applicable to their problems. Treatment completers tended to have reductions in somatic complaints and health anxiety. There were no changes in a wait-list control group.

Bouman (2002) conducted an open trial of group psychoeducation for patients with hypochondriasis. Treatment was administered in a community setting. Twenty-two percent of participants dropped out. Two main reasons for dropping out were identified: (1) very high expectations about the benefits of the program (thereby leading to disappointment when expectations were unmet), and (2) inability to combine attendance with other personal obligations. The latter underscores the importance of timing in choosing when to begin treatment. For treatment completers, the intervention was effective in reducing hypochondriasis, including a mean reduction of 40% in the frequency of medical service utilization (as indicated by a comparison of the frequency of physician visits 6 months before vs. 6 months after treatment). Participants reported that they valued the opportunity to share their concerns, and most were relieved to learn that they were not the only ones suffering from excessive health anxiety.

The role of bibliotherapy as a psychoeducational tool remains to be investigated. Written psychoeducational materials, such as the handouts included in later chapters of this book, can be used in conjunction with routine medical management. These materials might be especially useful in reducing mild health anxiety, and also would be a useful component in more intensive psychoeducational programs.

Explanatory Therapy

Developed by Kellner (1979), explanatory therapy includes a number of interventions intended to persuade the patient that there is nothing wrong with her or his physical health. It involves repeated physical examination, whenever the patient requests one, or when new bodily complaints arise. Patients are also repeatedly told that there is nothing wrong with them. Thus, the approach is based primarily on a good deal of bland reassurance, along with anxiolytic medication when the patient becomes anxious. It also contains psychoeducation similar to that described in the previous section. The following case illustrates explanatory therapy for a patient with hypochondriasis who feared that she was infected with genital herpes:

> Her understanding of herpes and venereal disease was assessed, and a written summary of all of her questions regarding her health was compiled. A 3-hour consultation was held with an infectious disease fellow and one of the authors . . . to present understandable, accurate information, to persuade the patient that her conviction was false. This information was repeated many times in subsequent sessions along with facts, such as the high frequency of minor somatic symptoms in normal people, and that anxiety leads to a vicious cycle generating selective perception that creates more anxiety etc. Diazepam was prescribed when needed for episodes of severe anxiety. (Romanik & Kellner, 1985, p. 543)

Patients are encouraged to keep a diary in which they record their disease fears and beliefs. They are also encouraged to write alternative interpretations for their somatic sensations. The therapist then provides feedback. Explanatory therapy does not contain the extensive cognitive restructuring exercises used in cognitive and cognitive-behavioral therapies.

A case study, one uncontrolled trial, and a controlled study suggest that explanatory therapy can reduce hypochondriasis (Fava, Grandi, Rafanelli, Fabbri, & Cazzaro, 2000; Kellner, 1982; Romanik & Kellner, 1985). It is superior to a wait-list control and is associated with a reasonably low dropout rate (approximately 16%; see Table 5.2 on p. 81).

The benefits of explanatory therapy may be primarily due to the use of psychoeducation and rudimentary cognitive restructuring exercises. The value of reassurance is questionable. Some clinicians advocate the use of reassurance (including repeated physical examinations) because they see these strategies as a form of cognitive restructuring (Kellner, 1992; Starcevic, & Lipsitt, 2001). However, we, along with many others, consider it counterproductive to repeatedly tell the patient that there is nothing wrong with him or her (Barsky, 1996; Leonhard, 1961; Warwick & Salkovskis, 1985). Patients with health anxiety disorders typically fail to benefit from reassurance (APA, 2000). Studies using single-case designs have shown that hypochondriasis persists when patients receive reassurance and abates when reassurance seeking is discouraged (Salkovskis & Warwick, 1986). Reassurance can also lead to other problems:

> The difficulty in reassuring hypochondriacal patients is often compounded by the task they set for their physicians: that of disproving a negative. Instead of asking whether or not they have cancer, for example, these patients may inquire: "How do you know I don't have cancer?" The physician's attempt to answer that question can generate a series of increasingly complicated, dangerous, and expensive tests, the primary purpose of which may be reassurance, rather than diagnosis. (Slavney, 1987, p. 302)

Another concern with persistently giving reassurance is that it may encourage the patient to be dependent on the advice of his or her therapist. It would be preferable to teach patients to assure themselves about the significance of their bodily sensations.

Exposure and Response Prevention

Hypochondriasis is often characterized by phobic avoidance. This observation led some clinicians to investigate the merits of using *in vivo*, interoceptive, or imaginal exposure to reduce health anxiety. *In vivo* exposure entails exposure to harmless but distressing disease-related objects or situations (e.g., hospitals, physicians, videotapes on medical topics). Interoceptive exposure involves the induction of feared bodily sensations (e.g., inducing palpitations by jogging, for patients who are frightened of having heart attacks). Imaginal exposure consists of imagining feared health-related outcomes (e.g., imagining that one has developed cancer). Exposure is conducted within the treatment sessions and as homework assignments. Hypnosis has been occasionally used to purportedly increase the vividness of imaginal exposure (O'Donnell, 1978).

A number of case reports suggest that exposure-based interventions may be useful in reducing health anxiety (Furst & Cooper, 1970; O'Donnell, 1978; Rifkin, 1968; Scrignar, 1974; Tearnan, Goetsch, & Adams, 1985). But exposure is unlikely to be sufficient. There is much more to hypochondriasis than phobic avoidance. Repetitive checking and reassurance seeking are prominent features. Exposure may not reduce these behaviors. Indeed, disease exposure without response prevention might lead to an increase in checking and reassurance seeking. Similar effects have been observed for obsessive–compulsive disorder in those cases in which patients are exposed to feared stimuli but their compulsive rituals are not blocked (Foa, Steketee, & Milby, 1980).

Accordingly, treatments for health anxiety disorders were devised to include exposure *and* response prevention. Disease-related exposure is used in combination with strategies to reduce or block checking and reassurance seeking. It is often necessary for the therapist to instruct family members how to refrain from giving reassurance (e.g., "Hospital instructions are that I do not give you reassurance").

To our knowledge, the earliest published account of exposure and response prevention for hypochondriasis was published by Leonhard (1961), who anecdotally reported that treatment was rapidly successful in many cases. The following is his description of the treatment of a case in which fear of heart attacks was a prominent feature.

> Among the principles that guide me in the therapy of hypochondriac neurosis, the most important one is *to expect from the patient exactly what he himself in his state of fear feels incapable of doing.* Under these circumstances it is of advantage that many hypochondriacs maintain that they are suffering from a heart complaint, because the heart can easily be put under strain. In other words, we can call upon the patient to do things he himself dares not do. It is surprising to see how rapidly even those hypochondriacs, who were most afraid of walking, take part in games and sports, in spite of the strain on their heart. The psychotherapist, however, has to join the patient at first to make him feel sure that his state of health is watched over carefully during his sporting activities. In most cases hypochondriacs are glad to leave the responsibility to the doctor and they will do what is demanded of them willingly. I think that any heart-hypochondriac, no matter of what degree, whose confidence I enjoy, will perform without special preparations ten knee-bends, provided that I join him in doing so and assure him that I will take the whole responsibility. These demands may be increased very rapidly and soon the self-styled heart-sufferer will spend several hours a day straining his heart with games, sports, and gymnastics. . . . While the patient gradually feels capable of doing what can be expected only from healthy people, he regains his confidence in his own body." (pp. 130–131; emphasis in original)

> If permitted to do so, hypochondriacs will talk incessantly about their fears and complaints. Whenever there are [doctor] visits they wish to tell everything, merely repeating all that they have told you many times before to ensure that their complaints are properly attended to. *These constant discussions must be stopped at all costs.* There will always remain points to be talked about from the patient's life, and therefore psychotherapeutic talks between the doctor and the patient will never cease. But once the hypochondriac phenomenon has been thoroughly discussed, and its origin has been made clear, there should be no more discussions about it whatsoever. . . . Provisions must be made to ensure that the patient who has given up telling the doctor the same thing over and over again, does not go on talking about it to other patients or to his family. . . . Usually this is successful, because at this stage of the therapy hypochondriacs will already believe in their

recovery provided they comply with the instructions given to them. (p. 131; emphasis in original)

These days clinicians would not take such an authoritarian approach in making patients perform exposure and response prevention exercises. The interventions would be negotiated and implemented gradually, and treatment engagement strategies would be used (as described in Chapter 7). Nevertheless, Leonhard's pioneering contribution is noteworthy, particularly because it was developed in the 1950s and 1960s, at a time when the common treatments for hypochondriasis (e.g., psychodynamic psychotherapy) were largely ineffective. Leonhard's use of therapeutic modeling (i.e., the therapist performing the exposure exercises) was also ahead of its time. This intervention is routinely used today.

But Leonhard's valuable contribution was largely overlooked, and it was not until the mid-1980s that exposure and response prevention was rediscovered, principally by investigators at London's Maudsley Hospital. Case studies and uncontrolled trials indicated that this treatment is often successful in producing enduring reductions in all facets of health anxiety (including disease conviction), even for people with chronic hypochondriasis (Logsdail, Lovell, Warwick, & Marks, 1991; Visser & Bouman, 1992; Warwick & Marks, 1988). In a controlled study, Visser and Bowman (2001) found exposure and response prevention to be effective, and superior to a wait-list control, with gains maintained at 7-month follow-up. The proportion of dropouts tends to be low (around 14%; see Table 5.2), suggesting that treatment is generally acceptable to patients.

Cognitive-Behavioral Therapy

Several uncontrolled trials suggest that a course of cognitive-behavioral therapy (CBT), such as 8–16 weekly sessions, can effectively reduce health anxiety in people suffering from full or abridged hypochondriasis (Furer, Walker, & Freeston, 2001; House, 1989; Miller, Acton, & Hedge, 1988; Stern & Fernandez, 1991). Trials comparing CBT to wait-list controls or other treatment conditions have produced similarly encouraging results (Clark et al., 1998; Speckens et al., 1995; Warwick, Clark, Cobb, & Salkovskis, 1996). Most CBT studies have implemented therapy on an individual (one-to-one) basis, although Stern and Fernandez (1991) found that group treatment was effective. In addition to being economical, group treatment for hypochondriasis can foster a sense of acceptance and social support (Bouman, 2002; Brown & Vaillant, 1981). For patients living far from treatment centers, CBT can be effectively delivered by telephone (McLaren, 1992).

The dropout rate for CBT tends to be about 10% (Table 5.2), suggesting that this intervention is acceptable to most patients entering treatment. Some clinicians have attempted to enhance treatment acceptability by emphasizing the role of stress in producing unwanted bodily sensations: "The concept of stress has become widely known among the general public, and for this reason patients are likely to accept a course of therapy labeled stress management, although they would probably refuse a psychiatric referral" (Stern & Fernandez, 1991, p. 1229).

CBT is more effective than routine medical management from the patient's primary care physician. This was demonstrated by Speckens et al.'s (1995) comparison of CBT to "optimized" medical care. The latter was routine management by primary care physicians who received additional training in identifying psychiatric disorders. CBT proved superior to optimized medical care in reducing health anxiety. Although most patients in CBT studies have chronic health anxiety, typically lasting many years, treatment gains are generally maintained at follow-ups of 3–12 months (Clark et al., 1998; Miller et al., 1988; Speckens et al., 1995; Warwick et al., 1996).

In one of the most sophisticated studies of health anxiety treatments, Clark et al. (1998) compared three conditions: CBT, behavioral stress management (BSM), and wait-list control. BSM was intended as an equally credible alternative treatment. It is based on the rationale that some people react to stress by becoming worried about their health. BSM did not focus directly on health anxiety. Instead, it was used to train patients in ways of managing the stress in their lives which, in turn, would reduce arousal-related bodily sensations and thereby enhance their sense of health.

Unlike previous authors of studies, Clark and colleagues reported a detailed assessment of treatment fidelity, and provided data indicating that CBT and BSM actually did differ in the components they were supposed to contain (i.e., treatments were delivered as intended). Although BSM was intended as a control condition (e.g., controlling for nonspecific treatment factors), it proved to be effective. Both it and CBT were effective, compared to the wait-list control. At posttreatment, CBT tended to be more effective than BSM, although the advantages of CBT were lost over time, to the point that there was little difference in the efficacy of the two at 12-month follow-up. Patients in both conditions had less health anxiety at follow-up compared to their pretreatment levels. Thus, both treatments were useful, although CBT had the advantage of reducing health anxiety more rapidly.

CBT and BSM did not differ in their mean credibility ratings, although some patients may be more likely to go along with a BSM rationale and others to accept CBT. Accordingly, both treatments have their place. An advantage of BSM may lie in its nonspecificity: it focuses largely on helping patients manage stress, rather than on health-related beliefs. BSM might be particularly useful for patients with comorbid disorders, such as hypochondriasis co-occurring with a mood disorder, an anxiety disorder, or behavioral medicine problems (e.g., recurrent tension headaches). As with hypochondriasis, symptoms of anxiety, depression, and pain are exacerbated by stress (Asmundson et al., 2001; Oltmanns, Emery, & Taylor, 2002; Taylor, 2000). BSM can reduce all of these problems, and therefore might be useful for patients with complex mixtures of symptoms and disorders. Alternatively, for patients with severe health anxiety as their primary problem, a course of CBT could be implemented first. If comorbid problems remain at the end of treatment, then a course of BSM could be considered.

Component Studies

Several studies have looked at the merits of the various CBT components. On the basis of their experiences using the full CBT package, Warwick et al. (1996) thought that an important ingredient was providing patients with clear-cut evidence that their problem was one of health anxiety, rather than getting into debates about the validity of negative test results. Extensive use of behavioral experiments also seemed helpful. Emphasis on modifying dysfunctional assumptions may have helped prevent patients from switching to a new disease preoccupation once treatment had dealt with their current fears. These clinical impressions suggest that a number of CBT techniques could be useful by themselves. Recent research supports this conjecture.

Applied relaxation training and cognitive restructuring are each effective in reducing hypochondriasis (Bouman & Visser, 1998; Johansson & Öst, 1981; Visser & Bouman, 2001). Case reports suggest that thought stopping combined with relaxation training can also reduce hypochondriasis (Kumar & Wilkinson, 1971). The latter authors proposed that repeated practice in thought stopping, which involved replacing disease-related thoughts with pleasant thoughts, gradually strengthened the inhibition of unwanted thoughts. Alternatively, thought stopping might work as a distancing strategy because repeated practice at deliberately dismissing upsetting disease-related thoughts might eventually help patients realize that such thoughts are not to be taken seriously. In other words, the patient comes to understand that these thoughts can be safely ignored without any harmful consequences.

Attention training exercises (see Chapter 9), which teach the patient to reduce bodily scrutiny, are often used in CBT. Case studies by Papageorgiou and Wells (1998) suggest that these exercises are effective in reducing hypochondriasis. With practice, patients are able to spend less time dwelling on their own bodily functions. Such exercises are also useful in reducing dysfunctional disease-related beliefs because the exercises teach patients that the tendency to frequently experience "symptoms" (bodily sensations) can arise largely from the tendency to focus excessively on one's body.

PHARMACOTHERAPIES FOR NONDELUSIONAL HEALTH ANXIETY

Early views that hypochondriasis was a form of "masked depression" (Lesse, 1967) led to the use of antidepressant medications to treat health anxiety. Subsequent research did not support the masked depression hypothesis (see Chapter 1). Moreover, it is not necessary for a person to have depression (masked or otherwise) in order to benefit from antidepressants. Such medications, including tricyclics and selective serotonin reuptake inhibitors, are useful in treating a variety of disorders, such as anxiety disorders and eating disorders, regardless of whether the person is depressed (Oltmanns et al., 2002; Taylor, 2000). These medications reduce dysfunctional beliefs in anxiety disorders and in mood disorders (Fava, Bless, Otto, Pava, & Rosenbaum, 1994; Simons, Garfield, & Murphy, 1984; Taylor, 1999, 2000), and therefore might be useful in reducing disease convictions and fears. Several studies support this supposition. Case studies and open trials suggest that the following medications (at the doses so far studied) are often helpful in reducing hypochondriasis:

- Clomipramine (25–225 mg per day: Kamlana & Gray, 1988; Stone, 1993).
- Imipramine (125–150 mg per day: Lippert, 1986; Wesner & Noyes, 1991).
- Fluoxetine (20–80 mg per day: Fallon, 1999; Fallon, Jovitch, Hollander, & Liebowitz, 1991; Fallon et al., 1993, 1996; Viswanathan & Paradis, 1991).
- Fluvoxamine (300 mg per day: Fallon, 2001; Fallon et al., 1996).
- Paroxetine (up to 60 mg per day: Oosterbaan, van Balkom, van Boeijen, de Meij, & van Dyck, 2001).
- Nefazodone (200–500 mg per day: Kjernisted, Enns, & Lander, 2002).

These medications can reduce all aspects of hypochondriasis, including disease fears and beliefs, pervasive anxiety, somatic symptoms, avoidance, and reassurance seeking (Fallon, 2001; Wesner & Noyes, 1991). The drugs can be effective even for patients who don't have comorbid major depression (Fallon et al., 1993; Wesner & Noyes, 1991). Little is know about whether these medications are helpful for patients with circumscribed types of health anxiety disorders, such as disease phobia. Little is also known about the long-term effects. There are reports of patients relapsing when medications are discontinued (e.g., Viswanathan & Paradis, 1991).

Despite the promising effects of these drugs, there are several problems in using pharmacotherapy to treat hypochondriasis and other health anxiety disorders. No medication is universally effective. There are numerous case reports of health-anxious patients failing to benefit from one or more of these drugs (Fallon, 1999; Stone, 1993; Viswanathan & Paradis, 1991). Even for short (8–12 week) drug trials, 13–21% of patients drop out of treatment, even for drugs with few side effects, such as nefazodone (Fallon, 2001; Fallon et al., 1993, 1996; Kjernisted et al., 2002; Oosterbaan et al., 2001; Wesner & Noyes, 1991). Some patients become preoccupied with side effects (Keeley, Smith, & Miller, 2000; Stone, 1993; Wesner & Noyes, 1991), as illustrated by the following observations:

> Our . . . subjects seemed especially sensitive to the initial side effects of imipramine. Their vigilance and scanning for cues of illness contributed to concern about the meaning of new bodily sensations. This fearful reaction to side effects may have contributed to a decision to stop medication. (Wesner & Noyes, 1991, p. 46)

> The use of psychotropic medications in primary hypochondriasis poses a dilemma. . . . In general, these agents are not markedly beneficial, as the patients often react with bothersome side effects or with new symptoms. In addition, the hypochondriacal patient often views the prescription of medication as a paltry and unsatisfactory substitute for the personal interest and attention of the physician. (Barsky, 1996, p. 51)

In some cases, health anxiety worsens during drug treatment as patients become alarmed by side effects like gastrointestinal discomfort (Fallon, 2001; Oosterbaan et al., 2001). A further issue is whether the drug effects are due to specific properties of the medications or whether they are due to nonspecific (placebo) factors, such as expectancy for improvement. There has been only one placebo-controlled pharmacotherapy study (Fallon et al., 1996). The full report has not yet been published, but the 1996 interim report stated that 20 patients with hypochondriasis were randomized either to fluoxetine or placebo. Four patients (20%) dropped out. There was no significant difference in the proportion of responders in either condition (in part due to low statistical power), although there were trends favoring fluoxetine (e.g., for patients completing 12 weeks of treatment, 80% of fluoxetine patients were classified as responders, compared to 60% of placebo patients). Fallon's more recent results, based on an increased sample size, indicate that fluoxetine is superior to placebo, both in terms of outcome after 12 weeks and at 9-month follow-up (B. A. Fallon, personal communication, September 10, 2002).

    Treatment dropout or poor adherence to drug regimens is especially likely if the patient is not given a good explanation about the need for psychotropic drugs. Some pharmacotherapists offer their patients an explanation similar to those used in CBT. For example, some have adopted the practice of informing patients that they are suffering from a hypersensitivity to experience unpleasant but harmless bodily sensations, and that medication will reduce this sensitivity (Enns, Kjernisted, & Lander 2001). Possible side effects should be carefully explained in advance to limit the chances of patients catastrophically misinterpreting these effects (Barsky, 2001).

META-ANALYTIC COMPARISON OF TREATMENTS FOR NONDELUSIONAL HEALTH ANXIETY

The available data from controlled and uncontrolled studies allow us to perform a preliminary meta-analysis of treatments for health anxiety, in order to gauge the relative efficacy of these interventions. This was done by using the methods of our previous meta-analyses (Fedoroff & Taylor, 2001; Taylor, 1995, 1996; van Etten & Taylor, 1998). For trials having five or more patients per treatment condition, we computed the within-trial effect size, using a variant of Cohen's (1988) d statistic. For each trial the magnitude of change from pre- to posttreatment was defined as $(M_{pre} - M_{post})/SD_{pooled}$, where $SD_{pooled} = \sqrt{[SD_{pre}^2 + SD_{post}^2)/2]}$.

The magnitude of change from pretreatment to follow-up was defined by replacing M_{post} with $M_{follow-up}$, and SD_{post} with $SD_{follow-up}$. Positive effect sizes represent improvements in symptoms (i.e., reductions in problem severity), whereas negative effect sizes indicate a worsening of symptoms. The larger the effect size, the greater the magnitude of treatment-related reductions in symptoms.

Effect sizes were based on completer analyses rather than intent-to-treat analyses. In other words, effect sizes were based on pre- and posttreatment data for participants completing each trial. This approach was necessary because many trials only reported data for treatment completers.

There are a number of different formulae for computing effect sizes and none has been established as a gold standard. We selected the above-mentioned effect size because the same or very similar effect size formulae are commonly used and because it provides an effect size for each trial, rather than an effect size defined as the posttreatment difference between a treatment and a control trial. Thus, we were able to include uncontrolled studies in the meta-analysis, thereby increasing the number of trials. One should not interpret in isolation an effect size for a given treatment. The meaning of the effect size is determined by comparing it to effect sizes for other treatments.

For a variety of disorders and outcome variables it has been found that interviewer-rated scales tend to yield larger effect sizes than self-report scales (e.g., Lambert, Hatch, Kingston, & Edwards, 1986; Taylor, 1995; van Etten & Taylor, 1998). This may reflect the greater sensitivity of interviewer-rated scales, or it may be an artifact of interviewer bias (i.e., the interviewer typically knows whether or not the assessment is a pre- or posttreatment evaluation, and therefore may be biased to expect comparatively lower symptom scores at posttreatment). Systematic bias in computing effect sizes can occur if some types of treatments are evaluated with interviewer-rated measures (e.g., drug therapies) and others with self-report measures (e.g., psychological therapies). Due to the shortage of studies using interview measures, we computed effect sizes only for self-report measures. Effect sizes for health anxiety measures were based on measures of global hypochondriasis (e.g., the Whiteley Index). Where two or more measures were used in a given trial (e.g., the Whiteley Index and the total score on the Illness Attitude Scales), we computed the mean of these effect sizes for that trial. If a trial reported results only for components of hypochondriasis (e.g., scores on subscales of the Illness Attitude Scales), then the health anxiety effect size for that trial was based on the mean of the effect sizes across the subscales.

As shown in Table 5.2, a total of 25 trials contained sufficient data for the purpose of computing effect sizes or for assessing the proportion of dropouts. These trials were based on data from 15 studies (Avia et al., 1996; Bouman, 2002; Bouman & Visser, 1998; Clark et al., 1998; Fallon, 2001; Fallon et al., 1993, 1996; Fava et al., 2000; Kjernisted et al., 2002; Lidbeck, 1997; Oosterbaan et al., 2001; Speckens et al., 1995; Stern & Fernandez, 1991; Visser & Bouman, 2001; Warwick et al., 1996). Participants in these studies either had full or abridged hypochondriasis. They were typically aged in their 30s or 40s, and approximately two-thirds were female. The duration of health anxiety, when reported, was typically several years. Patients in drug trials were on their medications at the time of the posttreatment assessment.

Table 5.2 shows that there were few trials per treatment condition and that samples sizes tended to be small. Accordingly, the results need to be interpreted with caution. The findings suggest that the proportion of dropouts for psychosocial treatments tend to be higher than those for control conditions, but similar to the proportions of dropouts from medication trials. Of the psychosocial and drug treatments, cognitive therapy, CBT, and BSM tend to have the lowest proportions of dropouts, particularly in studies of patients with full-blown hypochondriasis. This suggests that these treatments may be somewhat more acceptable to patients than other interventions.

For studies of full-blown hypochondriasis, the pre–posttreatment effect sizes for measures of hypochondriasis suggests that CBT and fluoxetine yield the largest effects for treatment completers. These effects are substantially larger than the effects of control conditions. The effect size for CBT and fluoxetine are broadly similar to one another. For studies using mixes of full

TABLE 5.2. Comparative Efficacy of Treatments for Health Anxiety

Treatment condition	No. of trials	Mean no. of treatment completers	Mean treatment duration (weeks)	Mean no. of therapy hours	Mean % dropout	Mean follow-up duration (months)	Mean pre–post effect size: Hypochon.	Mean pre–follow-up effect size: Hypochon.	Mean pre–post effect size: Anxiety	Mean pre–post effect size: Depression
Studies of patients with hypochondriasis										
Control conditions										
Wait-list control	3	17	15	—	0	—	0.29	—	0.23	0.10
Pill placebo	1	6	12	—	25	—	—	—	—	—
Psychosocial treatments										
Psychoeducation	1	21	6	12	22	6	1.05	1.27	0.08	0.89
Explanatory therapy	2	8	16	4	16	6	0.91	0.88	—	—
Cognitive therapy	1	8	12	12	11	1	0.83	0.96	—	0.37
Exposure and response prevention	2	16	12	12	14	4	1.00	1.19	—	0.42
Cognitive-behavioral therapy	4	16	13	15	10	7	2.05	1.74	1.90	1.36
Behavioral stress management	1	23	15	15	4	12	1.59	1.25	1.75	1.44
Drug treatments										
Paroxetine	1	9	12	—	18	—	1.34	—	—	—
Fluoxetine	2	12	12	—	15	—	1.92	—	—	—
Fluvoxamine	1	11	12	—	21	—	—	—	—	—
Nefazodone	1	9	8	—	18	—	1.07	—	—	1.01
Studies of mixed samples: Full and abridged hypochondriasis										
Wait-list control	1	17	8	—	0	3	0.19	0.18	0.00	0.03
"Optimized" medical care	1	40	21	—	0	6	0.20	0.30	0.02	−0.06
Psychoeducation	2	23	7	17	2	8	0.74	0.87	0.19	0.05
Cognitive-behavioral therapy	1	39	21	21	13	6	0.51	0.61	0.31	0.41

and abridged hypochondriasis, the effect sizes are uniformly smaller than those of studies of full hypochondriasis. The differences are probably due to range restriction. Patients who enter treatment with mild symptoms, compared to those entering with severe symptoms, have a smaller range in which their scores can decrease on measures of symptoms. Even so, for studies of mixed samples, the results suggest that psychoeducation and CBT tend to yield larger effects on measures of hypochondriasis, compared to wait-list controls and optimized medical care.

Pretreatment to follow-up effect sizes for measures of hypochondriasis could not be calculated for drug studies because follow-ups were not reported. The available follow-up results suggest that CBT has the largest effect sizes in studies of full hypochondriasis, and psychoeducation and CBT have the largest effects in studies of mixed full and abridged hypochondriasis.

For pre- to posttreatment effect sizes of measures of depression and general anxiety, data from drug studies were generally lacking. The available data indicates that, for studies of full hypochondriasis, the largest effects on depression and general anxiety are obtained from CBT and BSM. For studies of mixed samples, the largest effects on measures of depression and anxiety are associated with CBT. The depression results are noteworthy because CBT for hypochondriasis does not directly target depression. Presumably the effects on depression are secondary: a reduction in the patient's primary problem (hypochondriasis) may reduce the patient's dysphoria about having hypochondriasis.

To summarize, the meta-analysis suggests the following:

- For measures of hypochondriasis, all of the psychosocial and drug treatments had larger effect sizes than wait-list controls. This suggests that the clinician has several useful tools at his or her disposal.
- When treatment acceptability, and strength, breadth, and durability of effects are taken into consideration, CBT appears to be the treatment of choice for full hypochondriasis.
- For patients preferring medication, fluoxetine appears to be particularly promising, although little is known about whether the benefits are maintained when the drug is discontinued.
- The studies of mixed full and abridged hypochondriasis suggest that psychoeducation might be sufficient for many patients with mild health anxiety, particularly if the person is not depressed. If depression is present in cases of abridged hypochondriasis, then CBT (for health anxiety) may be more appropriate because it appears to be superior to psychoeducation in reducing depression.

There was insufficient data to include other treatments in the meta-analysis, such as psychodynamic psychotherapies. These treatments remain to be fully evaluated, although the reports summarized earlier in this chapter cast doubt upon their value. There was also insufficient information to assess the merits of treatment modality (group vs. individual) and treatment setting (e.g., mental health clinic vs. community or general medical settings). Group treatment may be more economical, and treatments based outside of mental health settings may be less stigmatizing.

Because there has been only one placebo-controlled study, little is known about nonspecific treatment factors. The benefits of psychosocial treatments appear to be maintained at follow-ups of 3–12 months. Such gains would not be expected if treatments were simply placebos. Moreover, CBT is more effective than optimized medical care (Speckens et al., 1995; see Table 5.2). These findings further suggest that cognitive-behavioral and related interventions offer more than nonspecific effects.

A complication of all the follow-up studies is that patients may have sought additional treatment during the follow-up period. This was rarely assessed and, to our knowledge, no studies have attempted to control for the effects of additional treatment seeking. Not only would this blur comparisons between treatments, but it also may paint an overly rosy picture of the durability of the interventions. However, we expect that additional treatment seeking would be more likely to occur for patients who had initially received relatively weak interventions (e.g., explanatory therapy) compared to those initially receiving stronger treatments (e.g., CBT).

The merits of combining drug and psychosocial treatments remain to be investigated. Given the pattern of results in Table 5.2, it would be particularly interesting to see whether outcome is improved when CBT is combined with fluoxetine. Combination treatments might be especially useful for very severe hypochondriasis.

TREATMENTS FOR DELUSIONAL DISORDER (SOMATIC TYPE)

Delusional disorder (somatic type) was once considered rare. Its prevalence was underestimated because sufferers usually do not present to mental health clinics (Zomer, de Wit, Van Bronswijk, Nabarro, & van Vloten, 1998). Instead, they tend to seek help from other professionals. People with delusions of parasitic infestation, for example, commonly seek help from dermatologists or, in some cases, turn to zoology departments for help (Koo & Lee, 2001; Needham, 2000). Delusional disorder is often chronic in the absence of treatment, sometimes leading to suicide (Munro & Chmara, 1982).

Antipsychotic Medications

Case reports suggest that typical antipsychotic medications, such as halo-peridol, thioridazine, and trifluoperazine, can treat delusional disorder (so-matic type) (Andrews, Bellard, & Walter-Ryan, 1986; Fishbain, Barsky, & Goldberg, 1992; Gould & Gragg, 1976; Scarone & Gambini, 1991). Pimozide is currently the medication with the greatest research support for its efficacy. Case reports and two small controlled trials suggest that pimozide is effective in treating delusions of parasitic infestation (e.g., Hamann & Avnstorp, 1982; Ungvari & Vladar, 1986; Zomer et al., 1998). In a meta-analysis of 1,223 of these patients, pimozide treatment led to full remission in 50% of cases (Trabert, 1995).

Pimozide's mechanism of action is a topic of speculation. It is an opiate antagonist that can act as a central suppressor of abnormal peripheral sensations (Johnson & Anton, 1983). In other words, it reduces bothersome cutaneous sensations such as itching. The benefit of pimozide may lie primarily in these antipruritic effects. Once the unwanted sensations are reduced, the patient may come to believe that he or she is no longer infested with parasites (Johnson & Anton, 1983). Consistent with this view, studies have found that patients treated with pimozide report reductions in bothersome skin sensa-tions, but most fail to gain insight that they were never infested with parasites (Koblenzer, 1997; Munro & Chmara, 1982).

Pimozide doses of 1–10 mg per day can be effective in reducing delu-sional disorder (somatic type) (Koblenzer, 1997). In some cases doses as high as 20 mg per day have been required (Opler & Feinberg, 1991). Until recently, pimozide was widely considered to be the treatment of choice for delusions of parasitic infestation (Elmer et al., 2000). However, it can have unpleasant and sometimes serious side effects. The most common are extrapyramidal symptoms such as stiffness and, less frequently, an inner sense of restlessness (akathisia). Extrapyramidal reactions can be managed with benztropine or diphenhydramine. The lowest effective dosage of pimozide should be used for the shortest possible duration to minimize the risk of tardive dyskinesia developing in these patients (Koo & Lee, 2001). A further concern is that pimozide can produce cardiac arrhythmia, particularly at doses over 10 mg per day (Phillips, 1991). As a precaution it is necessary to perform an ECG before starting pimozide and periodically throughout treatment (Opler & Feinberg, 1991).

Case reports suggest that so-called atypical antipsychotic medications, such as risperidone, clozapine, olanzapine, and sertindole, may be used effectively instead of pimozide (Atmaca, Kulogu, Tezcan, & Unal, 2002; Cetin, Ebrinc, Agargun, & Yigit, 1999; Fawcett, 2002; Gallucci & Beard, 1995; Safer, Wenegrat, & Roth, 1997; Songer & Roman, 1996; Weintraub & Robinson, 2000; Yorston, 1997). Atypical antipsychotics have the advantage of having fewer side effects (Koo & Lee, 2001), and some clinicians currently consider these to be the first-line treatments for delusional disorder (somatic type) (Elmer, George, & Peterson, 2000). However, there is little information on the optimal doses, benefits, and risks of atypical antipsychotics for treating delusional disorder (somatic type).

Antidepressant Medications

Antidepressants have been used to treat somatic delusions, even in undepressed patients. Such drugs include tricyclic antidepressants, monoamine oxidase inhibitors, and selective serotonin reuptake inhibitors. Case studies suggest that these medications can be useful in treating delusional disorder (somatic type) (e.g., Brotman & Jenike, 1984; Pylko & Sicignan, 1985; Roberts & Roberts, 1977; Ross, Siddiqui, & Matas, 1987). These drugs are sometimes useful for patients who have failed to benefit from pimozide (Brotman & Jenike, 1984; Pylko & Sicignan, 1985; Ross et al., 1987).

The available evidence, although limited to case reports, suggests that antidepressant medications may be less likely to be effective for patients with delusions of parasitic infestation. These medications appear to be more promising for patients with other somatic delusions (Enns et al., 2001), as illustrated by the following case:

> Mr. B . . . complained of an "anal odor" of 1 year's duration that had begun after his lover of 7 years left him. . . . The results of multiple medical evaluations, including a complete gastrointestinal workup, were normal. He left his job because of embarrassment, wore several pairs of underwear, showered at least three times a day, and checked his anal area for seepage several times a day. He had no other evidence of thought disorder. The results of an EEG after sleep deprivation, thyroid function studies, a CBC, serum electrolyte measurements, and a DST were all normal. Mr. B had no history of drug or alcohol abuse and . . . did not meet the DSM-III criteria for depression. (Brotman & Jenike, 1984, p. 1608)

Mr. B. had been unsuccessfully treated with a variety of interventions, including psychodynamic psychotherapy, amitryptiline, alprazolam, haloperidol, and tranylcypromine. He finally responded to 250 mg per day of imipramine. His symptoms abated, his checking and showering rituals ceased, and he began seeing friends again. Occasionally he detected an anal odor when he was stressed, although it no longer affected his daily life.

Walter (1991) described a case report of a man with delusional disorder (somatic type) characterized by the belief that he had a urethral stricture (narrowing). The patient could not explain why he believed he had a stricture, and reported having no urinary problems. On a number of occasions his belief led him to insert a knitting needle into his urethra in an attempt to correct the stricture. This caused pain and bloody urine, which prompted him to seek medical attention. On each occasion he was successfully treated with amitriptyline (up to 200 mg per day), improving after 3–4 weeks, and later relapsing after stopping his medication.

Much remains to be learned about the mechanisms of change for antidepressant treatments for delusional disorder (somatic type). Unlike pimozide, which seems to work by reducing bodily sensations (without changing delusional beliefs), it is likely that antidepressant medications work primarily by changing beliefs. As mentioned earlier in this chapter, such medications reduce dysfunctional beliefs in a range of disorders, including major depression, panic disorder, and nondelusional hypochondriasis. It is likely that these medications work the same way in reducing somatic delusions. It seems unlikely that the effects of these medications arise from their antidepressant properties because, as illustrated in the above-mentioned example of Mr. B., these treatments are effective in reducing delusions in undepressed patients.

Psychosocial Interventions

It is unknown whether cognitive-behavioral interventions can be used to effectively treat delusional disorder (somatic type), or whether treatment outcome is enhanced by combining CBT with medications. There are a few cases in which delusions of infestation have been "cured" simply by persuasion from a dermatologist that there is no infestation (Jibiki & Yamaguchi, 1992; Sheppard et al., 1986). These would appear to be in the minority of cases because people with somatic delusions are notoriously resistant to reassurance (Zomer et al., 1998). Indeed, Kellner (1983) reported that a patient with "paranoia hypochondriaca" (delusional disorder, somatic type) failed to benefit from his explanatory therapy. Nevertheless, it is possible that other psychosocial methods could be helpful.

CBT protocols have been successfully developed for treating other types of delusions, such as bizarre delusions in people with schizophrenia (Chadwick et al., 1996). There are at least three ways in which CBT might be helpful for delusional disorder (somatic type). First, cognitive-behavioral interventions, such as treatment engagement strategies (see Chapter 8), might persuade patients to agree to a trial of medication. It can be difficult to persuade delusional patients to take psychotropic medications. Zomer et al.

(1998), for example, were unable to convince 25% of their 24 patients to take pimozide:

> The principal difficulty in management is convincing patients to take the drug. When patients read on the instruction leaflet that the drug is used for psychiatric disorders they are often reluctant to take it. (Zomer et al., 1998, p. 1031)

Second, CBT might be useful in treating delusions that have failed to respond to medications (as used by Chadwick and colleagues [1996] in treating people with schizophrenia). Third, the periodic use of skills learned in CBT, such as cognitive restructuring exercises and behavioral experiments, could ward off relapse. It is not uncommon for patients to relapse when medications are withdrawn (Lyell, 1983; Munro & Chmara, 1982; Ungvari & Vladar, 1986).

ISSUES IN TREATMENT EVALUATION AND SELECTION

Treatment Acceptability

The available research suggests that we have effective psychosocial and drug treatments for many forms of health anxiety, and that many patients with these disorders can be persuaded to try these interventions, conducted by psychologists or psychiatrists either in a mental health clinic or other settings. Patients with hypochondriasis often know that they are overly concerned with illness, and they are often reminded of this by their family and friends (Fallon, 1999). Yet it is unclear whether the majority of health-anxious patients are willing to receive such treatments (Ben-Tovim & Esterman, 1998). If only, say, 30% of patients with hypochondriasis are willing to accept these treatments, then we would not be reaching most of the people who need help. Surprisingly little is known about this issue. To our knowledge there have been no rigorous studies on the proportion of patients who refuse referrals from their primary care physicians for treatment of health anxiety. Some health-anxious patients perceive a mental health referral as an accusation that they are imagining or fabricating their symptoms, or that their primary care physician is trying to get rid of them (Barsky, 2001). Patients with somatic delusions are particularly difficult to engage in treatment.

How can we improve treatment acceptability for patients reluctant to undergo a course of therapy for health anxiety disorders? Patients may be more likely to accept a referral to a mental health professional if the latter delivers treatment in a medical clinic rather than in a mental health setting.

Tyrer, Seivewright, and Behr's (1999) clinical impression, along with our own, suggests that many patients with hypochondriasis can be persuaded to accept treatment under these conditions:

> We are piloting this [cognitive-behavioral] approach in genitourinary clinics and our initial impressions are favourable. Not only are hypochondriacal patients accepting that they have excessive fears about their health, but are willing to accept a short course of treatment which they know has nothing to do with the investigation of disease and is designed to change their attitudes about it. This approach, possibly simplified and shortened by a bibliotherapy component, would be feasible for the large number of people with hypochondriacal symptoms seen in clinical practice. (Tyrer et al., 1999, p. 672)

Is one form of treatment more acceptable than others? Walker, Vincent, Furer, Cox, and Kjernisted (1999) presented balanced written descriptions of CBT and pharmacotherapy for "intense illness worries" to a community-based sample of 23 people with hypochondriasis who were interested in seeking treatment for their health anxiety. The descriptions outlined the time commitment and the major advantages and disadvantages of each treatment. Most preferred CBT. This was the first choice of 74% of participants; 48% said they would only accept this form of treatment. Given that CBT and some medications may be roughly equivalent in efficacy, at least in the short term (Table 5.2), and that there is no evidence that one treatment works any faster than another, some clinicians let the patient choose between the two (Enns et al., 2001). The availability of such choices might enhance treatment acceptability and adherence. Patients failing to benefit from one intervention could be placed on another.

Prognostic Factors

With the exception of delusional disorder, for which antipsychotic medication can be useful, there is little evidence that specific characteristics of health anxiety indicate that specific treatments should be used. Patients with a strong preference for one type of treatment (e.g., CBT) may have a worse prognosis if offered some other type of treatment (e.g., medication) because the odds of dropping out may be higher if they receive a nonpreferred treatment. Otherwise, the bulk of useful prognostic factors appear to predict outcome for a range of treatments, including medications and psychosocial interventions. The following tend to be good prognostic signs, as identified by various sources (APA, 2000; Barsky, 1996; Barsky et al., 1998b; Fallon et al., 1993; House, 1989; Kellner, 1983; Noyes et al., 1994a; Pilowsky, 1968; Speckens et al., 1997):

- Acute onset.
- Short duration of health anxiety.
- Mild symptoms of health anxiety.
- Absence of strongly held (overvalued or delusional) hypochondriacal beliefs.
- Absence of personality disorder.
- Absence of a comorbid general medical condition (e.g., chronic bronchitis, emphysema, angina).
- Absence of contingencies ("secondary gains") that reinforce health anxiety or illness behavior.
- Absence of accompanying stressful life events.

In other words, a good prognosis is associated with mild, short-lived health anxiety that is not associated with any complicating factors. This comes as cold comfort to the mental health professional, who is typically referred severe cases of health anxiety. "Good prognosis" cases are less likely to require a mental health consultation. It may be sufficient to provide them with simple psychoeducation (e.g., bibliotherapy) about the causes of health anxiety.

Some variables are uncertain prognostic predictors. According to some sources, comorbid Axis I disorders are poor prognostic indicators (APA, 2000; Barsky et al., 1998b; Noyes et al., 1994a), whereas other sources report that prominent, comorbid anxiety and depression is associated with good outcome (House, 1989; Pilowsky, 1968) or is unrelated to outcome (Kellner, 1983). Similarly, some sources report that good outcome is associated with young age at presentation for treatment (Barsky, 1996; House, 1989), while other sources have found that age is unrelated to outcome (Kellner, 1983; Speckens et al., 1997). The inconsistencies could be due to any of a variety of reasons, including the possibility that particular variables predict outcome for some treatments but not others. Another possibility is that the inconsistent findings indicate that the variables are only weak (unreliable) predictors of outcome.

Pilowsky (1968) studied outcome in 147 patients with hypochondriasis treated with a range of interventions, including psychotherapy, medications, and electroconvulsive therapy (ECT). He identified a number of sex-specific prognostic factors. Poor outcome among men was associated with being older, resentful, especially resistant to reassurance, and lack of response to ECT (which was often administered on the assumption that hypochondriasis was a "depression equivalent" and would therefore respond to treatments for depression). Poor outcome for women was associated with being younger, having a "hysterical" personality, and having seen a variety of nonpsychiatric consultants before finally being referred to a psychiatric service. To our knowledge there have been no efforts to replicate Pilowsky's findings, and so their clinical value remains uncertain.

Special Populations

Little is known about how treatment protocols need to be adapted or modified for special populations of health-anxious people, such as particular age groups, cultural groups, or groups with severe general medical conditions. Such individuals need to be considered on a case-by-case basis. For health-anxious children, interventions should be consistent with the child's developmental level (e.g., cognitive restructuring exercises would be simplified or omitted). For patients with comorbid general medical conditions, some medications or medication doses are contraindicated (e.g., pimozide would be used sparingly, if at all, for delusional patients with heart disease). For cognitively impaired (e.g., dementing) patients, simple behavioral programs might be most effective, such as contingency management programs (Williamson, 1984; Wooley, Blackwell, & Winget, 1978) where patients are reinforced for adaptive behaviors (e.g., engaging in health activities, talking about topics other than their health), and not rewarded for maladaptive behaviors (e.g., complaining about symptoms). For the cognitively intact elderly, it is our impression, and that of others (e.g., Logsdon & Hyer, 1999; Snyder & Stanley, 2001) that cognitive-behavioral interventions can be useful in treating health anxiety disorders.

SUMMARY AND CONCLUSIONS

Despite the pessimistic assertions of some clinicians, research has shown that we have several effective methods for treating health anxiety disorders. For mild or short-lived health anxiety, psychoeducation may be sufficient, delivered either by the primary care physician or in the form of educational courses. If that does not prove effective, or if the patient has full-blown hypochondriasis, then more intensive interventions could be considered.

For patients with delusional disorder (somatic type), pimozide and atypical antipsychotics are currently the treatments of choice. It remains to be seen whether cognitive-behavioral methods are helpful in these cases. Among the most promising psychosocial interventions for nondelusional hypochondriasis are CBT and BSM. For patients preferring medications, a number of selective serotonin reuptake inhibitors are effective. Preliminary research suggests that fluoxetine is the most promising of these drugs. However, it is unclear whether the gains from medications are maintained when drug treatments are discontinued. Research suggests that the gains from psychosocial treatments tend to be maintained at follow-up. Medications can take several weeks to exert their therapeutic effects and do not seem to work any more rapidly than CBT. Much remains to be learned about the mechanisms of action of treatments. It is possible that many psychosocial and drug treatments work in much the same way: by reducing the strength of dysfunctional beliefs.

The principal challenge in treating health anxiety disorders is to find ways of making treatments acceptable to people who are reluctant to acknowledge that their health concerns are excessive. Research suggests that many health-anxious patients are willing to accept such treatment, but are these the majority of health-anxious people? Conducting treatment in a nonpsychiatric setting may improve treatment acceptability.

6

Assessment and Case Formulation

In this chapter we outline the purposes and scope of assessment, discuss various assessment methods, and suggest ways of using assessment to develop a case formulation. The formulation, which is used to devise a treatment plan, is a working model of the four Ps of clinical causation: *predisposing*, *precipitating*, *perpetuating*, and *protective* factors. For purposes of illustration we will refer to the case of Alexander P. throughout this chapter.

> Alexander P. was a 32-year-old junior partner in an architectural firm. He was married with two sons, ages 9 and 11. His primary care physician referred him for psychological assessment and treatment because of Alexander's persistent fear that recent headaches, associated episodes of dizziness, and general clumsiness meant that he was going to have a stroke. A comprehensive medical evaluation, including a neurological investigation, revealed no evidence of a general medical condition that might account for his problems.

PURPOSE AND SCOPE OF ASSESSMENT

Assessment Targets

Assessment is, in part, a conceptually driven venture, where theories of the causes and treatment of health anxiety determine what is important to evaluate. Our approach is based on the cognitive-behavioral conceptualization of health anxiety described in Chapters 2–4. For patients referred for cognitive-behavioral therapy (CBT), an assessment is conducted by the CBT practitioner to develop a formulation of the causes of the patient's problems. The practitioner draws information from the patient's general medical evaluation to rule out general medical conditions that might account for the presenting problems. The targets of a comprehensive assessment are listed in Table 6.1. A good treatment plan depends on a detailed initial assessment. Assessment then continues throughout CBT to monitor treatment progress, to collect further information to test, and, if necessary, to revise the case formulation.

Therapeutic Relationship

The initial assessment with the CBT practitioner provides an opportunity to establish a sound working relationship, in which the therapist conveys the message that she or he is taking the patient's problems seriously.

> Alexander was told on several occasions by various doctors, including his primary care physician and his neurologist, that his troubling bodily sensations were "not physical" and that he had nothing to worry about. Alexander was not satisfied with this explanation because it didn't tell him what was causing his problems. He worried that the doctors were not taking him seriously, and that they thought his problems were "all in his head." Alexander firmly believed that his symptoms were real, not imaginary. He was relieved to see that the CBT practitioner was con-

---

TABLE 6.1. Comprehensive Assessment of Health Anxiety Disorders

1. General medical evaluation
2. Current Axes I and II diagnoses
3. History
4. Specific features of health anxiety
   - Troubling bodily changes (e.g., rashes, blemishes) or sensations (e.g., pains)
   - Disease fears and associated avoidance
   - Dysfunctional beliefs and strength of conviction
   - Safety signals and safety behaviors
5. Living circumstances
   - Social functioning and relationship with significant others (e.g., do they provide reassurance?)
   - Occupational functioning
   - Health habits
   - Stressors
6. Reasons for seeking psychological treatment
7. Prognostic indicators

---

ducting an in-depth assessment of his problems, including a detailed review of his bodily concerns. Although Alexander was skeptical about whether CBT could help him, he was pleased that the CBT practitioner was taking his concerns seriously. Thus, he began to feel comfortable working with the cognitive-behavioral therapist.

Medical Mimics

Health anxiety disorders are diagnosed only when general medical conditions are ruled out as sufficient causes of the patient's health anxiety. To this end, the CBT practitioner should obtain a copy of the patient's medical history and a list of current medications. Approximately 2% of patients presenting for CBT are misdiagnosed with a health anxiety disorder when, in fact, they have a general medical condition (Warwick et al., 1996). On occasion, the CBT practitioner might therefore request that further medical evaluations be conducted before starting a course of CBT. We have encountered patients who were initially considered by their physicians to have hypochondriasis, but who subsequently turned out to have general medical conditions, such as multiple sclerosis (MS). In these cases the patient's anxiety about his or her bodily changes and sensations turned out to be justified. Fallon (2001) similarly reported a case of a patient initially misdiagnosed as having hypochondriasis. The patient did not respond to drug treatment (fluvoxamine) for this disorder. A subsequent medical evaluation indicated a diagnosis of Lyme disease. Once the latter was treated, the patient's health anxiety abated.

Medical tests are rarely, if ever, 100% accurate. So when can we say that a general medical condition has been sufficiently ruled out as the cause of a patient's health anxiety? Complete certainty is not a realistic goal. The clinician must rely on the balance of probabilities to decide whether a patient suffers from a health anxiety disorder. The odds of the latter are higher if:

- Repeated medical investigations conducted by more than one physician consistently reveal no evidence of a general medical condition that would explain the patient's problems.
- The patient has multiple, shifting physical complaints that are more consistent with a health anxiety disorder than with a general medical condition.
- The troubling bodily changes (e.g., rashes, blemishes) or sensations (e.g., coughs, pains) are not progressive; they do not worsen over time or develop into a more sinister, debilitating condition.
- Evidence is obtained that cognitive or behavioral factors contribute to the troubling bodily changes or sensations—for example evidence

might suggest that swelling and tenderness of the lymph glands is simply the result of repeatedly checking (palpating) the glands.

Alexander had worried about having a stroke for several years, initially after his father, now 65, had had a stroke 10 years earlier. His father blamed his doctor for not giving him proper treatment. At the time, his father went to his doctor complaining of headache, lightheadedness, and feeling unsteady. His doctor said the symptoms would probably pass and that the father should go home to rest. However, the symptoms became progressively worse, to the point that his father collapsed and was rushed to the hospital. Fortunately, he was successfully treated and was left with only minor residual problems. This near-tragic experience led Alexander to worry about the competence of medical practitioners in looking after his own health. His worry worsened 3 years ago when a 33-year-old neighbor died suddenly and unexpectedly from a ruptured cerebral aneurysm. Alexander worried that he too might one day have a brain hemorrhage. According to a neurological report provided to the CBT practitioner, Alexander made repeated visits to three hospital emergency departments, for which he had growing hospital charts. All evaluations were consistent in finding no evidence of medical abnormalities. Medical records indicated that he had no history of cerebrovascular disease. He did not have hypertension or hyperlipidemia, was a nonsmoker, and was not overweight. He was not currently taking any prescription medications. Hospital records mentioned that Alexander's headaches, dizziness, and feelings of clumsiness were most intense during stressful periods at work, suggesting that stress may be a cause of his troubling bodily reactions.

CLINICAL INTERVIEWS

The Importance of Diagnostic Interviews

The task of assessing DSM-IV Axes I and II disorders encourages the clinician to look beyond the patient's most salient problems to identify psychiatric problems that might otherwise be missed (Wittchen, 1996). A combination of structured, open-ended questioning and empathic listening, used in the context of a structured inquiry about specific events and symptoms, yields the most complete and accurate diagnostic information (American Psychiatric Association [APA], 1995).

Structured interviews have become the gold standard for diagnostic evaluation. They are "structured" in that they comprise a series of questions that directly correspond to the diagnostic criteria for a given psychiatric disorder. The interviewer is encouraged to ask additional questions to clarify ambiguous or inconsistent responses, and to probe particular areas in more detail.

Structured Clinical Interview for DSM-IV

The Structured Clinical Interview for DSM-IV (SCID-IV; First, Spitzer, Gibbon, & Williams, 1996) is among the most widely used structured interviews. It assesses a range of Axis I disorders and is available in formats for assessing current and lifetime disorders. The SCID-IV takes 1.5–2 hours to complete, depending on the complexity and number of presenting problems, and the person's ability to articulate his or her problems. The SCID-IV somatoform disorders module is used to assess hypochondriasis. Disease phobia is assessed using the specific phobia section of the anxiety disorders module. Delusional disorder (somatic type) is assessed using the psychotic disorders module. Time permitting, the SCID-II can be added to the assessment package to assess Axis II disorders (First et al., 1994). The SCID-IV and SCID-II have adequate reliability for the diagnosis of most of the disorders they assess (Taylor, 2000; Williams et al., 1992).

A comprehensive structured clinical interview like the SCID-IV can be used to assess clinical problems that may be comorbid with a health anxiety disorder. Information on comorbidity is relevant for understanding and treatment planning. If the assessment reveals that hypochondriasis is comorbid with, say, major depressive disorder, then it may be necessary to treat the depression first, particularly if the person is at imminent risk of suicide. On the other hand, if the person became mildly depressed after developing severe hypochondriasis, then the depression might be a consequence of hypochondriasis. That is, the depression may be a product of secondary demoralization due to the functional impairments associated with hypochondriasis. Here, the treatment of hypochondriasis may result in an improvement in mood.

Structured Diagnostic Interview for Hypochondriasis

The Structured Diagnostic Interview for Hypochondriasis (SDIH; Barsky et al., 1992) was designed to diagnose hypochondriasis defined by DSM-III-R criteria. The interview has good diagnostic reliability (Barsky et al., 1992) and performs well on various indices of validity (Spekens, 2001; Stewart & Watt, 2001). The SDIH was originally designed to be a module of the somatoform disorder section of the SCID for DSM-III-R. At the time, the only somatoform disorder assessed in the SCID was somatization disorder. Ultimately, the SDIH was not incorporated into the SCID for DSM-III-R or the SCID-IV. Instead, a shorter hypochondriasis section was used. A limitation of the SDIH is that it does not assess DSM-IV criteria for hypochondriasis, whereas the SCID-IV does. (The criteria for hypochondriasis were changed slightly from DSM-III-R to DSM-IV; see Asmundson et al., 2001, for details.)

Health Anxiety Interview

We developed the Health Anxiety Interview (HAI) to provide a detailed assessment of all the DSM-IV health anxiety disorders—hypochondriasis, disease phobia, and delusional disorder (somatic type)—along with milder forms of health anxiety. The HAI also assesses the circumstances in which the person's health anxiety arose. The HAI was designed as a supplement to the SCID-IV, replacing the SCID-IV sections assessing health anxiety disorders. The HAI has the advantage of assessing health anxiety in more detail than the SCID-IV, including information that is used to develop a formulation of the causes of the person's health anxiety (e.g., learning history). The HAI is reproduced in Appendix 1. It requires about 30 minutes to administer. Reliability data are currently unavailable. The format and content of the HAI is similar to that of the SCID-IV, so the psychometric properties of the former may be much the same as the latter.

> Alexander's responses to the SCID-IV and HAI indicated a diagnosis of hypochondriasis. His mood was mildly depressed, but not to the point of having a mood disorder. Alexander was deeply concerned that he was going to have a stroke, despite negative medical findings and reassurance from his doctor. He worried about his health for several hours each day, and worried that his doctors may have missed something important. Alexander believed that repeated medical tests were needed because the greater the number of tests, the greater the chances of identifying the source of his symptoms. Whenever he had headache, dizziness, or feelings of clumsiness he feared that his blood vessels were about to burst. Alexander's preoccupation with his health interfered with his relationships and work productivity. Although his hypochondriasis was severe and debilitating, he had some insight into the psychological nature of his problems. In his calmer moments Alexander recognized that his health concerns were excessive. Therefore, he was not diagnosed as having the poor-insight form of hypochondriasis.

Expanding the Clinical Interview

During the structured interview the clinician can include additional questions to comprehensively assess the patient's problems and the circumstances in which the problems arose. Importantly, questions can be added to assess safety signals and safety behaviors. Recall that *safety signals* are stimuli that the person believes will be associated with the absence of feared outcomes. *Safety behaviors* are things the person does to avert danger, such as avoidance, checking, and reassurance seeking. Safety signals and safety behaviors are important to identify because they maintain health anxiety (see Chapter 3). A goal of treatment is to fade out safety signals and reduce the patient's reliance on safety behaviors. Questions for assessing safety signals and safety behaviors are as follows:

- Is there anything that you avoid in order to protect your health?
- When you feel anxious about your health, what do you do? Follow-up questions: Do you seek reassurance from others? Do you check your body for signs of illness, such as by checking your pulse? Do you check medical texts or the Internet for information about health and disease?
- Do you carry anything with you in order to feel safe about your health? Follow-up questions: Do you carry things to use in the event of a medical emergency, such as a cell phone, a Medic Alert bracelet, or phone numbers and addresses of local hospitals?

Alexander developed a number of safety behaviors that he thought would reduce the risk of a cerebrovascular accident. He avoided many formerly enjoyable activities, including hiking, biking, and playing with his sons, for fear that physical exertion might strain his blood vessels. Although he continued to work, Alexander spent increasing amounts of time surfing the Internet for information about stroke and other medical conditions that might account for his symptoms. He purchased a portable blood pressure monitor that he carried with him in order to check whether he was having a "hypertensive crisis" that would warrant immediate medical attention. Alexander also repeatedly visited a local pharmacy to check his blood pressure on a "more accurate" device.

Patients may be embarrassed to reveal their safety behaviors (e.g., checking stools each day for "irregularities"). If patients do not volunteer information about safety behaviors, the therapist can make a direct inquiry (e.g., "It's not unusual for health-anxious people to check their bodily products, such as the color of their saliva or urine. Is that something that you do?").

The clinical interview can also be used to obtain information about the patient's personal and family history of psychiatric disorders and general medical conditions. The clinician can assess the patient's current living circumstances. What is the nature of the patient's social support network and relationship with family, friends, and coworkers? This information is used to assess whether significant others are reinforcing or facilitating the patient's health anxiety. Significant others can be directly interviewed, with the patient's consent, to assess how they interact with the health-anxious patient. If the significant others are playing a reinforcing or facilitating role, then they need to be considered in the treatment plan.

> Alexander readily consented to the CBT practitioner's request to interview his wife. He reasoned that the more information the practitioner obtained, the greater the chances of correctly identifying the source of his problems. In a separate interview with Alexander's wife, Claire, the practitioner learned that Alexander often asked her for reassurance that he didn't look pale. He also would ask her to check the readings on his blood pressure monitor, in case he had misread the results. Claire was frustrated with Alexander's reassurance seeking. She was particularly troubled when Alexander began to ask his sons for reassurance about whether he looked pale. Alexander hadn't mentioned this to the CBT practitioner, probably out of embarrassment. Claire said she wanted to stop giving Alexander reassurance, but found it easier to give in to his repeated requests.

The practitioner should also assess the patient's treatment history. How many specialists have she or he seen, and for what reason? How frequently does he or she visit his or her primary care physician? What has she or he been told by the referring physician regarding the purpose of the referral to the CBT practitioner? This provides an inroad to eliciting attitudes toward psychological treatment.

> Alexander said that he had reluctantly accepted the CBT referral. His doctors had told him that his problems were due to stress, but Alexander couldn't see how that would cause headaches, dizziness, and clumsiness. Alexander agreed to try CBT only at the urging of his wife and doctor. "I figure I might as well," he said, "I expect we'll be able to prove to my wife and doctor that my problems aren't 'all in my head.'"

As noted in previous chapters, stressful life events have been implicated in the development and persistence of health anxiety disorders. Current and past stressors can be assessed during the interview. The initial interview can be used to obtain a preliminary picture of the role of stressors in triggering and maintaining health anxiety. A more detailed measure of daily stressors can be used during treatment to help the patient understand the role of these events in producing troubling bodily changes (e.g., rashes) or sensations (e.g., palpitations). This fine-grained assessment is discussed in Chapter 11.

Alexander reported that he has some major problems at work. He worked in a large architectural firm that was experiencing financial problems. There were rumors that staff would be laid off, so Alexander felt pressured to excel at his work, to convince the senior partners that he was indispensable. Accordingly, he worked long hours and made sure that each of his projects was completed on schedule. To keep up his performance level, he drank a lot of coffee throughout his long days at the office.

The interview also provides information on treatment-related variables such the factors influencing whether the patient will enter treatment and the factors predicting treatment response (as discussed in Chapter 5). These include situational variables that affect the patient's ability to attend scheduled appointments, negative attitudes about being treated by a cognitive-behavioral therapist for something she or he believes to be principally related to organic pathology, and her or his reasons for attending therapy.

Although Alexander believed he had an undiagnosed general medical condition, he was willing to explore the possibility that health anxiety might be his main problem. This was a good prognostic sign for him entering treatment. His wife and primary care physician strongly encouraged him to seek CBT, which was also considered to be a good prognostic sign. On the other hand, his health anxiety was severe, which was not a good sign. Accordingly, the prognosis was guarded.

The Downward-Arrow Method

The downward-arrow method (Burns, 1980) is one of the most useful ways of identifying dysfunctional thoughts (and associated images) about death and disease. This brief interview method elicits much more detail about beliefs than can be obtained from self-report questionnaires or structured diagnostic interviews. To assess beliefs relevant to understanding health anxiety disorders, the clinician can ask the patient to describe a recent episode of health anxiety. Systematic questioning is then used to identify what the patient regards as the worst part of the event, and why he or she thinks that is bad. Questions such as the following are asked:

- "What was most upsetting about _____?"
- "Supposing _____ did happen, why would that be bad?"
- "If _____ was true, what would that mean to you?"
- "What could happen if _____ did occur?"

The following transcript illustrates the downward-arrow method. Questioning reveals a number of idiosyncratic beliefs about the consequences of death, which would be important to address in treatment (e.g., by cognitive restructuring).

THERAPIST: You've mentioned that you have a number of bodily concerns. Which is your biggest problem right now?

ALEXANDER: I'm worried about my headaches.

THERAPIST: What worries you the most about them?

ALEXANDER: I'm worried that I might have something wrong with my brain. Maybe an arteriovenus malformation, which I read about on the Internet.

THERAPIST: If that was true, what would that mean to you?

ALEXANDER: It means I'd surely die.

THERAPIST: What do you think will happen after you die? What's the worst thing you imagine?

ALEXANDER: I'm frightened that death will bring nothingness—oblivion.

THERAPIST: What would be bad about that?

ALEXANDER: I'd lose everything—myself, my family, everything—all that I've striven to have.

THERAPIST: And what would be the worst thing about that?

ALEXANDER: I don't know really. I guess that's the worst of it—to lose everything, including my existence. That would be horrible.

The downward-arrow method can also be used to identify dysfunctional beliefs about the effects of safety signals and safety behaviors. The CBT practitioner asked Alexander to imagine what would happen if he stopped performing some of his safety behaviors. Although this is an intervention often used in treatment, it is also a valuable assessment tool.

THERAPIST: Alexander, imagine for a moment that you stopped searching the Internet for medical information. What do you think would happen?

ALEXANDER: If I stopped searching, then I might miss out on the latest information on the treatment of brain problems.

THERAPIST: What would be upsetting about not having the information?

ALEXANDER: Well, I wouldn't be able to prepare my doctor with vital information about how to take care of me.

THERAPIST: And if you didn't give him this information, what would happen?

ALEXANDER: He wouldn't use the best treatment and I could die.

THERAPIST: OK, so to summarize, you believe checking the Internet is important for getting the latest information, and getting this information is important so that your doctor can prevent you from dying. So, it sounds like an important thing that motivates you to check the Internet is the belief that your doctor is incompetent to take care of you without expert information that you are responsible for providing. Is that an accurate summary?

ALEXANDER: Yes, I guess it is.

SELF-REPORT QUESTIONNAIRES

Uses and Limitations

Self-report questionnaires provide supplementary information that complement, but do not replace, the need for a good clinical interview. No amount of questionnaire data can exceed the value of careful questioning by a skilled clinician. Questionnaire results need to be interpreted with caution. Elevated scores can be obtained not only by people with health anxiety disorders, but also by those with general medical conditions, or those with psychiatric conditions in which health concerns are an associated but not a central feature (e.g., major depression, generalized anxiety disorder). Accordingly, scores on the self-report questionnaires need to be interpreted in light of findings from a clinical interview. Self-report questionnaires, when used for clinical purposes, are most valuable when used in the following ways:

- To corroborate information obtained from the clinical interview. This is especially useful for novitiate clinicians who are not experienced in assessing the many facets of health anxiety disorders. Questionnaires would be used for this purpose if they were given to the patient at the end of the interview, for completion as a homework assignment.
- If questionnaires are administered prior to the initial interview, then they could be used for screening purposes. Questionnaire responses can be reviewed before starting the interview, to determine whether the clinician needs to conduct a detailed assessment of health anxiety disorders.
- To monitor treatment progress. Short questionnaires can be completed periodically throughout the course of treatment. The patient, for example, could complete a questionnaire in the waiting room prior to

the CBT appointment. The session could then begin with a review of the responses.

As a resource for readers, all of the self-report inventories reviewed in the following sections are presented in the Appendices, along with their scoring keys. As we will see, some inventories are well suited for clinical purposes, while others are better suited for research purposes.

Whiteley Index

This measure was developed by Pilowsky (1967) to assess the core features of hypochondriasis. Respondents are asked to answer *yes* or *no* to each of 14 questions, including items such as "Do you often worry about the possibility that you have a serious illness?" and "Is it hard for you to believe the doctor when he tells you there is nothing to worry about?" The Whiteley Index and scoring key appears in Appendices 2a and 2b. Scores can be derived for a total scale and for three subscales: disease fear, disease conviction, and bodily preoccupation. The Whiteley Index has generally good reliability and validity, and predicts treatment outcome and health care utilization (Barsky et al., 1992; Noyes et al., 1994a; Pålsson, 1988; Pilowsky, 1967; Speckens, Spinhoven, Sloekers, Bolk, & van Hemert, 1996). Norms for various patient samples, as well as screening cutoff scores, are available (Pilowsky & Spence, 1994). Given the brevity of this questionnaire, it can be readily used as a brief screen for health anxiety or as a means of monitoring treatment response.

Illness Behavior Questionnaire

This questionnaire was developed to assess maladaptive or inappropriate ways of responding to illness. Although originally comprising 52 items, including all 14 items from the Whiteley Index, its most recent format has been expanded to include 62 items. It is available in formats for clinical and nonclinical settings, with the latter using wording that does not assume the presence of illness (e.g., "Does your illness interfere with your life a great deal?" vs. "Do you have an illness that interferes with your life a great deal?"). The questionnaire contains seven subscales:

- Phobic concern about having an illness. This is labeled "general hypochondriasis," although it could be called "disease fear."
- Disease conviction.
- Perception of illness—whether illness is perceived as somatic or psychological in origin.
- Affective inhibition.

- Affective disturbance (anxiety and depression).
- Denial of stress.
- Irritability.

Appendices 3a and 3b contain the Illness Behavior Questionnaire for clinical settings and the scoring key. The questionnaire performs well on various indices of reliability and validity, and high subscale scores (particularly disease conviction) predict poor treatment outcome (Pilowsky, Chapman, & Bonica, 1977; Pilowsky, Murrell, & Gordon, 1979; Wilson et al., 1994; Zonderman, Heft, & Costa, 1985).

Factor analytic research suggests that the seven subscales can be reduced to two factors: affective state and disease affirmation. Detailed norms are available for the subscales and for the factor scores (Pilowsky & Spence, 1994). The Illness Behavior Questionnaire has the advantage of being broad in its assessment by measuring features that are commonly associated with health anxiety disorders, such as depression and irritability. A weakness of the questionnaire is that it's lengthy.

Illness Attitude Scales

This inventory, which appears along with the scoring keys in Appendices 4a–4c, was developed to comprehensively measure the central facets of health anxiety (Kellner, 1986, 1987). It contains nine 3-item subscales, which can be tallied to yield a total scale score. The subscales are as follows:

- Worry about illness.
- Concerns about pain.
- Health habits.
- Hypochondriacal beliefs.
- Thanatophobia (fear of death).
- Disease phobia.
- Bodily preoccupation.
- Treatment experience.
- Effects of symptoms.

The subscales have performed generally well on indices of reliability and validity (Speckens, 2001; Stewart & Watt, 2001). Norms are available in the manual (Kellner, 1987). The subscales are correlated with one another, which is consistent with the observation that the features of health anxiety naturally tend to co-occur (e.g., strong disease conviction typically co-occurs with, or leads to, difficulty accepting reassurance that one's health is fine; see Chapter 1).

Factor analytic studies suggest that the nine subscales can be reduced to a smaller set of scales. Hadjistavropoulos et al. (1999), for example, found that the Illness Attitude Scales contains four factors: (1) fear of illness, disease, pain, and death; (2) symptoms interference with lifestyle; (3) treatment experience; and (4) disease conviction. One has the option of scoring the original nine subscales or the smaller set of factorially derived subscales. The latter may be sufficient for assessing the global severity of health anxiety. The original subscales may be preferable for a detailed assessment of treatment response. Although the nine subscales are correlated, the correlations are far from perfect. Treatments may not reduce scores on all subscales to the same degree. An assessment of scores on the nine subscales provides information on which aspects of health anxiety have responded to therapy and which aspects require further treatment.

Health Anxiety Questionnaire

This questionnaire contains four subscales assessing (1) worry and health preoccupation, (2) fear of illness and death, (3) reassurance seeking, and (4) interference in functioning due to bodily concerns. The subscales were derived using an empirical clustering procedure and follow-up factor analysis (Lucock & Morley, 1996). The questionnaire and scoring keys appear in Appendices 5a and 5b. Preliminary research suggests good reliability and validity (Lucock & Morley, 1996; Lucock et al., 1998). A strength of the Health Anxiety Questionnaire is that it balances breadth (four scales) with brevity (21 items), making it an attractive option for assessing health anxiety. However, additional psychometric evaluation is needed and norms are not available, which undermines the questionnaire's usefulness as a clinical tool.

Reassurance Questionnaire

As its name suggests, this questionnaire specifically assesses the extent to which the respondent feels reassured by medical information provided by a physician (Speckens et al., 2000). The current version of the scale and a scoring key appear in Appendices 6a and 6b. Preliminary research suggests encouraging reliability and validity (Speckens, Spinhoven, van Hemert, & Bolk, 2000). A problem, however, is that the scale confounds the patient's tendency to be reassured ("reassurability") with the physician's skill in providing reassurance. Some patients, particularly those with poor-insight hypochondriasis or delusional disorder (somatic type), are very difficult to reassure. Patients with milder health anxiety may respond more readily to reassurance. Similarly, some physicians may not be very skilled at providing convincing reassurance, while others may be highly persuasive. The Reassurance Questionnaire fails to disentangle these factors, which thereby limits its usefulness. Further revisions to this scale may rectify this problem. Other questionnaires, such as those reviewed earlier, assess the patient's general tendency to have difficulty accepting reassurance. A further limitation is that no norms are available for the Reassurance Questionnaire.

Somatosensory Amplification Scale

Health anxiety is associated with a tendency to perceive bodily changes and sensations as intense, noxious, and distressing (see Chapter 2). Barsky et al. (1988b) called this tendency *somatosensory amplification*, which is measured with the Somatosensory Amplification Scale (Appendices 7a and 7b). This short, 10-item questionnaire measures the person's response to mild somatic experiences that are unpleasant but not typically symptomatic of disease (e.g., "I sometimes can feel the blood flowing in my body"). The psychometric properties of the Somatosensory Amplification Scale are generally sound (Speckens, 2001; Stewart & Watt, 2001). Normative data are available from several sources (e.g., Barsky et al., 1988a, 1990a, 1990b, 1994a).

Selecting Self-Report Instruments

Which questionnaires are most useful for assessment and treatment planning? The questionnaires differ in several ways, including breadth of assessment, time required for administration and scoring, availability of norms, and the amount of research on their reliability and validity. The choice of scale depends partly on the purpose of the assessment. If the clinician requires a quick assessment of health anxiety, then the Whiteley Index is a particularly good choice because, unlike other brief measures such as the Health Anxiety Questionnaire, norms and screening cutoff scores are available. The Whiteley index is short enough for periodically readministering it throughout treatment to monitor progress.

　　If a more detailed assessment of the various facets of health anxiety is desired, then the Illness Attitude Scales would be a good choice, particularly because it is easy to score, there are a good deal of data on its reliability and validity, and norms are available. The Illness Attitude Scales don't assess all aspects of health anxiety, such as somatosensory amplification or illness-related irritability and depression. Depending on the time available for an assessment, a battery of questionnaires (for which norms are available) could be administered, such as the Illness Attitude Scales and the subscales of the Illness Behavior Questionnaire that do not overlap with those of the Illness Attitude Scales.

During the intake evaluation, the CBT practitioner conducted an extensive assessment of Alexander's problems using the SCID-IV and HAI. A battery of questionnaires was deemed unnecessary because it would be time-consuming for Alexander and probably would not add much new information. Alexander was asked to complete the Whiteley Index, primarily for the purpose of monitoring treatment progress. As expected, Alexander obtained near-maximum scores on all the subscales: disease fear, disease conviction, and bodily preoccupation. The results were shared with Alexander, to help him understand that health anxiety was a major problem for him. The therapist planned to initiate a course of CBT and to administer the questionnaire every 2 weeks in order to monitor treatment progress. When Alexander was asked to complete the questionnaire throughout treatment, he was asked to base his responses on how things had been over the past 2 weeks.

PROSPECTIVE MONITORING

Clinicians working with health-anxious patients often use some form of prospective monitoring to gather detailed information on bodily changes or sensations, dysfunctional beliefs, and safety signals and safety behaviors. Prospective monitoring involves the use of a daily diary or checklist, such as the one in Appendix 8. Patients can be asked to complete the diary each day for 1 or 2 weeks prior to treatment. This provides a wealth of information about daily episodes of health anxiety, which can be enlightening for the patient.

After completing the intake evaluation, Alexander completed the diary for 2 weeks and then returned for his first treatment session. Results of the diary corroborated the questionnaire and interview data. Alexander found the diary to be useful because it helped him realize the extent to which health anxiety was a problem for him: "The diary helped me realize that I freak out every time I have a headache, thinking, 'This time for sure it's a stroke.' I'm starting to think that I might be worrying way too much about my health."

DEVELOPING A CASE FORMULATION
AND TREATMENT PLAN

Formulation

The case formulation is constructed from all the available information in an attempt to develop a working model of the patient's problems. There are several different ways of developing a case formulation (Taylor, 2000). One simple but useful method is to list the patient's main problems and then, based on the cognitive-behavioral approach to health anxiety (see Chapters 2–4), to develop hypotheses about the predisposing, precipitating, perpetuating, and protective factors.

Alexander's problem list consists of troubling bodily changes and sensations (headaches, dizziness, feelings of clumsiness) associated with a diagnosis of hypochondriasis. The latter disorder was the overarching problem, for which the CBT practitioner developed a case formulation. The main elements of Alexander's case formulation and the links between elements appear in Figure 6.1.

His father's stroke and the neighbor's unexpected aneurysm were salient learning experiences that predisposed Alexander to become anxious about his health. The stroke and aneurysm appear to have taught Alexander that (1) headache, dizziness, and feelings of clumsiness can be precursors of life-threatening cerebrovascular problems; (2) these problems can strike at any

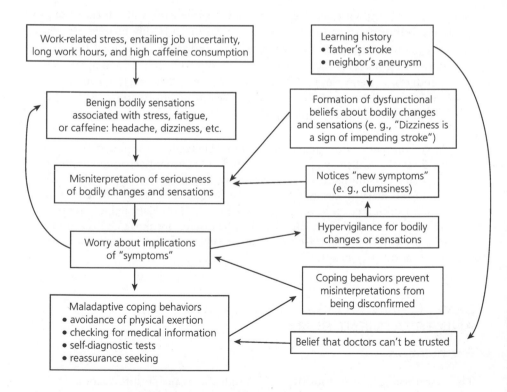

FIGURE 6.1. Case formulation for Alexander P.

time, even in people of his own age group, such as his 33-year-old neighbor; and (3) doctors aren't to be trusted, particularly when it comes to serious diseases. These learning experiences predisposed Alexander to become alarmed by benign bodily changes or sensations, and to be resistant to medical reassurance that the bodily events are harmless.

Alexander's hypochondriasis appears to have been precipitated by work-related stressors, entailing job uncertainty, long work hours, and compensatory overuse of caffeine. As a result, he experienced arousal-related bodily sensations such as tension headaches and dizziness. The latter may have been a somatic feature of anxiety or may have been due to fatigue. Given his learning history, Alexander misinterpreted the bodily sensations as signs of a severe threat to his health, thus triggering extreme worry about the implications of the sensations and difficulty accepting reassurance that they were benign.

The assessment suggests an interplay of factors that contributed to the perpetuation or maintenance of Alexander's health anxiety. His worry about the implications of the bodily sensations lead him to become anxiously aroused, thereby intensifying and prolonging his arousal-related bodily changes and sensations. His avoidance of physical exertion prevented him from learning that his blood vessels would not "burst." Avoidance therefore perpetuated Alexander's worry that his health was in jeopardy. Checking for medical information exposed him to a myriad of rare, lethal, and frequently unrecognized causes of cerebrovascular problems. This added fuel to his health concerns. Self-diagnostic tests (blood pressure monitoring) were frequently performed and produced the occasional false-positive result. Alexander took those results as "proof" that his health was under threat.

Alexander's belief that doctors can't be trusted led him to repeatedly seek reassurance and second opinions in the hope that the cause of his problems would eventually be identified. Continual reassurance seeking from his doctors, wife, and children constantly reminded him of his perceived health problems, thereby perpetuating his health anxiety.

Worry about his health led him to be hypervigilant for bodily changes or sensations. He began to notice and misinterpret bodily events that he hadn't noticed before. He became aware that occasionally he was clumsy. Alexander misinterpreted this as a "new symptom"—general clumsiness—which he misinterpreted as "further evidence" of cerebrovascular problems.

Protective factors are not present in every case formulation. Alexander's wife and primary care physician both believed that his health anxiety was excessive, and both encouraged him to seek psychological treatment. The urging of his wife and doctor are protective in the sense that they protected Alexander's health anxiety from becoming worse. If his wife had colluded in

Alexander's belief that his health was at risk, then this may have strengthened his disease conviction.

Using the Formulation to Develop a Treatment Plan

Most of the elements in Alexander's case formulation (Figure 6.1) are perpetuating factors, leading his health anxiety to become chronic. The identification of these factors is important because CBT works, in part, by reducing the factors that perpetuate health anxiety. The formulation would be shared with Alexander for the purpose of psychoeducation and to correct any errors in the formulation (e.g., there may have been other salient learning experiences that were overlooked). The formulation suggests the following interventions:

- Reduce Alexander's caffeine intake to test the idea that some of his bodily sensations are simply due to caffeine overuse.
- Track the pattern of headaches and dizziness to test whether they're more likely to occur on stressful days.
- Increase versus decrease attention to his body to assess whether these are associated with any changes in perceived "clumsiness."
- Increase physical activity (e.g., exercise regularly) so that Alexander can prove to himself that he is not at risk for stroke. (Alexander should be warned beforehand that physical activity may lead to tiredness and muscle soreness because his exercise avoidance has probably led to physical deconditioning.)
- Reduce reassurance seeking, checking for medical information, and self-diagnostic tests to reduce health preoccupation to see if this results in a reduction in health-related worry. Alternatively, Alexander could increase these activities to demonstrate that they contribute to or worsen his worries.
- Enlist the support of his wife and primary care physician in not providing reassurance.
- Consider interviewing his father, who believed that his stroke was due to medical mismanagement. Does his father believe that Alexander's concerns are excessive? What was the pattern of the father's prodromal symptoms of stroke? Were these clearly different from Alexander's episodes of headache, dizziness, and clumsiness? If so, then this could further weaken Alexander's belief that his health is at risk.
- Once Alexander no longer fears that his health is at risk, stress management methods could be used to help him better cope with the demands of his job (e.g., training in time management).

SUMMARY AND CONCLUSIONS

Assessment is used for several related purposes, including accurate diagnosis, strengthening the therapist–patient relationship, developing a case formulation, and then using the formulation to develop a plan for treatment. Assessment of health anxiety disorders begins by ruling out general medical conditions that could account for the patient's problems. Once this is done, the CBT practitioner can conduct a clinical interview for the purpose of DSM-IV diagnosis and for collecting information for constructing a case formulation. The clinical interview is the most important component of a good psychological assessment. The downward-arrow interview, consultations with the patient's significant other(s), and prospective monitoring also provide useful information. Several self-report questionnaires are available. These can be used for preinterview screening purposes or to corroborate interview data. Brief questionnaires are also useful for monitoring treatment progress. In summary, assessment and treatment are closely intertwined; initial assessment leads to a treatment plan, and ongoing assessment enables the therapist to monitor treatment progress and to modify the treatment plan if problems arise.

7

Cognitive-Behavioral Therapy

An Overview

There are several interventions used in cognitive-behavioral therapy (CBT) for health anxiety disorders:

- Liaison with other clinicians to ensure consistent, appropriate care.
- Treatment engagement strategies.
- Psychoeducation.
- Goal setting.
- Cognitive restructuring.
- Behavioral exercises.
- Stress management techniques.
- Relapse prevention methods.

Many of these are ways of helping patients to discard dysfunctional beliefs and to embrace more adaptive ways of thinking about health and disease. *Psychoeducation* provides information about the nature and treatment of health anxiety, based in part on the case formulation (see Chapter 6) of the patient's presenting problems. *Treatment engagement strategies* are methods principally intended to enhance treatment motivation, although they also encourage more adaptive thinking about health and disease. *Cognitive restructuring*, as used in the present context, refers to methods aimed specifically at altering disease-related beliefs. *Behavioral exercises* are additional vehicles of belief change, which include exposure, response prevention, and other strategies. *Stress management techniques* are intended to reduce anxiety and arousal-related bodily sensations, thereby helping patients discover whether troubling bodily changes or sensations are simply the effects of stress. *Relapse prevention methods* are strategies for maintaining and extending treatment gains, including methods for dealing with future episodes of health anxiety.

COGNITIVE-BEHAVIORAL PROCEDURES

Multidisciplinary Liaison

Primary care physicians play a particularly important role in encouraging patients to try a course of CBT for their health anxiety (Visser & Bouman, 2001). Patients referred for CBT are typically those who have failed to respond to simpler interventions, such as assurance that their health is fine. The CBT practitioner can offer the referring physician information about the general approaches used in managing health anxiety disorders, such as those listed in Table 7.1. This list was derived from our clinical experience and those of others (Barsky, 1996; Salkovskis, 1989; Sharpe, Bass, & Mayou, 1995; Warwick & Salkovskis, 2001; Wells, 1997). (The physician could also give the patient Handout 7.1, presented later in this chapter.) Depending on the time available in primary care consultations, the physician may be able to implement some or many of the methods in Table 7.1. The physician can also furnish valuable information to the CBT practitioner on the patient's medical status, details on the need—or lack of need—for further medical tests and examinations, and information on the nature and frequency of the patient's efforts at seeking medical assurance.

Psychoeducation

Psychoeducation, provided by either the CBT practitioner or the primary care physician, is important for patients with hypochondriasis because these patients fail to appreciate the benign causes of their bodily changes or sensations. For patients with disease phobia, education is simpler and briefer, because these patients typically recognize that they have a problem with excessive fear, and usually have at least a rudimentary understanding of how exposure can reduce fears.

The "noisy body" analogy is a useful psychoeducational tool for introducing severely health-anxious patients to a cognitive-behavioral approach. Here, troubling sensations are relabeled as harmless "bodily noise" rather than

TABLE 7.1. Strategies for Managing Health Anxiety Disorders

Things to do

- Express empathy and concern for the patient's suffering.
- Acknowledge the reality of the patient's bodily concerns.
- Uncover the patient's reasons for holding particular disease beliefs.
- Provide an alternative, noncatastrophic explanation of the causes of the patient's bodily changes or sensations.
- Openly acknowledge any doubts the patient may have about the role of psychological factors. Present the issue of psychological factors as something to be investigated.
- Check the patient's understanding of the formulation of the problem, and correct any misconceptions.
- Discuss the pitfalls of "doctor shopping."
- Present CBT as a "no lose" option that can help the patient learn about the causes of bodily concerns.
- Emphasize that even if bodily concerns are due to a general medical condition, CBT can enhance the patient's ability to cope.

Things to avoid

- Medically unnecessary physical exams and lab tests.
- Repeated assurances that there is "nothing wrong."
- Telling the patient that the bodily changes or sensations are simply "all in the mind" or "just nerves."
- Placating the patient by prescribing placebos.
- Argumentative or confrontational interactions with the patient. Treatment should be collaborative.
- Irregular, "symptom-driven" appointments. Consultations should be scheduled as regular (e.g., monthly) check-ins.
- Cutting the patient's consultation short, leaving him or her feeling that you are not taking his or her problems seriously.

indications of physical dysfunction. The therapist does not push this idea vigorously because that can provoke patient resistance (see Chapter 8). Rather, the therapist simply asks the patient to consider the notion of a "noisy body" and prompts her or him to collect some data on whether the idea has merit.

To limit misunderstanding, psychoeducation should be put in simple terms and the patient's understanding should be checked. For example, the therapist could say:

"It's important that we have the same understanding about your back pain. Could you please tell me, in your own words, what I've said about the causes of your pain?"

Where possible, formulation of the patient's problems should be phrased in positive terms—what it *is*, rather than focusing exclusively on what it *isn't* (Salkovskis, 1989; Sharpe et al., 1995). Instead of saying, for example, "No, you don't have cancer," something like the following might be said:

"The lab tests, physical examinations, and my assessment indicate that you do have a problem, but it isn't cancer. The problem has to do with excessive anxiety about your health. Many people suffer from health anxiety. It occurs when you detect bodily changes or sensations and conclude they are dangerous. Like the pain on your left side, which led you to think you had liver cancer, or when you noticed that your tongue was yellow, which led you to worry that you had oral cancer. All of these bodily changes and sensations are real, but harmless. I think it would be helpful if we could talk about the things that cause them. What do you think?"

Whenever possible, explanation should include physiological and psychological factors, to help patients understand that their "symptoms" are real, arising from normal bodily processes (Sharpe et al., 1995). Health-anxious people often doubt the competence of their physicians if the reality of the bodily changes or sensations is questioned (Peters et al., 1998). One should acknowledge the reality of the bodily concerns, avoiding any implication that they are "just nerves" or "all in one's head."

An explanation of the benign sources of bodily changes and sensations may be most credible if the patient and therapist discuss how beliefs, emotions, and bodily changes and sensations are interconnected (Smith, 1985). The patient's experiences can be reviewed to make this point. Here are some common examples:

- Thinking that you have done something foolish or inappropriate → feeling embarrassed → blushing, sweating, and feeling hot all over.
- Thinking that you can't cope with work responsibilities → feeling anxious → experiencing nausea and diarrhea.
- Thinking that somebody has done something wrong to you → feeling very angry → experiencing pulse throbbing in neck, flushed face, and, later, headache.
- Thinking about the loss of a loved one → sadness → experiencing tearfulness, chest tightness, and a lump in the throat.
- Seeing a TV program on endometriosis → focusing more attention on one's abdomen → increasing one's chances of detecting harmless sensations such as minor muscle twinges.

Health-anxious people may feel embarrassed if they have to admit to family or employers that their feared symptoms are actually harmless. To help these patients "save face" and thereby improve their chances of accepting the CBT formulation, it is useful to provide a meaningful but benign somatic explanation for their problems (e.g., excessive muscle tension, muscle strain, chest wall muscle spasm) (Smith, 1985).

Self-monitoring of bodily changes and sensations, thoughts, and emotions provides material for education about the role of beliefs and thoughts in health anxiety. Self-monitoring also helps to demonstrate to the patient that the sequence of events postulated in his or her formulation actually occurs in his or her daily life. This can make CBT more credible to the patient (Warwick, 1995). For example, after reviewing Joan B.'s self-monitoring of headaches, the therapist asked:

"If your headaches are always worse after your weekly meetings with your supervisor, then what might be causing them? Would you expect this pattern of pain from a brain tumor?"

Reviewing the impact of reassurance is also an important psychoeducational tool (Wells, 1997): "If reassurance relieves your symptoms, then what does this tell you about their cause?"

A psychoeducational handout can be given to the patient, along with a brief written formulation of his or her problems. This will help the patient remember what was discussed. An example of a generic psychoeducational handout appears in Handout 7.1. To facilitate learning, sessions can be audiotaped and reviewed by the patient in between sessions.

Therapy Style and Treatment Engagement

The CBT practitioner should try to steer clear of extreme reactions to the health-anxious patient. On the one hand, this means avoiding the extreme of encouraging overinvestigation of patient complaints by recommending further lab tests and physical examinations. The essence of the approach is captured in the expression "Don't just do something, stand there!" (Drossman, 1978, p. 370). On the other hand, the therapist should strive to avoid the other extreme of dismissing patient complaints out of hand. If one trivializes patient complaints, then there will be deterioration in the therapeutic relationship, the patient will feel that he or she is not being taken seriously, and the patient may come to worry about the quality of care and thus seek out other health care providers. Attention and empathy are important in establishing a trusting therapeutic relationship, thereby making the patient more amenable to treatment of health anxiety.

HEALTH ANXIETY: A COMMON, TREATABLE PROBLEM

What is health anxiety?

Health anxiety is characterized by excessive worry or fears about disease, despite the fact that you have had medical tests and checkups that have ruled out physical disease. Some health-anxious people are mainly worried about *having* a dreaded disease such as cancer, while other health-anxious people are primarily worried that they *could catch* a serious disease by coming into contact with sick people, hospitals, or other sources of germs.

Where do my symptoms come from?

People with health anxiety experience a lot of physical symptoms. The symptoms are *real* but harmless. They are caused by many different things. You and your therapist can work together to help understand why you experience unwanted bodily changes or sensations. In some cases the sensations are part of the body's anxiety response. Anxiety is associated with many harmless bodily changes or sensations, including stomach upset (e.g., nausea, bloating), fatigue, flushing and hot flashes, shortness of breath, chest tightness, racing or pounding heart, dizziness, and diarrhea. If you notice these changes or sensations and start to worry about them, then you will become more anxious and these bodily reactions will persist. These reactions may be inconvenient but are completely harmless.

Do healthy people experience physical symptoms?

People who are perfectly healthy experience many bodily changes and sensations. Most people don't notice them because they don't pay much attention to their bodies. People with health anxiety tend to be preoccupied with their bodies. They focus a lot of their attention on their bodies, and so they are more likely to notice and worry about harmless bodily sensations. This can happen because some people have particularly "noisy" bodies, in the same way that a rattling car can be mechanically fine.

Should I seek reassurance or discuss my symptoms with other people (aside from my therapist)?

No. Once your doctor has ruled out physical disease, then there is no need to seek further reassurance. In fact, *seeking reassurance and discussing symptoms can make your health anxiety worse*. Reassurance seeking has the following effects:

♦ It puts you in a passive, dependent role, which prevents you from proving to yourself that the bodily changes or sensations are harmless.
♦ It encourages you to become preoccupied with your body, which means that you will continue to notice harmless changes or sensations and become alarmed by them.
♦ It encourages the incorrect belief that you are physically sick.

(continued)

Once your doctor has ruled out a harmful physical disease, then we strongly recommend that you try to stop seeking reassurance, and stop discussing your health with friends, family members, and others. We also strongly recommend that you do not check up on symptoms by reading medical articles or textbooks or by searching for medical information on the Internet. These activities will make your health anxiety worse.

How do I know my symptoms are caused by something harmless, like anxiety?

By collecting evidence. No doubt you have been to your doctor to look for evidence of a physical disease, but have you looked for evidence that your bodily concerns are due to something harmless, like anxiety? Most people with health anxiety fail to do this. If your bodily concerns are due to anxiety, then it would be important to prove to yourself that this is the case.

How would someone overcome a fear of getting sick?

This is called *disease phobia*. It can be treated in the same way that other fears are treated, by gradually and systematically confronting the thing that you fear. You and your therapist can discuss ways that this can be done, in a way that is not too difficult for you.

A further challenge is that health-anxious patients may resist the notion that their symptoms are influenced by psychosocial factors. They might even become angry and indignant when this possibility is raised. This can lead the therapist to focus primarily on the physical symptoms, which can reinforce the patient's belief that he or she has a serious medical condition, while downplaying the significance of emotional factors (Barsky, 1996). Chapter 8 describes a series of treatment engagement strategies than can be useful in addressing these problems.

Goal Setting

The health-anxious patient's goals often differ from those of the CBT practitioner. The patient may wish to have his or her bodily concerns diagnosed, explained, and remedied. The therapist's goals may be the reduction of her or his health anxiety and improved tolerance of bodily changes and sensations. When the goals of patient and therapist are in conflict, nonadherence and treatment dropout are likely. Therefore, an important aim of treatment is to encourage the patient to explore the possibility that his or her problem is health anxiety rather than an occult (undiagnosed) disease. Treatment engagement strategies are used to achieve this goal.

The therapist and patient should work collaboratively to develop a formulation of the patient's problems. The formulation must be developed and presented in a credible fashion:

> [The formulation] must not diverge from the patient's previous experience and, with time, must survive his or her future experience. For example, patients may be told that their symptoms are due to stress, but they are unable to fit their symptoms and signs with their understanding of stress. This discordant experience will lead to rapid disconfirmation of the explanation and to persistence of the health concerns in the patient. It may also lead to feelings of mistrust in medical opinions. (Warwick & Salkovskis, 2001, p. 317)

Treatment goals and methods for achieving these goals are derived from the case formulation. Health-anxious patients often worry that no one can help them with their problems, and so it can be heartening for them to hear that health anxiety is not uncommon and that effective treatments are available (Warwick & Salkovskis, 2001). Although goals can vary from one patient to another, there are a number of commonalties, as listed in Table 7.2 (Barsky, 1996; Mayou, 1993; Salkovskis, 1989; Smith, 1985; Warwick & Salkovskis, 2001). The purpose of CBT is not to eliminate all bodily changes or sensations. A more realistic goal is to reduce the patient's tendency to misinterpret

TABLE 7.2. Common Treatment Goals
for Health Anxiety Disorders

- Decreased disease conviction, without necessarily reducing "symptoms" (bodily changes or sensations).
- Decreased health-related worry.
- Decreased medical utilization, including reduced frequency of doctor shopping and reassurance seeking.
- Decreased reassurance seeking from significant others.
- Decreased bodily checking.
- Reduction in comorbid mental health problems (e.g., depression).
- Increased ability to cope with the occurrence of new "symptoms."
- Strengthened adaptive beliefs about health and disease (e.g., strengthening of the conviction that even healthy people frequently have bodily sensations).
- Improved occupational and role functioning.
- Improved social relations (e.g., social interactions should no longer be centered on the patient's health concerns).
- Improved health habits.
- Improved overall quality of life.

---

the dangerousness of bodily events. Behavioral stress management techniques (see Chapter 11) can reduce, to some extent, bothersome bodily sensations, particularly arousal-related sensations such as palpitations, gastrointestinal upset, and tension-induced pain. However, these techniques cannot eliminate all bodily changes and sensations. Indeed, these are normal features of a healthy body. If behavioral stress management methods are used, then it is important that the patient understand that these techniques reduce bothersome but harmless bodily changes and sensations. The therapist should ensure that the patient is not using these methods as a way of avoiding bodily concerns.

Once treatment goals are identified, the therapist and the patient can review the extent that previous (medical) treatment has achieved these goals. Given that the patient presenting for CBT is still experiencing upsetting bodily changes or sensations and is still preoccupied with health, chances are that the patient's treatment goals have been largely unmet. The therapist can then suggest that perhaps it's time to consider a different approach to treatment. The patient can be led to understand that the goal of being "symptom-free" is unrealistic because everyone (including healthy people) experiences bodily sensations. Socratic dialogue and information gathering can be used to help convey this point.

THERAPIST: Do you think it's ever possible to be completely free of bodily sensations, such as aches and pains?

PATIENT: I hope so.

THERAPIST: Do you think that healthy people experience these sensations?

PATIENT: I don't see why that would happen to a healthy person.

THERAPIST: Let's draw an analogy. Have you ever had a noisy car?

PATIENT: No, but my refrigerator is very noisy. It keeps me awake at night.

THERAPIST: And is it working properly?

PATIENT: Yes, it's fine. I've had it checked and the repairman says that there is nothing wrong.

THERAPIST: So you can have a fridge that's noisy, even though it's in good working order?

PATIENT: Yes.

THERAPIST: Do you think the same thing could apply to human bodies? That is, do you think that some people have "noisy bodies," which produce a lot of sensations even though they're physically healthy?

PATIENT: I don't see how that could be. I think it's unlikely.

THERAPIST: OK, I appreciate you telling me that. But if this "noisy body" idea turned out to be true, how would that make you feel?

PATIENT: I guess I wouldn't get so upset when I noticed a symptom.

THERAPIST: Right. So it sounds like the "noisy body" idea is something that's important to check out. How could we go about collecting evidence to see if this idea is true? . . .

Cognitive Restructuring and Behavioral Exercises

Treatment should be tailored to the specifics of his or her patient and their problems. The importance of tailored treatment for health anxiety disorders has long been recognized. In 1730, for example, Bernard Mandeville observed that "for as the symptoms differ, so I alter my method; and I never saw yet two hypochondriacal cases exactly alike" (1976, p. 343). Although the details of treatment protocols often vary from case to case, there are a number of commonalities. For a patient suffering primarily from disease phobia, for example, treatment is commonly delivered in the following sequence:

- *Initial sessions*: Assessment, review of treatment goals, treatment engagement strategies.

• *Later sessions*: Planning and implementation of imaginal and *in vivo* exposure exercises. These are typically implemented hierarchically, beginning with the least distressing stimuli. Exposure exercises can be framed as behavioral experiments to test dysfunctional and adaptive beliefs about the feared stimuli. For example, one of our patients believed that she would contract germs by walking past a funeral home, resulting in a serious illness. Exposure exercises were developed that involved walking increasingly closer to and eventually entering a funeral home. The prediction that she would become seriously ill (defined as requiring hospital admission) was contrasted with our prediction that her health would not be harmed.

• *Other interventions*: Response prevention exercises could be used for disease phobic people who engage in repeated checking or reassurance seeking. Interoceptive exposure could be used for people with prominent fears of bodily sensations. Coping techniques such as breathing exercises could be used to make it easier for the person to encounter fear-evoking stimuli. These techniques would be faded out over time, so the patient would not become dependent on them. Relapse prevention methods would also be implemented.

A similar sequence of interventions could be used for full-blown hypochondriasis. The therapist would typically need to devote more time to treatment engagement strategies because hypochondriasis is characterized by stronger disease conviction, compared to disease phobia. Weekly self-monitoring of bodily concerns, beliefs, and emotions would be used to help the patient learn about the various factors that can account for the detection of bodily changes and sensations, such as selective attention, muscle tension, mood, misinterpretations, and environmental factors.

Cognitive restructuring exercises could be employed to challenge disease-related beliefs—that is, to promote the development of alternative, nonthreatening explanations of bodily events (Warwick, 1995). Cognitive restructuring can also facilitate adherence to exposure and response prevention exercises. Behavioral stress management methods can be used for patients suffering from recurrent arousal-related symptoms such as headaches. Depending on the patient's goals, therapy can also work on improving the patient's health habits, comorbid disorders, and overall quality of life.

As stated above, it is important to coordinate CBT with medical management. If the patient's primary care physician is relying on reassurance, then the CBT practitioner and the physician should discuss the possibility of suspending reassurance, at least in the short term, in order to assess the effects on health anxiety. Family members can also be encouraged to refrain from giving reassurance.

The treatment of delusional disorder (somatic type) can be more challenging than the treatment of other health anxiety disorders. Psychotropic medication such as pimozide is often required, and patient engagement strategies are essential to ensure medication adherence. The engagement strategies can be implemented by a clinician experienced in CBT, while medication is prescribed by a specialist physician such as a dermatologist. If family members are available, then it also can be useful to involve them in treatment to encourage medication adherence. Some family members inadvertently reinforce or encourage the patient's beliefs about parasitic infestation. In these circumstances treatment is unlikely to be successful unless these family members can be persuaded to participate in therapy.

MODE OF TREATMENT DELIVERY

Treatment Format

CBT can be readily applied in either group or individual formats. Psychoeducation, by virtue of its didactic style, is readily amenable to a group format of, for example, 8–10 participants. There is little evidence to determine which health-anxious people are most likely to benefit from individual or group treatment. Important considerations include patient preference and the availability of a sufficient number of people to form a group. Clinics in large medical centers, compared to smaller clinics and private practices, may have enough health-anxious patients to form treatment groups. Group treatment may work best when the participants have similar disorders of similar severity (e.g., a group of patients suffering from disease phobia or a group suffering from hypochondriasis). Participants with somatic delusions may be inappropriate for group treatment, given their extreme illness convictions, along with the fact that their disease beliefs are often quite different from the beliefs held by people with nondelusional hypochondriasis. People with somatic delusions commonly believe they are infested with parasites, whereas nondelusional health anxiety is associated with other concerns, such as concerns about cancer, heart disease, or viral infection. Consequently, the content of discussion with these patients is typically quite different.

Treatment Setting

Some clinicians argue that health anxiety disorders should be treated in general hospitals or other nonpsychiatric medical settings because health-anxious patients may resist the idea that their problem is anxiety rather than disease. An advantage of the CBT practitioner delivering treatment in a general medical setting is that the patient is being treated in a familiar setting (e.g., his or her primary care clinic).

Health-anxious patients commonly present to medical specialty clinics, such as those dealing with sexually transmitted diseases, genitourinary problems, or dermatological conditions (e.g., Koo & Lee, 2001; Miller et al., 1988a; Tyrer et al., 1999; Zomer et al., 1998). In such cases, it may be easier for a health-anxious patient to accept a referral for CBT if it is delivered in a medical specialty clinic as opposed to a psychiatric setting.

Health-anxious patients are sometimes willing to accept a referral to a mental health setting. In other cases, it may be most appropriate for patients to be treated in a community setting. Some health-anxious patients have prominent disease phobias and thereby strive to avoid all things associated with disease, including hospitals and physicians. Such patients might be best treated in university settings, such as psychology clinics, or in community settings offering psychoeducational courses for health anxiety.

USING COGNITIVE-BEHAVIORAL THERAPY TO FACILITATE MEDICAL MANAGEMENT

Medication Adherence

For patients choosing to receive pharmacotherapy (with or without a formal course of CBT), the cognitive-behavioral therapist can play an important role in facilitating compliance with drug treatment. The patient and CBT practitioner could have a few sessions in which the patient's beliefs about medications are explored. The following beliefs, all of which can interfere with medication adherence, are often encountered:

- "Medications are needed only when I have symptoms."
- "If medication doesn't work immediately, then it's useless."
- "I can't stand side effects."
- "I have to be sure to be on the very best medication, at the perfect dose."

Health-anxious patients who elect to be treated with drugs may ruminate about their medications, sometimes to the point that this becomes the focus of their health concerns. Sometimes simple education about the nature of psychotropic medication is sufficient to alleviate their concerns. Side effects can often be managed by slowly increasing the dose, and by informing the patient that any side effects are harmless and typically transient (Enns et al., 2001).

If these simple approaches don't work, then catastrophic misinterpretations of the significance of benign side effects, such as mild jitteriness, can be challenged in the same way that one can challenge other misinterpretations of bodily sensations (see Chapter 9). Beliefs about the need for the perfect medication at the perfect dose can similarly be treated with cognitive restructuring.

PATIENT: Despite what my doctor tells me, I worry I'm not on the right drug.

THERAPIST: Please tell me about your concerns.

PATIENT: If my problem really is health anxiety, then I should be on the best medication. I searched the Internet and there are all kinds of anxiety drugs. But what if I'm not on the right one?

THERAPIST: What do you think would happen?

PATIENT: Maybe I wouldn't get better, or maybe the wrong drug would make me worse.

THERAPIST: I can see why that thought would be upsetting. Are you still taking your medication?

PATIENT: Yes.

THERAPIST: How come?

PATIENT: Well, I try to tell myself that my doctor knows best. [Here the therapist encourages the patient to generate reasons why she should not worry about her medication.]

THERAPIST: So you tell yourself that your doctor knows best. Why do you think that?

PATIENT: She says she's had a lot of success treating anxiety with this medication.

THERAPIST: Then it's worthwhile to stay on the drug for the time being?

PATIENT: Yes, I guess so.

THERAPIST: How will you know whether the drug is the one for you?

PATIENT: I suppose I'll have to wait and see.

THERAPIST: I agree. Only time will tell. If this one doesn't work, then there are lots of other treatment options. By the way, let me ask you, is it helpful for you to be spending your time checking the Internet for drug information? Does this make you less anxious? [Here the therapist encourages the patient to think about the adaptiveness of checking.]

PATIENT: At first it seemed reassuring, but I started to worry more and more as I learned of so many different drugs and their side effects.

THERAPIST: So checking was helpful at first, but then started to make things worse. I wonder if it would be worth seeing what would happen if you stopped checking, at least for a little while. . . . (*The patient and therapist then proceed to discuss a behavioral experiment for testing the effects of not checking.*)

Planning for General Medical Consultations

It is important to devise, with the input of patients and their medical doctors, an appropriate plan for ongoing medical care. Most patients, particularly the medically ill and the elderly, will require periodic medical investigations (e.g., assessing a patient's thyroid level). Appropriate guidelines should be negotiated regarding the frequency of these investigations. Guidelines can also be devised to determine when the patient should or shouldn't seek additional medical attention. The cognitive-behavioral therapist and patient could develop a list of "symptoms" that *do not* warrant immediate consultation with a medical doctor. The CBT practitioner and patient might come up with examples such as bloodshot eyes, transient stomach pain, minor rashes, and so forth. If the patient notices such bodily changes and experiences an urge to consult a physician, then he or she could be encouraged to write down the "symptom" (e.g., on a self-monitoring form) and then wait a week before deciding on whether or not to consult a physician. Writing down the bodily concern circumvents the problem of patients worrying that they might expose themselves to harm by forgetting about important symptoms (Wells, 1997).

During the delay period the patient should not check the troublesome symptoms (e.g., refrain from palpating lumps or picking at skin blemishes) and should not engage in any other form of checking behavior. This intervention can be conceptualized as a behavioral experiment because it encourages the patient to collect information on the meaning of the symptom (i.e., by waiting for 1 week he or she will learn whether the minor ailments are transient and innocuous). The CBT practitioner and patient could also draw up a list of symptoms that *do* warrant prompt medical attention (e.g., crushing chest pain, bloody stools, broken bones). The goal is to help the patient to use medical resources in an appropriate, responsible manner.

SUMMARY AND CONCLUSIONS

On the basis of a careful assessment and case formulation, the therapist and the patient devise a set of treatment goals and methods for attaining these goals. Commonly used CBT interventions include psychoeducation, treatment engagement strategies, cognitive restructuring, behavioral experiments, stress management methods, and relapse prevention procedures. These are implemented in an integrated fashion. For example, treatment engagement strategies lay the foundation for cognitive restructuring of disease beliefs, and cognitive restructuring helps patients understand why behavioral exercises are important to perform. The CBT practitioner can liaise with the patient's primary care physician to ensure optimal treatment outcome. The patient's family members and other significant people can also be usefully involved in treatment. The following chapters describe, in more detail, each of these approaches to treating health anxiety disorders.

8

Treatment Engagement Strategies

How can cognitive-behavioral therapists introduce their health-anxious patients to cognitive-behavioral therapy (CBT) in a way that engages the patient in therapy? Health-anxious people present for CBT for all sorts of reasons. Some realize that they have an anxiety problem that needs to be treated. Others are persuaded or even coerced into taking CBT by their family or physicians. Such patients may reluctantly enter treatment with the agenda of proving that their problems are not "all in their head" and that they are not mentally ill (Warwick, 1995). These individuals are reluctant to fully participate in therapy, believing that they need medical rather than psychological help. Providing strategies for overcoming health anxiety, such as exposure and response prevention, is premature when there is insufficient treatment motivation. Treatment engagement strategies are often a vital prerequisite. These strategies complement general CBT methods, such as psychoeducation and cognitive restructuring. General CBT methods for health anxiety are used for the dual purpose of promoting treatment engagement and directly reducing health anxiety. The treatment engagement strategies discussed in this chapter are primarily intended to enhance treatment motivation, and are especially important for reluctant or ambivalent patients.

Our discussion draws on the methods of motivational interviewing (MI; Miller & Rollnick, 2002), which are used for enhancing the odds that the patient will (1) enter CBT, (2) remain in treatment for a sufficient period of time, and (3) actively participate by, for example, completing homework assignments. MI was originally developed to enhance treatment motivation for people with substance-use disorders, for which it has been shown to be effective (Miller & Rollnick, 2002; Walitzer, Derman, & Connors, 1999). A small but growing body of research shows that MI can be usefully applied to increase treatment motivation for other clinical problems such as eating disorders (Feld, Woodside, Kaplan, Omsted, & Carter, 2001; Humfress et al., 2002; Resnicow et al., 2001). To our knowledge, however, this chapter represents the first published account of how MI can be used in the treatment of health anxiety disorders. One or two treatment sessions may be devoted primarily to enhancing treatment motivation for health-anxious people, and the MI style can be used throughout CBT, particularly when motivational issues arise, such as problems with treatment resistance or nonadherence.

MOTIVATIONAL INTERVIEWING FOR HEALTH ANXIETY DISORDERS

Rationale: Ambivalence and Change

MI is more a style of doing therapy than a collection of techniques. Its focus on enhancing treatment motivation is a distinct advantage that makes it useful to incorporate into CBT for health anxiety disorders. MI involves the use of open-ended questions, reflective listening, summary statements, and differential reinforcement of the patient's utterances in order to elicit self-motivating statements.

People are often ambivalent about important issues in their lives. Health-anxious people can hold inconsistent attitudes about the causes and cures of their problems. They believe they have a serious disease but also would like to think this is not true. Periods of doubt typically occur: "Maybe my night sweating is due to anxiety instead of a metabolic imbalance." Doubts may be fleeting but nevertheless suggest that the person has a belief, even if weakly held, that he or she does not have a dreaded disease. Health-anxious patients may also hold inconsistent beliefs about the value of checking and reassurance seeking. At times they may believe that these behaviors are crucial to their health, while at other times they may recognize that the behaviors create more problems than they solve. Health-anxious people also can be ambivalent about the value of treatments, sometimes believing that medical intervention is essential and at other times seeing it as worthless.

It can be useful for the therapist to *amplify* the patient's ambivalence (Miller & Rollnick, 2002). It is often helpful to make health-anxious people increasingly aware of the inconsistencies in their beliefs ("I have undiagnosed cancer" vs. "I don't have cancer because the tests are negative"). This induces a form of cognitive dissonance, which the person seeks to resolve. The state of ambivalence motivates efforts to change. The therapist can, therefore, strengthen ambivalence to motivate health-anxious patients to test their beliefs about disease.

Attempts to force resolution in a particular direction, such as by force-fully telling a health-anxious person that she or he worries too much about her or his health, can sometimes lead to a paradoxical response, even strength-ening the very beliefs or behaviors that the therapist is seeking to diminish (Miller & Rollnick, 2002). This phenomenon is known as *reactance* (Brehm, 1962). When the therapist forcefully presents one side of an issue ("You worry too much"), the ambivalent patient may respond by thinking of the ar-guments for the other side of the issue, associated with "Yes, but . . . " re-sponses ("Yes, but worry keeps me on the lookout for the first sign of illness. I could get really sick if I don't worry"). Rather than forcefully trying to con-vince patients to change their attitudes, therapists are more effective when they elicit arguments for change from the patients themselves (Emmons & Rollnick, 2001). This can be done in several ways, as illustrated in the following sections.

Open-Ended Questions and Reflective Listening

Open-ended questions are those that do not involve yes/no or similarly cir-cumscribed sets of responses. Open-ended questions encourage patients to ex-plore their beliefs, feelings, and behaviors. Such questioning is useful in helping patients identify self-defeating beliefs and actions. Open-ended ques-tioning can be followed by reflective listening. In reflective listening the ther-apist reflects what the patient has said, but often in a slightly modified or reframed fashion. The reflection may include the patient's expressed or im-plied emotions. There are several advantages of reflective listening (Miller, 1995):

- It is unlikely to evoke resistance ("Yes, but . . . " responses) to what the therapist says.
- It can be used to encourage the patient to explore his or her thoughts and feelings about his or her health, thereby reinforcing the formula-tion that his or her problem is one of health anxiety.
- Reflective listening communicates the therapist's respect and caring for the patient, thereby contributing to a good working relationship. This is particularly important, given that health-anxious patients often be-lieve that doctors don't listen to them.
- It clarifies for the therapist exactly what the patient means.
- It can be used to reinforce self-motivating statements. Patients hear themselves making self-motivating statements, and then hear the thera-pist reflect them back (e.g., Therapist: "You're saying that you're will-

ing to work at reducing the amount of time you spend checking your body in the shower").

- Reflective listening can be used to selectively reinforce ideas expressed by the patient (e.g., Therapist: "I hear you saying that repeated surgical investigations have not helped you in the past and, in fact, have worsened your abdominal pain").

The last-mentioned point, selective reinforcement, should be used with caution because it can sometimes backfire, eliciting a "Yes, but . . . " response. If the patient is clearly ambivalent about, say, the effects of further medical testing, it is better to reflect both sides of the ambivalence (e.g., "You hope that further surgery will fix the problem, but you also recognize that surgery has in some ways worsened your pain").

Open-ended questions and reflective listening are good ways to increase patients' awareness of their ambivalence and to move them toward more adaptive thinking. This is illustrated in the following example:

PATIENT: My doctor doesn't listen to me. I'm sure I've got something seriously wrong with my bowels, given the way they gurgle and cramp.

THERAPIST: That must be very upsetting to you, to think that you've got a serious bowel disease. Have you ever tried to assure yourself that there's nothing wrong?

PATIENT: Yes, sometimes I try to tell myself it's just gas.

THERAPIST: What makes you think it could be gas?

PATIENT: Well, the gurgling and cramps often happen when I need to use the washroom, and I usually feel better afterward.

THERAPIST: OK, I can see why that would make you think it's gas. What else has made you think, even for a moment, that you don't have a serious disease?

PATIENT: The doctor says that all the tests are negative, but I worry that he's missed something.

THERAPIST: It sounds like you're in quite a dilemma. You would like to hold onto the belief that your health is fine, and sometimes you can stick to that belief for a while. But you also believe that you've got something seriously wrong with you. What's it like for you to hold these two contradictory beliefs?

PATIENT: I've never considered it before. Now that I think about it, I guess it is confusing.

THERAPIST: Would it be helpful if we could look at these beliefs in detail, to sort out which beliefs are most likely to be true? . . .

It's not the therapist's job to provide all the answers and generate all the solutions. Doing so, in fact, invites the patient to find flaws ("Yes, but . . . ") in each suggestion (Miller & Rollnick, 2002). Open-ended questioning and reflective listening are used to help patients generate answers for themselves.

PATIENT: I have these funny little bumps on my arm. (*Begins scratching.*)

THERAPIST: How does that make you feel?

PATIENT: I'm worried. Do you think I should see my doctor?

THERAPIST: Has that helped in the past?

PATIENT: No. She always tells me that there's nothing wrong.

THERAPIST: So you're expecting to hear that there's nothing wrong. I wonder how you could figure that out for yourself.

PATIENT: I don't know. What do you think I should do?

THERAPIST: What does your doctor tell you each time you have a health concern?

PATIENT: She says "wait and see."

THERAPIST: That suggests two options: you could go to your doctor and be told to "wait and see," or you could follow that advice without going to all the hassle of seeing your doctor. Should we look at the pros and cons of each option?

The patient in this example decided that it would be better not to see her primary care physician, because it would provide an opportunity to convince herself that in a healthy person, like herself, bodily changes and sensations simply come and go, without harmful consequences.

Open-ended questioning and reflective listening are also useful tools for exploring the patient's skepticism about the value of CBT. This can help to correct any misconceptions.

THERAPIST: From what you've said, you're skeptical that CBT will help you.

PATIENT: Yeah. My pain is in my back, not in my head. I don't see how a shrink can help me.

THERAPIST: I treat patients with all sorts of problems, including cancer pain, bowel diseases, diabetes, skin problems, and so forth. Why would these patients come to see me?

PATIENT: I don't know. . . . Maybe they have depression.

THERAPIST: Maybe. And how might depression influence a person's pain or his or her ability to cope with pain?

PATIENT: I guess it would make it worse.

THERAPIST: Right. And there are all sorts of things that can make a person's pain worse. That's how I help people—by helping them identify the things in their lives that either make their problems better or worse. Is it important to you to figure out the things that are affecting your back pain?

PATIENT: I suppose we could try a couple of sessions. The quacks at the hospital haven't helped me so far.

THERAPIST: OK, good. I'd be happy to work with you.

These sorts of questions, along with periodic summary statements, help patients reframe their problem as one of health anxiety. Open-ended questioning and reflective listening are used for initially engaging the patient in treatment, and are used throughout CBT in the various cognitive and behavioral interventions discussed in later chapters.

Eliciting Self-Motivating Statements and Strengthening Self-Efficacy for Change

An important goal of treatment is to have the patient voice adaptive responses because self-generated responses are more likely to be remembered by the patient, compared to responses provided by the therapist (Miller & Rollnick, 2002). This is the *generation effect*, first identified in memory experiments (Anderson, 1990). Self-generated responses are often more believable than those imposed by the therapist: "If I said it, and nobody forced me to say it, then I must believe it" (Miller, 1995). The therapist therefore assists patients in talking themselves into changing (Moyers & Rollnick, 2002).

In the treatment of health anxiety disorders, self-motivating statements are useful for encouraging the patient to try a course of CBT and, later in treatment, to encourage him or her to persist at homework assignments, such as behavioral experiments. The following example illustrates one useful strategy for eliciting self-motivating statements and for identifying motivational barriers (Miller & Rollnick, 2002; Resnicow et al., 2001):

THERAPIST: To help me understand your reasons for seeking help, I'd like to ask you a couple of things. On a scale of 1 to 10, with 10 being the highest, how motivated or interested are you in trying some CBT sessions to help you with your health concerns?

PATIENT: To be honest, I have my doubts about whether you can help me. My rating would be 3.

THERAPIST: OK, 3 out of 10. Thanks for being frank with me. What made you choose 3? Why not choose a lower number like 2 or 1?

PATIENT: My doctor and my wife keep telling me that I need psychological help.

THERAPIST: Are there any other reason for choosing 3 instead of 2 or 1?

PATIENT: . . . Well, nothing's helped me so far, so I might as well give it a try.

THERAPIST: OK. This sounds like a good reason. And why choose 3 instead of a higher number, like 9 or 10?

PATIENT: I feel that my problems are medical. I don't see how my symptoms could be caused by stress or nerves.

THERAPIST: What would it take to get you to a 9 or 10?

PATIENT: Hmmm. I'd need to see some proof that my problems are psychological.

THERAPIST: So, to summarize, you're saying that CBT might be worthwhile because your doctor and wife think so, and because nothing has worked so far. But for you to get really interested in CBT, we first need to look at whether psychological factors are contributing to your problems.

PATIENT: Yes, that sums it up.

THERAPIST: OK, good. Should we start by looking at some of the things that might be causing your symptoms?

PATIENT: OK.

The patient's self-efficacy about overcoming his or her problems can be enhanced by the therapist providing psychoeducational information, including information about the efficacy of CBT for health anxiety disorders. Also, simply telling the patient that you are genuinely pleased that she or he has attended the CBT session can enhance treatment engagement, especially for health-anxious patients who feel that they have been belittled or ridiculed by their physicians in the past. The latter unfortunately occurs when busy doctors, such as emergency room physicians, become frustrated by repeated visits by health-anxious patients who have failed to respond to reassurance. Later in treatment, the therapist can also strengthen the patient's treatment motivation by sincerely complementing (reinforcing) his or her efforts at completing CBT homework assignments.

Dealing with Resistance

Resistance to CBT can take many forms, such as the patient arguing with the therapist, repeatedly interrupting the therapist, and rejecting or ignoring the therapist's suggestions. This is important to address early in treatment, because it signals a treatment engagement problem that could escalate into treatment dropout. A general guideline is to avoid confronting resistance directly because that can escalate rather than reduce resistance (Moyers & Rollnick, 2002). There are three useful MI strategies for dealing with resistance early and throughout treatment (Humfress et al., 2002; Miller, 1995; Miller & Rollnick, 2002; Moyers & Rollnick, 2002):

- Amplified reflection.
- Double-sided reflection.
- Strategic responses to resistance.

Amplified Reflection

In an amplified reflection the therapist slightly overstates the patient's resistance, in a sincere, nonaccusatory fashion. This capitalizes on the natural tendency of the patient to speak against either side of an issue about which he or she is ambivalent. This induces the patient, rather than the therapist, to advance arguments for the desired change (Moyers & Rollnick, 2002).

PATIENT: Despite what the neurologist says, I worry that my headaches are caused by a brain tumor.

THERAPIST: To help me understand, can I ask whether you're saying that you're absolutely sure that you've got a brain tumor? Are you saying that it's impossible that there's another cause?

PATIENT: Well, no, the headaches could be due to stress.

THERAPIST: What makes you think it could be stress instead of a brain tumor? . . .

Double-Sided Reflection

When offering a double-sided reflection, the therapist voices arguments for and against a given issue, using the linking word "and." Such questions encourage the patient to examine the discrepancies between his or her beliefs.

THERAPIST: You'd like to stop worrying about your health because it disrupts your life, *and* you believe that worry helps to keep you on the lookout for disease.

PATIENT: Yes, I'm in a dilemma.

THERAPIST: What are some of the ways of solving the dilemma? . . .

Strategic Responses to Resistance

These involve shifting the direction of the discussion. The therapist might overtly shift focus by declining to argue about whether the patient's problem is one of health anxiety, and instead inquire about whether medical tests and physical examinations have been helpful. This can involve "agreeing with a twist," where the therapist offers initial agreement but with a slight twist or change of direction (Miller & Rollnick, 2002).

THERAPIST: Thanks for being open with me. It's important for me to know that you don't believe that your problems are due to health anxiety. Maybe you're right. But maybe not. Have your doctors found any evidence of a medical problem? Have they been able to help you understand your problems?

PATIENT: No, so far I've been to see lots of specialists and none have helped.

THERAPIST: That's a tough position to be in. Would you like to try a different approach? We could spend a few weeks looking at whether your problems are due to health anxiety. What have you got to lose?

THE INITIAL INTERVIEW

Engagement strategies can be implemented from the first session onward. A good place to start is to ensure that the patient is physically comfortable when he or she first comes into the office. If the patient has low back pain as a presenting problem, for example, then the therapist can inquire if the chair is comfortable. If the patient presents with globus, or throat tightening, as a feared symptom, then the therapist can offer to get the patient a glass of water. If the patient presents with gastrointestinal symptoms, then the therapist could orient the patient to the bathroom facilities. These are straightforward but often overlooked ways for the therapist to demonstrate to the patient that her or his distress is accepted as authentic and that there will be no attempt to prove that her or his problems are imaginary. As observed by Pilowsky (1997), "This approach to the patient's discomforts is likely to be more persuasive than any verbal guarantees of understanding and acceptance, and is a sine qua non to gaining the patient's confidence and trust" (p. 136).

The initial interview is also used to explore the patient's attitudes about receiving CBT. What was he or she told by his or her referring physician? Sometimes patients are told precious little. They are simply informed that they need to see another doctor for their problems, without being told that they have been referred to a mental health practitioner. Some patients are annoyed or angry about being referred for psychological treatment, and they may feel stigmatized about a mental health referral. Such treatment attitudes can be discussed in order to set the foundation for a collaborative therapeutic relationship. The therapist can address these concerns in an open, non-defensive manner. For example:

> "Some people in your position would be annoyed that their doctor says that their problems are due to health anxiety. Do you feel this way?"

The therapist could empathize with the patient's frustration (or anger) about the way that other health care professionals have dealt with him or her in the past. The therapist can emphasize that he or she believes that the patient's problems are not trivial, and that it is important to identify the source of the difficulties. This will help engage the patient in treatment. A detailed, unrushed initial inquiry about the patient's physical concerns can have a therapeutic effect. It may be the first time the patient has felt that a doctor is listening and taking him or her seriously (House, 1995).

The following is an example of how one can inquire about these issues in a way that engages the patient in treatment. Observe how the therapist uses open-ended questioning and other MI methods.

THERAPIST: I'd like to find out about your problems and to talk about the sorts of therapy I can offer, so we can figure out whether I can be of help. But first, tell me, what's your understanding of why you were referred by your doctor to see me?

PATIENT: The doctor thinks my symptoms are all in my head. So he said I should see a psychologist.

THERAPIST: How do you feel about that?

PATIENT: I feel annoyed. My pain is real! I'm not making it up. I can't sleep at night because of stomach cramps.

THERAPIST: That must be awful for you, to be in pain and to find that your doctor can't help. Maybe I can help you in finding the causes of your pain. What did your doctor tell you?

PATIENT: He said there's nothing physically wrong with me.

THERAPIST: And what do you believe?

PATIENT: I'm worried that I could have cancer.

THERAPIST: That would be bad news indeed if it was cancer. So I'm relieved that the medical tests haven't found any evidence of cancer. Do you have any thoughts about what else could be causing the pain?

PATIENT: My doctor thinks it's all in my head.

THERAPIST: But how could that be? The pain is in your stomach?

PATIENT: Right! That's what I believe.

THERAPIST: So, what else could be causing the pain? What have other people told you?

PATIENT: My wife says it's stress.

THERAPIST: What do you think of that idea?

PATIENT: I don't see how it could be.

THERAPIST: Have you had a thorough evaluation to see if it's stress-related?

PATIENT: No.

THERAPIST: Why not? You've had all sorts of other medical tests, even exploratory surgery. And you're still in pain. Don't you owe it to yourself to find out if it's stress?

PATIENT: I guess so.

THERAPIST: And how would you feel if you knew the pain was caused by stress rather than stomach cancer?

PATIENT: I'd be relieved.

THERAPIST: Right, that would be good news, because there are lots of ways of managing stress problems. So do you think we can spend a few sessions exploring whether stress or other emotional things influence your pain?

PATIENT: Yes, I suppose we could.

Notice that the patient in this example moved from initial reluctance concerning CBT to tentative engagement in CBT. This is a small but important step. With the use of additional treatment engagement strategies and other cognitive-behavioral interventions, the therapist aims to further strengthen the patient's commitment to trying a course of CBT. Sometimes it is useful to draw up a written treatment contract, in which the patient and therapist commit to trying CBT for a specified period of time, such as 3 months.

Once the patient has begun to consider—even provisionally—a cognitive-behavioral formulation of his or her problems, then additional restructuring exercises can be introduced to more directly target misinterpretations of bodily changes or sensations and associated dysfunctional beliefs (see Chapter 9).

CBT can also be made more palatable to the patient if treatment is aimed at important areas of emotional distress in the patient's life (Barsky, 1996). If depression presents in addition to health anxiety, the CBT practitioner could offer to first treat the depression, informing the patient that this should enhance his or her ability to cope with the bodily changes or sensations, and may even relieve somatic problems.

USING EXPERIENTIAL DEMONSTRATIONS AS ENGAGEMENT STRATEGIES

Behavioral experiments (see Chapter 10) provide patients with important information about the causes of their bodily changes or sensations. These interventions, particularly the more demanding exposure and response prevention exercises, are often used only after the patient has been fully engaged in treatment. Some behavioral exercises, however, can be used in the first session or two, to demonstrate how selective attention influences the detection of bodily sensations. The goal of these exercises is to show patients how the tendency to focus on one's body can increase the frequency of bodily sensations that are commonly misinterpreted as indications of disease. One could ask the patient to complete Raven's Progressive Matrices (Raven, 1998), and then describe the bodily sensations experienced during the task. Patients typically report few sensations because their attention is directed away from the body. Then the patient can be asked to complete a guided attention exercise, where he or she is asked to close his or her eyes and focus on his or her body. The therapist then reads a script, like the following, pausing for several seconds between each statement:

> "First I'd like you to focus on your breathing, noticing what it feels like as the air moves in and out of your throat . . . and how the air moves in and out through your nasal passages. . . . Now I'd like you to focus on the muscles in your jaws and around your eyes. . . . Now focus on your scalp, noticing how your skin feels. . . . Focus now on your fingertips and hands. . . . Focus now on your heart and your pulse. . . . Now focus your attention on your stomach and see what you notice."

The patient is then asked to describe the bodily sensations experienced during this exercise, and to compare these to the sensations experienced in the previous task. Patients typically report many more sensations during the guided attention exercise. These findings can then lead to a discussion of how selective attention can influence the occurrence of "symptoms."

SUMMARY AND CONCLUSIONS

There are several strategies for encouraging health-anxious people to try a course of CBT. Methods derived from MI can be particularly useful. These include the use of open-ended questions, reflective listening, summary statements, and differential reinforcement of the patient's utterances in order to elicit self-motivating statements. These approaches represent a style of therapy rather than a list of techniques to be mechanically applied. Treatment engagement strategies can be used in the first session and throughout treatment when motivational concerns arise. Treatment engagement strategies enhance the likelihood that health-anxious people will fully participate in other CBT interventions.

9

Cognitive Interventions

The distinction between cognitive and behavioral interventions is arbitrary, but provides a convenient way of parsing the material to be covered in this and the following chapter. Cognitive and behavioral exercises both provide patients with corrective information, and so both are vehicles of belief change. Both kinds of interventions help to correct the patient's beliefs about:

- Their bodily changes or sensations.
- Their state of health in general.
- Their vulnerability to disease.
- The effects of avoidance, repetitive checking, and reassurance seeking.

When challenging dysfunctional beliefs, the therapist can help the patient understand how his or her beliefs arose. Observational learning experiences provided by parents, actual experiences with disease, and information (and misinformation) from the media can all foster health anxiety. Such information reinforces the message that the patient's problem is primarily one of health anxiety rather than one of disease.

Behavioral exercises are often designed as behavioral experiments, intended to help patients further test adaptive and dysfunctional beliefs. Behavioral exercises, such as interoceptive ("symptom induction") tasks, can be difficult for patients to complete because the tasks often encourage patients to directly confront their fears. Cognitive interventions, such as those described in the present chapter, pave the way for behavioral exercises. That is, cognitive interventions can weaken dysfunctional beliefs (e.g., weaken the belief that "I'll get seriously ill if I go near sick people"), thereby making it easier for patients to complete behavioral exercises (e.g., a visit to a local hospital). Thus, behavioral interventions build on cognitive interventions. In turn, the cognitive methods described in this chapter build on the treatment engagement methods described in the previous chapter.

This chapter considers the verbal reattribution methods commonly used in treating health anxiety. Such methods include empirical and adaptive disputations, as well as distancing strategies and methods for regulating worry. Imagery methods for facilitating cognitive restructuring are considered, along with attention-focusing strategies.

VERBAL REATTRIBUTION METHODS

Overview

Verbal interventions are used to help patients identify and objectively evaluate their health-related beliefs, which are typically catastrophic in nature, and to generate plausible, noncatastrophic alternatives. These interventions provide patients with tools for use during therapy assignments and in their daily lives. Tools consist of questions they can ask themselves, statements of noncatastrophic beliefs, and short lists of evidence for and against particular beliefs. Cognitive restructuring can be implemented in the following sequence:

- Introduction to cognitive distortions. Handout 9.1 lists a number of common distortions exhibited by health-anxious people. The therapist can share this handout with the patient, and ask him or her to identify any errors in his or her own thinking.
- Begin prospective monitoring of health anxiety episodes, using Handout 9.2.
- Challenge dysfunctional beliefs and strengthen adaptive beliefs about the causes of bodily sensations or changes.

Restructuring begins by asking patients to identify their thinking errors and write them down in the "anxiety-provoking thoughts" column of Handout 9.2. In this way, patients learn to label their thoughts (e.g., "This thought is an example of catastrophizing"). This is a distancing strategy that helps patients view their thoughts as assumptions rather than as facts. The forms are reviewed during the treatment session, where further cognitive restructuring is conducted. If the patient's entries in the cognitive restructuring form contain a number of dysfunctional beliefs, the therapist might choose, during the session, to work first with the most weakly held belief because that one may be most amenable to change.

THINKING ERRORS THAT CREATE HEALTH ANXIETY

The following are common thinking errors that create excessive health anxiety and lead to associated problems, such as repeatedly checking one's body or repeatedly seeking medical reassurance. These categories of thinking errors overlap to some extent with one another, although they still can be useful for helping you understand how thinking patterns can influence anxiety about your health.

Which of the following thinking errors contribute to your health anxiety?

All-or-nothing thinking. Seeing things in black-and-white categories, ignoring the shades of gray. Examples of all-or-nothing thinking are: "I'm either healthy or seriously ill" and "Medical tests are worthless if they're not 100% accurate."

Overfocusing on the negatives. You pick out a single negative detail and ignore the positives. For example, if your doctor said "Your stomach cramps are probably due to a mild virus," you might start dwelling on the word "probably" and begin thinking about lethal causes of cramps, while ignoring the doctor's main message that there's no cause for concern.

Disqualifying the positives. Rejecting positive information. For example, if your doctor said "The test found no indications of cancer," you might reject the result by insisting that the positive result "doesn't count" because the test might be wrong. Similarly, you might discount nonserious explanations of bodily complaints (e.g., rejecting the idea that your shoulder soreness is the harmless result of stress).

Jumping to conclusions. For example, anticipating that results of a Pap smear will be bad news or jumping to the conclusion that a headache is caused by a brain tumor. Another example is the "fortune teller error," where you assume that your pessimistic expectation is already an established fact (e.g., "I would never recover if I got a serious disease," and "If I got sick, I would be in great pain and suffering").

Catastrophizing. Attributing horrible consequences to minor things. For example, "A breast lump means certain death," "My chest pain indicates a serious heart problem," and "Bodily complaints are always signs of disease."

Overgeneralization. Taking one example as "proof" for a general rule (e.g., "I feel tired today. I must have MS").

Emotional reasoning. Regarding your feelings as facts. For example, "There must be something medically wrong with me because otherwise I wouldn't feel so anxious."

(continued)

Intolerance of uncertainty. Refusing to accept that uncertainty is a part of everyday life, and insisting that perfect certainty can and should be obtained—for example, by insisting that "Doctors must rule out all possible diseases" and "I must be completely certain that I'm healthy."

Superstitious thinking. Assuming that something you do prevents bad things from happening because the bad events haven't happened so far—for example, "I take a seaweed extract pill each day and I haven't developed bowel cancer. Therefore the extract protects me from getting cancer." This is the same error as believing that garlic cloves ward off vampires: "I carry garlic cloves with me and I've never seen a vampire. Therefore the cloves must be working!"

HANDOUT 9.2. Cognitive Restructuring Form

Day and date	Health anxiety trigger (e.g., an event or bodily sensation)	Anxiety-provoking thoughts (and strength of belief, 0–100)	Intensity of anxiety (0–100)	Behaviors that may be calming in the short term, but create problems in the longer term	Rational responses and good coping responses
Example	*Saw a TV program on breast cancer*	*Worried that I might have cancer. (Believed it 100%.)*	*95%*	*Checked my body for lumps. Checked so much that my breasts became tender and sore.*	• *Told myself that I'm catastrophizing.* • *Reminded myself that repeated checking makes my anxiety worse.* • *Told myself that I only need to do a breast self exam once a month.* • *Went for a walk in the park to focus on something pleasant.*

Style of Questioning

Verbal interventions make use of *Socratic dialogue*, which consists of guided questioning to help patients identify whether their beliefs are accurate and adaptive. Socratic dialogue can be used in all stages of treatment, from the initial session onward. In contrast to the lecture approach, in which the patient is the passive recipient of information presented by the therapist, the Socratic approach encourages patients to do most of the work in questioning their own beliefs and in coming up with alternatives. The goal is not to provide patients with all the answers, but instead to help them think for themselves. This method is quite consistent with the treatment engagement methods described in Chapter 8. The following transcript illustrates Socratic dialogue, in which the therapist helps the patient understand the effects of reassurance seeking:

PATIENT: This morning I noticed that my saliva was a funny brown color.

THERAPIST: How does that make you feel?

PATIENT: I'm worried that I might be sick. Maybe I should see a doctor. What do you think?

THERAPIST: It sounds like you'd like me to reassure you. What do you think would happen if I offered some reassurance?

PATIENT: I'd feel better.

THERAPIST: Then what would happen? Would the effects be long-lasting?

PATIENT: It would help for a while, but then I'd start thinking that I should have some medical tests, to really make sure that there's nothing wrong.

THERAPIST: So the reassurance would offer temporary relief, but soon you'd be wanting more.

PATIENT: Yes.

THERAPIST: Do you ever feel like you're addicted to reassurance?

PATIENT: I hadn't thought of it like that before. But now that you mention it, yes, it's just like the time I was hooked on painkillers I was taking for headaches.

THERAPIST: In what way was that a problem for you?

PATIENT: Well, I was obsessed with getting the drugs—I couldn't think of anything else. I had to take more and more pills to get pain relief, because I'd built up a tolerance.

THERAPIST: How did you get over the problem?

PATIENT: My doctor told me that I was getting rebound headaches from the painkillers, so he gradually tapered me off them. Then the headaches went away.

THERAPIST: OK, I'm glad you solved that problem. Let me ask you, how is reassurance seeking similar to being hooked on painkillers?

PATIENT: I guess I can't get enough reassurance—I seem to need more and more to feel calm.

THERAPIST: And do you spend a lot of time thinking about reassurance?

PATIENT: When I'm worried about my health, yes. It's the first thing I think of.

THERAPIST: Do you think that reassurance seeking makes your health anxiety worse?

PATIENT: Maybe, but I'm not sure how.

THERAPIST: OK, let me rephrase that question. Does reassurance seeking help you feel happy and healthy, or does it make you feel fragile and dependent on other people?

PATIENT: It makes me feel weak and that I can't cope on my own.

THERAPIST: So reassurance is not good for you in the long run. How might we address this problem of reassurance addiction?

PATIENT: I guess I could try to wean myself off it.

Troubleshooting

The main problems with Socratic dialogue are twofold. The first is one of aimless questioning. This occurs when the therapist does not have a clear goal in mind. What conclusion would you like to lead your patient toward? Before initiating a sequence of questioning, the therapist needs to consider the sorts of conclusions that would be helpful for the patient to reach. In the above-mentioned example, questioning was initiated with the goal of helping the patient realize that reassurance seeking was counterproductive. Of course, there is nothing inherently wrong with goal-less questioning, but such questioning is better suited for assessment sessions. It is not an efficient method for cognitive restructuring.

The second common problem concerns the overuse of Socratic dialogue. Excessive questioning can make the patient feel as if she or her is being interrogated. Socratic questioning is best used in short sequences, interspersed with other kinds of dialogue. The latter include (1) capsule summaries of the material discussed so far, provided by either the patient or the therapist; (2) short sequences in which the therapist provides information; and (3) simply letting the patient recount some incident (e.g., an episode of heightened health anxiety) while the therapist engages in reflective listening.

Empirical Disputations: Examining the Evidence

Empirical disputations help health-anxious patients examine the evidence for and against their dysfunctional beliefs, such as catastrophic assumptions about the meaning of their bodily changes or sensations. Much of the patient's evidence for having a disease is idiosyncratic and faulty (Warwick & Salkovskis, 2001). Alternative, noncatastrophic beliefs are generated by the patient and the therapist, and the evidence for the alternatives is considered. Evidence is collected from the patient's own experiences and from other sources. For each dysfunctional belief, the therapist and the patient develop an adaptive (non-catastrophic), plausible, and accurate alternative belief statement. The evidence for and against each belief is then listed. There are several questions that patients can ask themselves to facilitate this process:

- What evidence do I have for this belief?
- Is there any evidence that is inconsistent with this belief?
- Is there another explanation or alternative way of looking at things?

Once the evidence is generated, the patient and the therapist decide which belief is best supported. To determine whether this exercise is persuasive, the patient can be asked to rate the strength (0–100) of the dysfunctional and alternative beliefs before and after reviewing the evidence. If the exercise is effective, then it should produce a substantial drop in the strength of the dysfunctional belief and a corresponding increase in the strength of the alternative. The key points from the exercises can be distilled into a pithy coping statement written on a card, which the patient carries with him or her and reviews as needed.

Some health-anxious patients have not spent much time thinking about noncatastrophic interpretations of bodily events. Instead, they jump to catastrophic conclusions. It can be salubrious for patients to spend time generating noncatastrophic interpretations during the treatment session so that these will come to mind during episodes of health anxiety. Patients can also be asked to look for information that supports noncatastrophic alternatives.

When conducting a seemingly successful disputation, the therapist can adopt the role of interested skeptic: "But would that be *really* convincing?" (Salkovskis, 1989). This approach is useful for identifying any lingering doubts held by the patient.

Empirical disputations can be conducted with the aid of Handout 9.3, which is used both during therapy sessions and as a homework assignment. These disputations are not only useful for people with full-blown hypochondriasis, they can also be fruitfully applied to people with other health anxiety disorders. People with disease phobia, for example, sometimes have

HANDOUT 9.3. Matrix Method for Challenging Dysfunctional Beliefs

	Evidence for the belief	Evidence against the belief
Frightening belief Example: "The spot on my hand is skin cancer."		
Alternative belief Example: "The spot on my hand is simply a freckle."		

unrealistic beliefs about the spread of disease. They might fear and avoid driving past funeral parlors, believing that the air is filled with germs from the deceased. Such beliefs can be addressed by collecting evidence—for example, by asking "What evidence do you have that you or other people become sick by being near funeral homes? Could we test this out by taking a walk to the hospital mortuary?" During the treatment session, the patient and the therapist can generate coping strategies and then the patient can expose him- or herself to the triggers. Consider the belief that "deadly germs are in the air near places in which there are dead people." An appropriate coping statement might be: "There's no evidence of deadly germs in the air. I can prove this to myself by walking past funeral homes and hospitals."

Troubleshooting

A problem that can arise when conducting empirical disputations concerns the issue of disproving the negative. A patient might say, "How do you know I don't have cancer?" These sorts of questions often contain an implicit demand for certainty. When they arise in the course of empirical disputations, the therapist can try using a disputation that challenges the demand for certainty (as discussed later in this chapter).

Another common obstacle to implementing empirical disputations is what frustrated clinicians have sometimes (disparagingly) called the "organ recital"—that is, the pressured, difficult-to-interrupt stream of information that some patients insist on presenting to the therapist. Bodily concerns are described in exquisite detail, interlaced with requests for reassurance. Once one concern is described, the patient jumps to another. The therapist may feel overwhelmed and powerless in the face of this deluge of information.

To deal with this problem, it is important to understand its causes. The therapist can extract themes for discussion from the patient's narration. Common themes include vulnerability, fear of health decline, and concerns about not being taken seriously. Feedback to the patient about these themes strengthens the therapeutic relationship and provides material for cognitive restructuring. Consider the following case.

> Helen C. had a 2-year history of full-blown hypochondriasis arising in the context of a long-standing history of milder health concerns. Her hypochondriasis became full-blown after her brother unexpectedly died from a myocardial infarction, followed a few months later by the sudden death of her husband from cancer. Helen believed that both deaths were partly the result of medical mismanagement. She presented for cognitive-behavioral therapy (CBT) rather reluctantly after a battery of investigations found no medical basis for her many health concerns.

During her initial CBT sessions, Helen was garrulous and difficult to interrupt, providing a detailed account of her many health concerns. The therapist dealt with this problem by addressing it directly: "We need to pause for a moment to consider what's happening here. It seems like you feel the need to give me a lot of information. Why is that?" The ensuing discussion revealed that Helen held the following beliefs:

- Doctors don't listen to me, so I have to take extra efforts to make sure that they know about my problems.
- Doctors can help me only if they know about *all* of my symptoms.

These sorts of beliefs are commonly seen in the difficult-to-interrupt patient. Treatment proceeded by the therapist and the patient agreeing to develop an agenda at the beginning of each session. It was agreed that Helen would have 20 minutes to discuss her bodily concerns. The therapist emphasized that he didn't need a complete list of her concerns. A summary of the major issues would suffice. The remaining 40 minutes of the session was devoted to discussing the above-listed beliefs. She was quite willing to discuss these because they were relevant to her health concerns. Helen had long believed she was not getting proper medical attention, and she was relieved that somebody was finally taking the time to listen to her. When appropriate, the therapist validated her concerns. There was a germ of truth to her beliefs: on several occasions doctors had cut her off within a few minutes of the medical consultation, refusing to listen to her long list of concerns. The CBT practitioner empathized with Helen's frustration. Thus, a good therapeutic relationship began to emerge with a patient who had initially been quite skeptical of CBT.

In later CBT sessions, Helen's mention of bodily changes or sensations was used by the therapist as an opportunity to revisit her belief that doctors need to know about all of her bodily concerns. The evidence and origin of this belief was considered. Helen realized that her experiences regarding the death of her brother and husband were contributory.

THERAPIST: Given your experiences I can see why you believe that doctors need to know about all of your bodily concerns. But I'm wondering if this belief is helpful for you.

PATIENT: Well, I think it's necessary for my health. The doctors didn't do proper examinations of my brother and husband, and now they're both dead.

THERAPIST: Those losses must make you feel very sad. But your insistence that doctors know about every detail about your health seems to be harming your relationship with them. Of the seven doctors you've seen over the past year, how have they reacted when you've tried to give a detailed description of your problems?

PATIENT: They usually seem impatient. In fact, Dr. Jones was downright rude. That's why I have to keep changing doctors, so I can find one who'll listen to me.

THERAPIST: So giving a detailed description of your problems is actually harming your relationship with your doctors? Would that be an accurate description of the situation?

PATIENT: Yes, I suppose it is.

THERAPIST: And what happens to the quality of your medical care as a result?

PATIENT: I don't get proper care.

THERAPIST: OK, so would it be accurate to say that the strategy of giving very detailed descriptions of your bodily concerns actually *impairs* the quality of your medical care?

PATIENT: Now that I think about it, I suppose you're right.

THERAPIST: Yes. It turns out that giving detailed lists of medical concerns is not a very good way of staying healthy. So what's another approach that you could take?

PATIENT: I'm not sure.

THERAPIST: We have plenty of time. Let's give ourselves a few minutes to see if we can figure out a better way of interacting with your doctors. . . .

In this way Helen eventually concluded that an alternative strategy would be to describe her two most troubling concerns, and to give the physician a written list of the others. This strategy improved her doctor–patient interactions and reduced the difficult-to-interrupt pattern of interaction with her CBT practitioner. Helen was less frequently trying to give detailed accounts of her bodily concerns, and was more receptive to working on the issue of health anxiety.

Empirical disputations are most effective when they focus on clearly defined beliefs. This permits the therapist and the patient to identify evidence that unambiguously supports or refutes these beliefs. Sometimes, however, patients may have difficulty articulating their beliefs. This can be for a number of reasons. Some patients have clearly defined beliefs that they describe vaguely, possibly because they are embarrassed about them or because discussing their beliefs makes them feel anxious. Deliberate evasiveness (avoidance) may be suspected when the patient is visibly distressed about discussing the beliefs and shifts the topic of conversation. The therapist can address this problem by directly but tactfully raising it with the patient and then collaboratively looking for solutions. The therapist should be mindful of the quality of the therapeutic relationship and the way in which the empirical disputations are implemented. Patients will be reluctant to disclose if they feel attacked or criticized for disclosing their beliefs.

In other cases the beliefs appear to be genuinely vague. Here too avoidance may play a role. Upsetting beliefs may be vague because the patient tries not to think about them. John D. believed that his stomachaches indicated that something was seriously wrong, but he wasn't sure what this might be. To explore and challenge this idea, the therapist encouraged John to think of examples of what might be wrong (e.g., stomach cancer, bleeding ulcers) and to also think of benign interpretations (e.g., stress-related increases in muscle tone). The evidence for and against these possibilities was then considered.

If these approaches are unsuccessful, then other cognitive restructuring methods can be considered, such as adaptive disputations.

Questioning the Mechanism

A useful form of empirical disputation is to help patients consider the mechanisms by which diseases cause bodily changes or sensations (Wells, 1997). For patients who believe that some bodily change or sensation signifies a serious disease, the therapist and the patient can explore whether the nature and pattern of "symptom" occurrence is consistent with the disease. Particular attention should be paid to evidence that is inconsistent with the disease. If a patient believed that headaches are a sign of stroke, for instance, one could examine the pattern of headache occurrence. Do the headaches come and go? Are they more likely to occur in some situations than others? Are they the only "symptom" experienced by the patient—do they occur in the absence of neurological signs of stroke, such as slurred speech or limb paralysis? A "yes" response to any of these questions provides evidence against the notion that the headaches are due to a stroke.

A further step is to develop a noncatastrophic mechanism to explain the bodily changes or sensations (e.g., headaches are due to a stress-related accumulation of muscle tension). Then the plausibility of the alternative is explored by examining its mechanism (e.g., identifying stressful situations and their relationship to headache frequency).

A commonly used intervention is to help patients consider the evidence for and against the idea that a stress-related mechanism is the source of their bodily concerns. Many health-anxious patients who consult a CBT practitioner have already been told by their physicians that their bodily concerns are due to stress. These patients are often skeptical of this explanation because they have not been sufficiently educated about how stress influences the body. The assessment and treatment of stress-related bodily reactions is discussed in further detail in Chapter 11.

In addition to looking for stressors as potential triggers of bodily changes or sensations, the therapist should also look for other potential triggers or exacerbants—for example, the extent to which the patient's environment is attention grabbing versus boring. Bodily events are more likely to be detected and misinterpreted in boring environments. Identification of these factors can help the patient understand that he or she has probably always had a "noisy" body, and the recent detection of troubling changes or sensations (e.g., floaters in the visual field) is likely a product of selective attention to one's body.

A review of the patient's dietary patterns can also help to identify benign mechanisms of bodily sensations or changes. There are several common links between foods and bodily reactions:

- Spicy foods and tomato products can give rise to gastric reflux.
- High-fiber foods such as dried fruits can cause gastrointestinal upset.
- Overuse of alcohol can cause withdrawal effects such as palpitations, headache, tremulousness, hot flushes, sweating, and gastrointestinal upset.
- Caffeine can cause tremulousness, headache, hot flashes, gastrointestinal upset, gastric reflux, and urinary difficulty (polyuria, and sometimes urinary hesitancy).
- Milk products can cause gastrointestinal problems in lactose-intolerant people.

Troubleshooting

A difficulty in testing the mechanism concerns the *gambler's fallacy*. Brian W. believed that his headaches were due to a stroke. The pattern of headache occurrence was inconsistent with this belief. The headaches came and went with stress, and were not associated with any other problems that might suggest a cerebrovascular event. Despite being presented with this evidence, Brian believed that every new headache meant that "this time" he was having a stroke. He believed that the odds of having a stroke were one in a thousand. He reasoned that since he must have had about a thousand headaches, the next one must surely be due to a stroke. This is the same as the gambler's reasoning that because a "six" did not appear in the past six rolls of a die, then the likelihood of rolling a six must be very high. This is known as the "gambler's fallacy." The gambler fails to realize that dice have no memory. The probability of rolling a six on a given roll remains unchanged, regardless of what occurred previously. Brian's thinking shows the same error: a thousand tension head-aches do not alter the likelihood that the next headache would be due to a stroke.

How should the therapist address this thinking error? Collecting evidence may be ineffective. In fact, it may be counterproductive. The more evidence collected to indicate that the headaches are tension-related may increase the patient's estimate that the next headache would be due to a stoke. To address this problem, the therapist discussed the gambler's fallacy with Brian. A die was produced and Brian was asked to estimate the probability of rolling a "three." Brian correctly responded that the odds were one in six. Then the therapist asked about the probability of rolling a three if a three hadn't turned up in the past five rolls. Brian erroneously thought the probability would increase. This error was discussed and the therapist pointed out how it was similar to Brian's estimate of the odds that his next headache would be due to a stroke.

The Pie Chart Method

The pie chart method is another useful method for challenging the likelihood of feared events. This method encourages patients to consider the evidence for the occurrence of events, such as the probability of skin cancer, given the occurrence of a new spot on one's hand. When treating health-anxious patients, the pie chart method can be used to achieve two goals: (1) to help patients consider a range of alternative, noncatastrophic interpretations of their feared bodily changes or sensations; and (2) to help them to more realistically estimate the likelihood of catastrophic outcomes, as compared to noncatastrophic ones. The general procedure is illustrated in the following example.

Susan J. experienced bouts of stuffy nose and chest congestion. She felt the urge to recurrently clear her throat of catarrh, and as a result her throat was often sore. Despite reassurance from her physician, Susan worried that she was developing a potentially fatal respiratory disease, "perhaps pneumonia or even lung cancer." The pie chart method was implemented, for which Susan and the therapist collaborated to list all the things that could plausibly cause her chest congestion and stuffy nose. The first item listed was "a potentially fatal disease." Note that all the serious diseases were grouped into a single category. This is done in order to encourage the patient to consider non-catastrophic possibilities—which are the most likely causes, given the negative medical tests—rather than dwelling on the many rare, fatal disorders associated with respiratory distress. The pie chart method can backfire if patients simply generate a long list of lethal causes because this can reinforce the belief that there is something dangerously wrong with them.

Susan and her therapist produced the following list of alternative benign causes for her chest congestion and stuffy nose: (1) a harmless infection, such as a cold; (2) a mild allergy, such as a pollen or dust allergy; (3) mild bronchitis caused by smoking (like many health-anxious people, Susan had several unhealthy habits, like smoking and overeating); and (4) rebound congestion due to repeated use of nasal spray decongestant. Several benign alternatives were generated because the pie chart method tends to be more convincing when many harmless possibilities are listed.

The next step in the pie chart method is to assign a rating of percent likelihood to each of the listed causes. The therapist began with the benign causes because these were the most probable reasons for Susan's bodily sensations, and so they should occupy the bulk of the pie chart. Given that the percentages must add up to 100, this typically means that the percent likelihood for the catastrophic cause will be very low. Susan's percentages are shown in Figure 9.1. Susan and her therapist then decomposed the category of "serious disease" into subcategories of diseases that (1) are associated with complete recovery, (2) have lingering but tolerable impairment (e.g., mild breathlessness that one can cope with), and (3) have lethal consequences. The last-mentioned subcategory is the only truly catastrophic outcome, which Susan

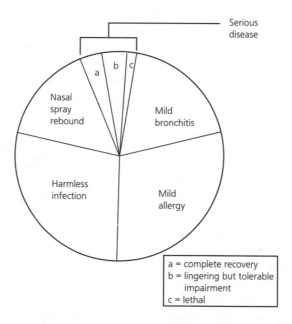

FIGURE 9.1. Example of the pie chart method: Causes of chest congestion and stuffy nose.

thought to have less than a 1% probability. Subcategories (1) and (2) are not catastrophic.

Once the percentages have been assigned, the patient and the therapist can further consider whether the rating for the catastrophic cause is accurate. Susan was asked to estimate the number of times that she and acquaintances in her age group had experienced a stuffy nose and congestion. She estimated that they had occurred thousands of times. Then she was asked how many of these episodes were due to a deadly disease. Susan recalled that none were lethal, which led her to conclude that the probability of lethal disease must be less than her initial estimate of 1%, and that benign causes were far more likely.

Troubleshooting

A common problem in using the pie chart method concerns the ability of the therapist and the patient to generate a sufficient number of categories. It is especially counterproductive if the patient and the therapist have trouble thinking of innocuous causes of bodily concerns. This would reinforce the patient's belief that she or he has a serious disease. To effectively implement the pie chart method (and other cognitive interventions), the CBT practitioner should have some general medical knowledge, or have access to medical texts and related resources (e.g., colleagues in general medical practice), in order to help the patient come up with noncatastrophic explanations of bodily changes and sensations. Some medical knowledge will also enhance the therapist's credibility with the patient.

Challenging the Cost (Badness) of Events

For patients who overestimate the cost, or badness, of diseases or bodily changes and sensations, the patient can be asked to consider the following:

- "Realistically, how bad would it be if _____ occurred? Am I overestimating how bad things would be? Example: Am I overestimating how bad it would be if I had irritable bowel syndrome?"
- "Am I overestimating how long _____ would last? Can I cope with _____ minutes of _____ in my day? Example: Am I overestimating how long my stomach cramps last?"
- Am I exaggerating how uncomfortable _____ would be? Have I been able to tolerate discomfort in the past? (These questions are useful when patients catastrophize about the unpleasantness of body sensations.) Example: Am I overestimating the intensity of my sinus pain?"

Troubleshooting

How can the CBT practitioner challenge beliefs about diseases resulting in death? Challenging the cost is unlikely to be fruitful. One way of coping with death is to develop an acceptable belief about what comes with death. The people who are most fearful of death are often those who harbor catastrophic expectations about death and dying (Wells & Hackmann, 1993). Sometimes these beliefs reveal what are probably overestimations of the badness of death. Some patients believe they will remain aware of their surroundings and body after death (Wells & Hackmann, 1993): "I'll be all alone in the cold earth, as my body decomposes." To challenge such metaphysical beliefs, patients can be asked about the evidence they have that this will occur, and whether there are less aversive possibilities of what will happen when they die (e.g., eternal sleep, passage to Heaven). This can help patients realize that although their beliefs can't be refuted, there is no evidence to support them, and that there are more plausible alternatives. Adaptive disputes can also be used. Catastrophic thoughts of death can be replaced with more adaptive cognitions: "I'll cross that bridge when I get to it. Worrying about it now is pointless." Exposure methods can also be used to address death concerns (see Chapter 10).

Adaptive Disputations

Highlighting the Cost of Dysfunctional Beliefs

Adaptive disputations involve an analysis of the costs and benefits of holding particular beliefs. Janet K. believed that she had multiple, potentially life-threatening food allergies. Over the years she had progressively cut many items from her diet, to the point that she lived almost exclusively on plain toast and tea. An evaluation by an allergist revealed no evidence of serious allergies, although she attended a seminar given by a "holistic naturopathic allergist," who led Janet to believe that almost everything is allergenic. The CBT practitioner attempted to help Janet test the idea that she had multiple allergies by encouraging her to gradually introduce various foods into her diet. This proved unsuccessful because Janet believed that virtually any bodily change or sensation could be an allergic reaction. She was anxious when she tried potentially "allergenic" foods, and believed her anxiety-related sensations (e.g., dry mouth, flushed face) indicated an allergic reaction. Janet also believed, after consulting a medical textbook, that allergic reactions come and go. Sometimes a particular food might cause a serious allergic reaction, sometimes not. These beliefs made it very difficult to test Janet's belief that she had multiple, serious food allergies. Accordingly, therapy shifted focus to help Janet consider the adaptiveness of her beliefs. The therapist and the patient considered the fact that medical allergy tests had revealed no evidence of allergies, and Janet was encouraged to consider all the harmless things that could be causing her so-called allergic reactions (e.g., mouth dryness arising from autonomic arousal). Janet was then asked to consider the adaptiveness of her beliefs by asking herself the following:

- "How does the belief 'I have multiple, serious allergies' impair my quality of life?"
- "What if I'm wrong about my allergies?"
- "Am I sacrificing my quality of life to an erroneous idea?"

Over the course of several CBT sessions Janet's beliefs gradually weakened and her dietary repertoire expanded. Not all patients have such a good outcome. Black (1996) documented cases in which allergists of questionable repute led patients to believe that they had multiple chemical sensitivities. It can be particularly difficult to correct misconceptions in such patients.

Challenging the Demand for Certainty

Even when the odds of an aversive event are very low, patients may still worry about the possibility of it happening. To illustrate, Jim J. worried that one day his chest pain might be due to a real heart attack instead of harmless spasms in his chest muscles. Of course, Jim's physicians could not guarantee that he would never have a heart attack. Jim took this lack of a guarantee as a justification for his fears. In such cases it can be useful to assess whether the patient has an unrealistic demand for certainty. The latter is reflected in beliefs such as "I can never relax so long as I know that _____ could happen." To challenge demands for certainty, the patient can consider the following questions:

- "Is it useful for me to worry about _____ or are my worries spoiling my life?"
- "How is worry relevant to my goals in life? What is more important for me, adding years to life, or adding life to years?"
- "What is so bad about the uncertainty? Am I making a mountain out of a molehill?"
- "Have I learned to tolerate other uncertainties? If so, then I can learn to tolerate this one."

The patient and therapist can review the daily low-probability "risks" that the patient already takes, such as driving or using pedestrian crosswalks. These examples can help patients learn that they already tolerate all kinds of

uncertainties, and therefore can learn to accept other low–probability uncertainties.

Challenging the Adaptiveness of Checking
and Reassurance Seeking

Careful questioning and reflective listening are useful in helping patients recognize the folly of repeated unnecessary checking and reassurance seeking.

THERAPIST: You mentioned that your boyfriend gets angry whenever you
ask him to check whether you look pale.

PATIENT: Yes, he's been getting quite annoyed.

THERAPIST: That must be stressful for you. Tell me, when you ask your boyfriend if you look pale does it help your relationship with him or harm it?

PATIENT: It definitely harms it.

THERAPIST: Then is there something you could do—or not do—that would
help your relationship?

PATIENT: I could stop asking him for reassurance.

THERAPIST: OK, good. And would there be any other benefits from not
checking on whether you're pale?

PATIENT: As you mentioned last session, I might be less preoccupied with my
health if I'm not constantly monitoring it.

THERAPIST: Right. So there are some important reasons for not seeking reassurance.

Troubleshooting

Sometimes patients readily acknowledge the maladaptiveness of their beliefs,
but insist that they can't help but worry. In these cases the therapist might
shift to an alternative cognitive intervention, such as an empirical disputation
to challenge the beliefs or a worry control strategy.

Devil's Advocate Method

Once the patient has become familiar with the process of questioning beliefs,
the therapist can consolidate belief change by using the "devil's advocate"
method. This is a form of role play in which the therapist voices one of the
patient's dysfunctional beliefs and the patient is asked to come up with evidence and arguments to refute the belief. The therapist then comes up with

counterarguments, which the patient tries to refute. Then the patient voices an adaptive alternative belief statement, which the therapist attempts to challenge. The patient's task is to defend this belief. Through this process the patient is induced to think deeply about the evidence and arguments for and against the beliefs.

Troubleshooting

The primary problems with the devil's advocate method concern timing and patient preparation. The method is unlikely to be helpful if patients are not able to come up with refutations for dysfunctional beliefs. Therefore, some other form of disputation needs to be done beforehand, such as an empirical dispute. The devil's advocate method also requires that patients are adequately informed about what is involved. They need to understand that the therapist is voicing arguments in favor of dysfunctional beliefs in order to help the patient to better develop counterarguments.

Distancing Strategies

Health-anxious patients tend to strongly believe their dysfunctional beliefs, particularly when they are feeling anxious. Distancing strategies (Beck & Emery, 1985; McMullin, 1986) are methods for helping patients view their beliefs objectively, as assumptions rather than as facts. There are several kinds of distancing strategies.

- *Observe, describe, but don't evaluate.* Patients can be asked to record the sequence of events during their episodes of health anxiety, objectively observing, as if they were scientists, the sequence of their symptoms, thoughts, feelings, and behaviors. The task is simply to observe and describe these events, without evaluating them as good or bad, and without trying to influence them.
- *Shift perspective.* This involves taking another person's perspective. "What would my dentist think about the fact that my gums sometimes bleed when I brush my teeth? I don't need to seek reassurance because I know she would tell me I have gingivitis, not oral cancer."
- In vivo *labeling of cognitions*. Here, patients are taught to label their beliefs. For example, if a patient believed that "my acid reflux will cause esophageal cancer," then the following self-statement could be used: "I'm simply having another catastrophic thought. I don't need to take it seriously." This intervention is particularly useful for patients who have too many catastrophic cognitions to individually challenge them all.

Troubleshooting

It requires a good deal of practice for patients to become adept at distancing themselves from their dysfunctional beliefs. This can be particularly difficult when the beliefs are strong. Failure experiences can be discouraging, and so it is often best to start practicing with mildly distressing beliefs. With practice, patients can often progress to successfully distancing themselves from more distressing cognitions.

Other Verbal Reattribution Methods

There are many other verbal reattribution methods that can be useful in treating health anxiety disorders (Salkovskis, 1989; Taylor, 2004; Warwick & Salkovskis, 2001; Wells, 1997). These are summarized as follows:

• *Delay plus time projection.* "How will I feel about this eyelid twitching next week? Will I still think I have Huntington's disease? Based on my experience, my worry is probably groundless. I can wait to see if the twitch goes away, instead of seeking immediate reassurance from my doctor."

• *The survey method.* "I'm worried that my popping and clicking joints are signs of bone degeneration. Are these normal for someone my age? I could survey some friends to find out." (Therapists need to be careful that this strategy is not misused by the patient for the purpose of reassurance seeking.)

• *Anticipatory coping.* This involves generating coping statements to be used in future anxiety-provoking situations. For example, "What are some things I can tell myself the next time I have pins and needles? How could I assure myself that I don't have a degenerative disease?"

• *Imagine new "symptoms."* The therapist asks the patient to imagine experiencing new "symptoms" (e.g., itchy feet, stomach pain, tight chest), and then to elicit and challenge catastrophic beliefs. This intervention is useful for targeting the general tendency to catastrophically misinterpret bodily changes and sensations.

WORRY MANAGEMENT

Worry consists of a chain of thoughts about threatening events along with attempts to think of ways of averting or dealing with these events. Some patients believe that worry about their health prevents them from becoming ill, and so they deliberately engage in this form of thinking (Wells, 2000). The adaptiveness of worry can be explored in therapy by considering the evidence for and against it usefulness. Behavioral experiments can be generated, ones in which patients compare their well-being on days that they did versus days that they didn't worry.

Once worry is initiated it can be are difficult to relinquish (Wells, 1997). Borkovec, Wilkinson, Folensbee, and Lerman's (1983) stimulus control method is among the most useful of exercises for reducing worry. The procedure is summarized in Handout 9.4.

Mary C. used the stimulus control method to control her worry about the consequences of a sexual encounter in which she had unprotected intercourse with a man who later turned out to have HIV. Although the encounter had taken place 2 years earlier, Mary persistently worried that she too might have caught the virus. She went over the sexual encounter again and again in her mind, trying to recall if there were any signs that her partner was infected at the time: "Did he have lesions on his body?" "Did he look pale?" "He coughed a couple of times during dinner; did he have a persistent cough?" Mary also ruminated over her own health: "Has my health changed since the encounter?" "Am I feeling more fatigued these days?" "Have I been getting more coughs and colds this year?" "My HIV test was negative, but maybe the virus is dormant—it might become active later."

Mary's worries were addressed in the following fashion. First, she and her therapist examined the adaptiveness of continually worrying about her risk of HIV. Mary readily acknowledged that this form of thinking was a source of great distress, and was not productive. After all, if she had the virus then there was nothing she could do about it. The therapist and Mary then discussed whether it was possible to determine, with absolute certainty, that she was completely healthy. After some discussion, Mary realized that this was impossible and that she had to learn to tolerate uncertainty in her life. She realized that just like everybody else she could accept life's uncertainties. She recognized that she accepted many other uncertainties in her life. For example, she drove her car even though there was some uncertainty about whether she would be involved in an accident. She went to banks to make financial transactions even though there was a possibility that she might be caught in the middle of a holdup. She walked outdoors even though there was a possibility that she might be struck by falling satellites or meteors. By generating a list of examples of life's uncertainties, the therapist was able to persuade Mary that she accepted a great many uncertainties in her life, and so there was no reason why she could not accept uncertainties about her health.

These interventions laid the ground work for the stimulus control exercise. Once Mary accepted the unnecessary, self-defeating nature of her worry, she was motivated to implement the stimulus control procedure described in Handout 9.4. After some practice Mary was able to substantially reduce the amount of time she spent worrying about HIV.

CONTROLLING YOUR WORRY

If you are troubled by needless worry, then try the following:

1. **Establish a worry period.** Set aside 30 minutes each day for worrying. Try to do all your worrying during that period. For example, you might decide that your worry period will be from 6:00 to 6:30 each night. Don't schedule the worry period too late in the evening, otherwise it might delay you from getting to sleep.

2. **Use a worry diary.** Write out all your worries during the worry period. Writing out your worries can help you view them more objectively. Use the "Thinking Errors" handout (Handout 9.1) to see if your worries contain any thinking errors. You might also decide to problem-solve some of your worries, or you might find that some worries can be simply dismissed because they are unrealistic.

3. **Postpone.** When you catch yourself worrying at other times, postpone the worry to your daily worry period. You might make a brief note of the worry in a notebook, and tell yourself "I'll worry about this later."

4. **Practice, practice, practice!** The more you practice these exercises, the better you will become at controlling your worry.

Troubleshooting

A primary problem with the stimulus control method is getting patients to consistently practice the exercise. Patients who "can't find time" to practice could be asked to consider the pros and cons of the procedure, and then to schedule a regular time for practice. Patients who believe that worry is adaptive may be reluctant to use the method. Here, it may first be necessary to implement other interventions (e.g., adaptive disputations and behavioral experiments) to highlight the maladaptiveness of excessive worry.

IMAGERY METHODS

Image Modification Strategies

Health-anxious patients may describe frightening cognitions in the form of fleeting images. These are sometimes evoked in response to bodily changes or sensations. Edward S. noticed that he had tinea (a fungal infection) between two of his toes. This discovery triggered a frightening image of fungal infection spreading all over his body. Cognitive restructuring can be used to challenge the probability or cost if the event depicted in the image came true. This can help the patient reappraise the meaning of the image. Guided imagery exercises also can be used to restructure catastrophic images. One method involves *imaginally altering the image* into something innocuous or amusing (Clark, 1999). In his response to the catastrophic image of fungus spreading over his body, Edward imagined himself turning into a goofy, brightly spotted talking mushroom, of the kind seen in children's TV programs. He found that this image modification robbed the catastrophic image of its emotional impact. In fact, he no longer took the catastrophic image seriously when it occurred.

Another method is to *"finish out" the image*, in which the patient is asked to provide a realistic, positive conclusion to a frightening image (Clark, 1999; Wells, 1997). This strategy is based on the observation that catastrophic images often stop at the worst point in the scenario (Beck & Emery, 1985). The finishing-out strategy is implemented by asking the patient to recall the feared image, then to hold it in mind until anxiety is experienced, and then to continue the image until there is a positive resolution. The patient may spontaneously come up with a realistic, positive outcome, or the therapist can guide the patient to arrive at such an outcome. Myrna F. was frightened of developing all kinds of cancer. She was particularly frightened of developing pancreatic cancer, which had recently claimed the life of one of her favorite movie stars. Myrna was plagued by recurrent images of herself lying in a hospital bed, dying of cancer. She was encouraged to practice finishing out the image by imagining herself being discharged from hospital after successful treatment.

Imaginal exposure (see Chapter 10) can reduce patients' anxiety reactions to catastrophic images. This can also alter patients' beliefs about the meaning of the images. Images that were formerly seen as harbingers of disaster are re-interpreted as "mental garbage." Imaginal exposure is discussed in the following chapter.

Troubleshooting

Some patients have difficulty generating sufficiently vivid images during the therapy session. This can happen if the images are primarily triggered by some environmental stimulus that is absent during the session. For instance, a patient troubled by catastrophic images of dying might have these images only when he or she encounters death-related stimuli. In this example the in-session elicitation of catastrophic images could be facilitated by asking the patient to read a newspaper obituary section. The patient could also be asked to write or draw a description of the image, or to produce a tape-recorded description. Patients should try to include all the elements that contribute to image vividness—all the sensory elements, thoughts, feelings, and behaviors that make up a given scenario.

ATTENTION MODIFICATION

Attention-Focusing Exercises

Various attention-focusing exercises can be used to show patients how their focus of attention can influence the detection of bodily changes or sensations. This can help patients learn that devoting excessive attention to one's body can be a source of bodily sensations or changes that may be misinterpreted as indications of disease. Patients can also learn that selective attention can ex-plain why they might experience more "symptoms" than other people. It is not the fact that they are more sickly, it is the fact that they focus so much at-tention on their bodies. The following are some useful 5-minutes exercises for illustrating the effects of attentional focus. These have been culled from vari-ous sources (Avia et al., 1996; Barsky, 1996; Furer & Walker, 2000; Salkovskis, 1989; Wells, 1997) and from our own clinical experience.

- Focus on one's throat sensations, noticing any itchiness, scratchiness, or dryness. This may lead to the need to cough or clear one's throat.
- Focus on one's scalp, noticing sensations such as tension, itchiness, or tingling.

- Direct one's attention to the external environment, and then review how one's body felt during that time. Was there any reduction in bodily sensations?
- Focus on and then distract yourself from an area of your body that concerns you. Notice any changes in bodily sensations.
- Focus on your eyes blinking. What sensations do you notice?

Patients can be reminded that we all have "noisy" bodies, and that bodily sensations and changes frequently occur, even in healthy people. The therapist can discuss how listening to music while jogging can reduce feelings of fatigue (as a result of distraction from one's muscles). Another example concerns soldiers who fail to notice injuries because they are intensely absorbed in combat. Patients can be asked to consider the effects of their environment on their detection of bodily sensations and changes. Do they notice more bodily sensations, for example, when they're in an unstimulating environment, as compared to an attentionally demanding situation?

Attention Training Technique

The attention training technique (Papageorgiou & Wells, 1998; Wells, 1997, 2000) is another method for reducing health anxiety by attentional means. Case studies provide encouraging evidence for the acceptability and efficacy of this intervention in reducing heath anxiety (see Chapter 5). The rationale is that although cognitive restructuring may alter dysfunctional beliefs, it may not necessarily change attentional styles. Therefore attention training is used to counter the tendency for health-anxious people to overfocus on their bod-ies and to improve their attentional control. The method consists of a number of 10-minute exercises first practiced in the session and then later as home-work. First, patients are trained in *selective attention* (e.g., focusing attention on the sounds in the room while ignoring outside noises). Then patients are trained in *attention switching* (shifting attention from one sound to another). Finally, patients practice *divided attention* (focusing on many things at the same time). Attention training is not intended as a distraction exercise or as a way of directly controlling anxiety or worries. Rather, it is used to help health-anxious patients to become proficient at ending episodes of somatic preoccupation. The following sample transcript, adapted from Wells (2000), illustrates the exercises, which are introduced once the rationale has been presented:

"I'm going to ask you to focus your gaze on a dot on the wall. I will sit slightly behind you so that I don't interfere with your fixed gaze. While you gaze at the dot I will be asking you to focus on different sounds. To begin, focus on the sound of my voice. Pay close attention to that sound, like no other sound matters. Try to give all your attention to the sound of my voice. No other sound matters, focus only on the sound of my voice.

"Now, while still gazing at the dot, focus your ears on the sound of me tapping on the table. Focus only on the tapping sound. No other sound matters. . . . (*pause*) Closely monitor the tapping sound. . . . If your attention begins to stray, refocus on the tapping. . . . Give all your attention to this sound. . . . Focus on the tapping sound and monitor this sound closely. Filter out all competing sounds, for they are not important. . . . Continue to monitor the tapping sound. . . . Focus all your attention on that sound. Try not to be distracted. . . .

"Now, while still gazing at the dot, focus your ears on the sound of the clock ticking. Focus all your attention on that sound. . . . Other sounds don't matter. Focus on the clock, paying close attention to it and not allowing yourself to be distracted. . . . This is the most important sound and no other sounds matter. . . . Give all your attention to that sound. . . . If your attention strays, refocus on the sound of the clock. . . . Focus only on the sound of the clock. . . . Give all your attention to that sound. . . . Continue to monitor that sound closely, pay full attention to it. . . . Try not to be distracted."

(*The same instructions are repeated for three sounds in the near distance—e.g., sounds of voices in the outside corridor, doors closing and opening, and the sound of the ventilation system—and then for three sounds in the far distance—e.g., outside traffic, birds chirping, voices outside of the building.*)

"Now that you have identified and focused on different sounds I would like you to rapidly shift your attention between the different sounds as I call them out. . . . First, focus on sound of the clock, no other sound matters, give all your attention to that sound. . . . Now focus on the sound of the sound of the ventilation system. Pay attention only to that sound. . . . Now switch your attention and focus on the sound of voices outside in the corridor. Focus only on that sound. No other sound matters. . . . Now switch your attention back to the sound of the clock. . . . Now focus on the sound of the road traffic. Focus back on the sound of the clock. . . . Now focus on the sound of birds outside. . . . Now focus on the road traffic. . . . Now focus on the clock. . . . [etc.]

"Finally, expand your attention, make it as broad and deep as possible and try to absorb all of the sounds simultaneously. Try to focus on and be aware of all the sounds, both within and outside this room at the same time. . . . Try to hear all the sounds simultaneously. Count the number of sounds you can hear at the same time. . . .

"This concludes the exercise. How many sounds were you aware of at the same time?"

The therapist emphasizes that the goal is not to remove all other material from consciousness, but to practice focusing attention in a particular way. The intervention can be delivered in a couple of treatment sessions, along with 15–20-minute homework exercises, to be practiced twice daily. The homework exercises are the same as those practiced in the sessions, adapted as necessary to the particulars of the patient's home environment.

To monitor treatment progress, patients are asked to rate their degree of self-attention on a 7-point scale (−3 = entirely externally focused, 0 = equal amounts; +3 = entirely self-focused). Failure to produce a reduction in self-attention over the course of treatment should be explored to identify the source of the problem. Although attention training can be used as a stand-alone treatment for health anxiety, this brief intervention can be readily integrated with other CBT interventions.

Troubleshooting

The attention training technique requires consistent practice. Patients should be advised that they will need to practice for a couple of weeks before they start to see benefits. Adherence problems may be encountered if the patient sees the exercise as irrelevant to his or her problems or finds it boring. In such cases the therapist can use the strategies for enhancing treatment motivation described in Chapter 8. Alternatively, the therapist might focus on other interventions that the patient finds more interesting. Fortunately, there are many cognitive interventions that can be selected for treating health anxiety, and so the patient and therapist can pick and choose to find the interventions that are most acceptable and effective for a given patient.

TREATING OVERVALUED IDEATION AND DELUSIONS

Regardless of the choice of intervention, it can be challenging for the therapist to alter dysfunctional beliefs that are held with particularly strong conviction. The small but growing literature on cognitive interventions for delusions (e.g., Chadwick et al., 1996) provides some suggestions about methods to consider and those to avoid. As in conventional cognitive restructuring for health anxiety, the therapist refrains from directly challenging or confronting delusions or overvalued beliefs because this can strengthen the beliefs (Brehm,

1962). This seems to occur because challenges to strongly held beliefs can cause people to generate belief-preserving counterarguments (see Chapter 8 for a discussion of how a similar process plays a role in treatment motivation). The following guidelines can be beneficial in treating overvalued and delusional health-related beliefs. These methods were adapted largely from Chadwick and colleagues (1996), who developed methods for treating delusions in general.

- If the patient has multiple overvalued or delusional beliefs, begin with the belief that is least important or least strongly held. This may be easier to alter than more strongly held beliefs.
- As in the treatment of health anxiety in general, challenge the evidence for the belief rather than the belief itself.
- Challenge the evidence for the belief in inverse order of the importance of the evidence. In other words, start with the weakest piece of the patient's evidence for the belief.
- Ask the patient if she or he is able to think of something that would create doubts about the validity of the belief.
- Present plausible hypothetical scenarios that are inconsistent with the patient's belief and ask the patient how such a scenario might alter the belief. This will give you an idea of the sorts of evidence that will or won't be persuasive.
- Capitalize on fluctuations in belief strength. The therapist can capitalize on naturally occurring fluctuations—for example, by identifying occasions in which the patient doubted (even for a moment) that he or she was ill. The therapist can then work to strengthen these doubts by building on the evidence that the patient found convincing.
- Reformulate the overvalued or delusional belief as being an understandable response to, and a way of making sense of, specific experience. The belief can be contrasted with a personally meaningful alternative—for example, "Given your skin sensations, I can understand why you'll feel like you're infested with bugs. But I wonder if there's another possible cause. . . . " The belief and its alternative are then evaluated, in a nonconfrontational manner, in light of the available information.

SUMMARY AND CONCLUSIONS

Many cognitive methods can be used to treat health anxiety, including verbal reattribution methods, imagery methods, worry control exercises, and attention training. The choice of interventions depends on a number of factors, including the nature of the patient's problems. Worry control methods, for instance, are indicated when excessive worry is a prominent part of the clinical picture. The therapist's expertise also needs to be considered. Some therapists have difficulty coming up with ways of empirically testing dysfunctional beliefs and are better skilled at other interventions. To successfully implement many of these interventions it is important for the therapist to have some general medical knowledge. Nonphysician therapists may need to do background reading about specific diseases, depending on the nature of the patient's concerns. For a patient concerned about contracting "flesh-eating disease" from cuts or scratches, for example, the therapist could become informed about this issue by reading about necrotizing fasciitis.

When implementing cognitive interventions, it is important to check the patient's understanding of what was covered in the session, so as to prevent misunderstanding (Salkovskis, 1989). It is also important that the therapist avoid being drawn into providing the patient with reassurance (Wells, 1997). If reassurance seeking occurs, this can be pointed out to the patient and the maladaptiveness of reassurance can be reviewed. With the patient's permission, significant others can be asked to refrain from giving reassurance.

Another important consideration concerns the patient's reactions to corrective information. It can be difficult to predict, a priori, the sort of intervention that will be most persuasive for a given patient. Some patients respond particularly well to empirical disputations, while others benefit more from distancing strategies and adaptive disputes. The most effective intervention can sometimes be identified by asking the patient questions like "What would it take for you to give up the idea that you're suffering from a serious disease?" An answer like "I'll give up the idea once I'm 100% certain that I'm healthy" would suggest that the therapist should target the patient's intolerance of uncertainty. An answer such as "I could give up the idea if someone could explain to me how my symptoms arise" suggests that the therapist would do well to develop a noncatastrophic explanation of the patient's bodily concerns, buttressed by clear, cogent evidence.

The selection of interventions also depends on the stage of therapy. Early in treatment it is often useful to focus on empirical disputations. Patients may be reluctant to accept adaptive disputations—such as "I should give up worrying about sickness because the worry is ruining my life"—until they have come to appreciate that the evidence does not support their dysfunctional beliefs.

10

Behavioral Methods

Behavioral methods play a prominent role in treating fear, avoidance, and maladaptive safety behaviors like excessive checking and reassurance seeking. Behavioral methods typically require the patient to be exposed to fear stimuli. This occurs in a systematic, controlled fashion. In this chapter we describe and illustrate four types of exposure exercises:

- Behavioral experiments that test the effects of beliefs and behaviors (e.g., testing the effects of performing vs. not performing safety behaviors).
- Situational exposure.
- Interoceptive exposure (sensation-inducing exercises).
- Imaginal exposure.

In practice, behavioral experiments overlap with the other exposure methods. Nevertheless, we have found it useful to distinguish between these methods in order to train clinicians in the components of behavioral treatment.

As with other cognitive-behavioral therapy (CBT) interventions, the exposure exercises are collaborative. Patient and therapist jointly decide on the exercises to be used. Behavioral exercises are vehicles for cognitive change, designed as "no lose" assignments, where something important is learned regardless of the outcome. Even exposure exercises for disease phobia can be seen as methods of introducing patients to corrective information—to help patients learn that their bodily sensations and related stimuli are not dangerous, or at least not as threatening as patients believe them to be. Corrective information includes within-session physiological habituation and information about the outcome of encountering the phobic object, both of which help the patient to realistically appraise the "threat value" of the stimulus (Foa & Kozak, 1986).

The choice of intervention depends, in part, on whether avoidance is active or passive. Active avoidance is characterized by the *commission* of some sort of behavior (e.g., avoiding an anticipated hypertensive crisis by compulsively checking one's blood pressure). Passive avoidance is defined largely by the *omission* of some behavior (e.g., refraining from visiting a friend in the hospital for fear of catching a disease). Exposure methods can be used for both forms of avoidance. Behavioral experiments are especially important for active avoidance, in which patients are encouraged to test the effects of dropping their safety behaviors (Bouman & Visser, 1998).

GENERAL CONSIDERATIONS

Indications and Contraindications

Before attempting exposure exercises, the patient should thoroughly understand their purpose and be willing to endure some degree of distress, at least in the short term ("short-term pain for long-term gain"). Exposure interventions can be gradually implemented, beginning with mildly distressing stimuli, in order to ensure that the exercises are not overwhelming. The patient's ways of coping with distress also need to be considered. If a person has a history of abusing alcohol during times of distress, then the therapist needs to ensure that the exposure exercises do not lead to an increase in alcohol misuse.

Interoceptive exercises are medically contraindicated in some cases. Patients with severe asthma, for example, may be medically unsuited for interoceptive exercises involving hyperventilation. Before attempting interoceptive exposure, the therapist should confer with the patient's primary care physician to learn whether there are any medical contraindications.

Preparation and Implementation

Patients should be informed beforehand about the side effects of behavioral exercises. These consist of transient increases in arousal, which may occur in the form of increased anxiety, irritability, or headache. We advise to patients not be alarmed by the side effects. These effects are typically mild, transient, and, importantly, are evidence that treatment is working. That is, side effects are evidence that the patient is being exposed to relevant health anxiety stimuli.

Exposure duration depends on the nature of the task. Behavioral experiments might range from 10 minutes to a day or more, depending on the type of information needed to test beliefs or to test the effects of checking and reassurance seeking. A full day of refraining from reassurance seeking might be needed to teach the patient that reassurance seeking perpetuates health preoccupation. Interoceptive exposure exercises typically consist of repeated 1- to 2-minute trials. Each situational and imaginal exposure exercise typically requires 30–45 minutes. Exposure exercises can be conducted during the treatment session and as homework assignments (e.g., daily homework). The therapist and the patient can review the results of homework during the treatment sessions, and the therapist can use the results as material for cognitive restructuring.

Fear reduction tends to be most complete and enduring if exposure—whether it be situational, interoceptive, or imaginal—is conducted across multiple contexts (Bouton, 2000). A person with cancer phobia, for example, could be exposed to harmless cancer-related stimuli in a variety of different circumstances, such as by visiting a number of different hospitals that treat cancer patients and viewing several different documentaries about cancer.

Facilitating Homework Completion

Homework is a vital aspect of all behavioral interventions. Homework should be reviewed in each session—in terms of what happened and what was or wasn't learned—and any difficulties should be addressed. Patients should be advised to practice the exercises regularly, regardless of how they feel. Structuring the exposure homework assignments in the following manner can improve adherence:

- Collaboratively plan each homework assignment so patients assume at least some responsibility.
- Ensure that the assignment is not too difficult. If necessary, break it up into manageable steps or subtasks.
- Ensure that patients understand the rationale for their homework assignments. Have them describe the rationale in their own words. If patients do not understand the rationale, then they may wonder why they should bother with the tasks. Cognitive restructuring can be used to persuade the patient to attempt the assignments.
- Provide patients with a written copy of each assignment so it is not forgotten.
- Use rating forms (e.g., Handout 10.1) so that patients can record details of their assignments. On the form the patient notes the day the ex-

HANDOUT 10.1. Monitoring Form for Behavioral Exercises

Day and date	Exercise	Peak anxiety (0–100)	What did you learn from the exercise?
Example 1	Spent 5 minutes feeling the lymph glands on neck to see if they were swollen	50	Repeated checking and squeezing makes my glands feel sore and swollen. Repeated checking creates problems—it makes me think my glands are swollen.
Example 2	Jogged around the block	70	I was worried that my body couldn't take the exertion. But I survived! Maybe I'm not as frail as I thought.
Example 3	Walked past a funeral home	65	Nothing bad happened. I can't get sick by being near dead bodies.

ercise was attempted, its duration, peak anxiety (0–100), and what was learned from the exercise.

- Ask patients to use weekly schedules or day planners to list all the tasks they will be performing during the following week (e.g., going to work, mowing the lawn, taking the children to football practice). The schedule is structured so that there is a specified time for the homework assignments. This strategy is particularly useful for patients who have difficulties with time management.

- Patients should be reinforced (and encouraged to self-reinforce) for their efforts.

- If patient adherence is an ongoing problem, employ a written contract. The contract specifies the nature of the assignment and outlines the responsibilities of the patient and the therapist. The contract may be written in the form: "I, [name of patient,] agree to practice [name of task] for [specified frequency and duration]. In return, I, [name of therapist,] agree to review progress and to consult on ways of maximizing the effectiveness of the task." This approach might seem unduly formal, but it has proved to be quite useful when adherence is a problem.

- Ask patients to make a commitment to their significant other(s) to perform the homework assignments.

BEHAVIORAL EXPERIMENTS

Testing the Effects of Safety Behaviors

Behavioral experiments can be used for a variety of purposes. Commonly, they are used to test the effects of safety behaviors such as reassurance seeking. The goal is to help patients learn whether their safety behaviors actually do keep them from harm and whether these behaviors create problems of their own (e.g., by maintaining the belief that one is in need of constant medical attention). Table 10.1 provides examples of these exercises.

Patients can be quite reluctant to give up their safety behaviors, so the exercises are typically performed after the patient has received sufficient cognitive restructuring to significantly weaken his or her belief in the usefulness of safety behaviors. Behavioral experiments can be supplemented by asking the patient to list the advantages and disadvantages of checking and reassurance seeking (Wells, 1997). The therapist can ask the patient to describe the disadvantages in detail, in order to strengthen patient motivation to drop these behaviors. The putative advantages can also be reviewed and challenged.

Another useful behavioral experiment is to ask patients to *increase* the fre-

TABLE 10.1. Sample Exercises for Testing the Effects
of Safety Behaviors

Safety behavior	Sample exercise	Learning objective
Bodily checking	Repeatedly checking lymph nodes by palpation (vs. not checking)	Repeated checking is a cause of bodily swelling and tenderness
Bodily checking	Checking throat by repeatedly swallowing (vs. not swallowing)	A feared sensation (lump in the throat) is caused by repeated swallowing
Pursuing special dietary regimens	Refraining, for 1 week, from using dietary supplements such as herbal preparations, vitamins, and tonics	Refraining from special dietary regimens has no adverse impact on one's health
Seeking medical reassurance	Seeking versus not seeking medical reassurance	Reassurance seeking perpetuates preoccupation with health
Seeking reassurance from family members	Asking family to refrain from giving reassurance	Health preoccupation declines when reassurance is not given
Cleaning	Refraining from excessive handwashing	Refraining from handwashing does not lead to illness

quency of their safety behaviors (e.g., increased checking of one's lymph glands) in order to demonstrate that these safety behaviors contribute to their problems (e.g., create swollen, sore glands) (Wells, 1997). These exercises are conducted within the treatment session and as homework. The results of homework assignments are recorded in a monitoring form (Handout 10.1).

Patients should be encouraged to give up their safety behaviors almost entirely. This includes reducing the frequency of medical consultations and bodily checking. The patient and the therapist should work together, along with the patient's primary care physician, to decide on the frequency of bodily checking and medical consultations. A patient might be encouraged, for instance, to perform one monthly breast self-examination instead of checking multiple times per day. An annual physical examination might be scheduled in place of monthly "checkups" used primarily as reassurance seeking. Patients should be encouraged to refrain from seeking reassurance from friends and family members and from checking medical information in textbooks, on the Internet, and from other sources.

Testing Interpretations of Bodily Sensations and Changes

Behavioral experiments can be used to teach patients that their bodily sensations or alterations are influenced by factors other than the ones they believe to be responsible (Salkovskis, 1989). For instance, Gina V. periodically experienced a mild tremor in her hands. She believed this was evidence of a neurological degenerative disease. A behavioral experiment was conducted to test an alternative interpretation that the tremor was a product of increased muscle tension due to job stress and high caffeine consumption. To test this alternative, Gina drank caffeinated coffee on some days and decaf on others. Gina tracked the frequency of tremulousness and the degree of stressfulness of each workday. She discovered that trembling was more likely to occur on stressful days in which she drank caffeinated coffee. Thus, she acquired evidence for a *benign* interpretation of her trembling.

Testing Interpretations of Environmental Stimuli

Behavioral experiments can be used to obtain information about the meaning or significance of environmental stimuli, as illustrated by the following case. The data is then used during subsequent cognitive restructuring.

> Arnold B. was unpacking boxes from a truck as part of his storeman duties. One of the boxes leaked red liquid over his hands. Arnold's immediate interpretation was that the liquid was HIV-contaminated blood. He became highly anxious, spent a good deal of time washing his hands, and left work early because he was feeling so frightened and nauseated. Upon arriving home he phoned his therapist, with the hope of receiving reassurance. Instead, the therapist asked Arnold to list the evidence for and against the idea that the red liquid was contaminated blood. Arnold's evidence was that the liquid "looked pink, like blood" and had a "weird, fleshy smell." The therapist then asked him to list the evidence *against* the catastrophic interpretation. Arnold recalled that the liquid was not in a container that one would expect for blood products (it was simply a cardboard box), and, to his knowledge, his warehouse did not store blood products. The therapist then asked Arnold, "Aside from blood, what else might the red liquid be?" To his surprise, Arnold realized that he hadn't thought about the alternatives. After some consideration, he said that perhaps the liquid was beet juice. In support of this interpretation, Arnold noted that his warehouse did stock supermarket products. To collect further evidence for this interpretation, the therapist encouraged Arnold to buy a tin of beet juice. Arnold discovered that the juice was the same color as the liquid that had spilled on him, and, importantly, also had a "weird, fleshy smell." The therapist also gave Arnold some

corrective information about the color and smell of blood. Thus, Arnold came to believe that he had not come into contact with HIV–contaminated blood.

The busy therapist might object that it takes time and effort to devise good behavioral experiments, particularly for patients who have a lot of different dysfunctional beliefs. Some might say that it would be quicker to simply say to Arnold: "It was probably a harmless liquid. Contaminated blood is not shipped to warehouses like yours." The problem with offering bland reassurance is that Arnold learns nothing about the *process* of questioning the evidence for his beliefs. If he had been simply reassured, Arnold would not have learned to distance himself from his catastrophic beliefs and to consider the evidence and alternatives. Bland reassurance is Band-Aid treatment. It does nothing to limit the likelihood of future catastrophic misinterpretations. In contrast, behavioral experiments, combined with the detailed review of the evidence, teach the patient to take on the role of scientist, questioning his or her assumptions and generating alternatives. For subsequent catastrophic misinterpretations the process of conducting behavioral experiments and empirical disputation was practiced again, until Arnold became adept at evaluating the evidence on his own. In this way he was able to reduce his fears of contracting a serious disease.

Troubleshooting

It can be difficult to devise behavioral experiments for some health–related beliefs. It is especially challenging to test beliefs about things that might not occur for decades. A patient might take "memory supplements" of questionable value (e.g., ginko biloba) to ward off future Alzheimer's disease. The patient might believe that the effects of the supplements won't be evident for years, if not decades. Simply refraining from using the substances for a month would therefore be a weak behavioral experiment because the effects would not be expected to be evident.

The therapist has several options for addressing this problem. He or she might ask: "Is a behavioral experiment worth conducting? Does it really matter that my patient takes an expensive but ineffective herbal supplement each day?" The therapist needs to consider how much the safety behavior contributes to the patient's health anxiety and whether it creates other problems. If, for example, the patient was getting into financial trouble because of taking expensive supplements, then the therapist may wish to encourage the patient to discontinue his or her consumption. Alternatively, the safety behavior might be determined to be insufficiently important to address.

If it is important for the patient to drop a safety behavior, and the effects of the behavior are difficult to test in a behavioral experiment, then the therapist could try some form of cognitive restructuring. Corrective information could be provided (e.g., medical references on the effects of ginko biloba on memory functioning). Adaptive disputes could be used (e.g., "Are you getting value for your money? Are the herbal remedies giving you results in your daily life now, or are they depriving you of money that you might devote to more important things, such as a college fund for your daughter?").

What should the therapist do for patients who are unable or unwilling to test the effects of not checking or reassurance seeking? The therapist could try to correct the source of the problem (e.g., correct any misconceptions about the homework assignment, or use other cognitive restructuring methods to challenge dysfunctional beliefs about the need to check or seek reassurance). If these methods meet with limited success, then the therapist and the patient could collaborate to identify assignments that are easier to implement. This might involve increasing, for gradually longer periods of time, the interval between the onset of the urge to consult a physician and the actual seeking of reassurance. The point at which the patient experiences the urge to check or seek reassurance can be used as a cue for implementing coping statements (e.g., "The urge to seek reassurance will soon pass, especially if I busy myself with something else").

For patients who yield to the urge to check or seek reassurance, then these activities can be used as learning experiences. The therapist might ask questions like the following:

> "Did you learn anything new by seeking reassurance again from your physician?"
> "Did your symptoms change once you obtained reassurance?"
> "If so, what does that tell you about their cause?"
> "Does it suggest that the sensations are due to anxiety?"

SITUATIONAL EXPOSURE

Guidelines

This method involves exposure to harmless but fear-evoking stimuli. Such exposure is particularly important for reducing fears of contracting diseases. Situational exposure is used when avoidance is a prominent feature of the patient's problems. If a person with a fear of contracting cancer avoided medical textbooks on cancer, then the phobia could be treated by gradual exposure to such texts. Such an approach would not be used if the person compulsively checked medical texts in order to gain reassurance that she or he was unlikely to develop cancer. In this case the patient would be encouraged to refrain from checking, or behavioral experiments would be used to test whether checking perpetuates her or his cancer fears.

The goal of situational exposure is to test patient beliefs, not to free the patient from distress. Situational exposure exercises should be ones that patients can realistically accomplish, given their current levels of functioning. Patients should not be asked to attempt exercises that they are too frightened to undertake.

Situational exposure assignments can be therapist-assisted, within-session exercises, or self-directed homework assignments. The former can be used for more difficult (distressing) exposures or when the therapist needs to collect information on what the patient actually does during exposures (e.g., to assess whether the patient is using distraction so that the effects of exposure are attenuated).

In selecting the appropriate difficulty level, the therapist can describe the exercise and ask the patient to rate his or her confidence about completing the task (0 = not at all confident, 100 = completely confident). Patients can be asked to complete tasks that they are quite confident of completing (confidence rating of 80 or higher).

Situational exposure exercises should be specific and well defined in terms of duration, situation, and what the patient must do (or not do). The exercises should be written down so they are not forgotten by either the patient or the therapist. Predictions based on the dysfunctional belief and its noncatastrophic alternative should be made beforehand. Situational exposure should be comprehensive, with different exercises covering different manifestations of the feared situations. Long, continuous periods of exposure tend to be more effective than short or interrupted periods (Chaplin & Levine, 1981; Marshall, 1985; Stern & Marks, 1973). Although short exposure sessions (e.g., 10–15 minutes) can be effective if they strongly disconfirm catastrophic predictions, longer sessions (20–60 minutes) are often necessary. The longer the exposure, the greater the opportunity of the patient learning that the feared consequences do not occur. If the exposure session is short (e.g., 10–15 minutes), the patient may conclude that the feared consequence *could* have occurred if exposure had lasted longer. With regard to the frequency of exposure exercises, patients should be encouraged to practice the exposure exercises as frequently as they reasonably can, depending on the type of exercise and on its logistic constraints.

Table 10.2 shows some examples of potentially relevant exposure stimuli for various disease-related fears. Handout 10.2 contains guidelines to help patients implement exposure. Patients are often idiosyncratic in the things they fear. For people with cancer phobia, for example, exposure to cancer textbooks might trigger fear in one person but not in another. Accordingly, the examples in Table 10.2 will work for some patients but not for others. The

TABLE 10.2. Examples of Situational Exposure Stimuli

Fear of contracting . . .	Potentially relevant exposure stimuli
Cancer	• Magazine photos of people who battled cancer • Illustrated textbooks on cancer • TV documentaries on cancer • Hospital cancer wards
Airborne germs	• Walking past funeral homes • Sitting in a hospital waiting room where sickly people have sat • The sight and sound of a person coughing (e.g., the therapist) • Talking to people who appear to be ill
HIV	• Illustrated articles on HIV • TV programs on HIV • Walking in a "gay" part of town • Volunteering at a hospice for HIV-positive people
Food poisoning	• Eating canned foods without washing the cans beforehand • Eating unusual or unfamiliar foods (e.g., exotic fruits that have been washed before consumption) • Cooking and eating chicken that is 1 day past the "use by" date • Dining in a "cheap-looking" café
Rabies	• Visiting a pet store and handling puppies • Walking in a park frequented by people walking their dogs • Looking at dogs in a local pound • Volunteering as a dog-walker at a pound

therapist and the patient need to work together to identify relevant fear stimuli.

Exposure and Response Prevention

Situation exposure is insufficient if the patient uses some form of safety signal or safety behavior during or after the exposure. Recall from Chapter 3 that *safety signals* are stimuli that the person associates with the absence of feared outcomes. Safety signals include bottles of vitamin pills, the proximity of hospitals, and good luck charms. *Safety behaviors* are things the person does to ward off feared events. Such behaviors include escape, avoidance, and other "coping" responses such as handwashing to eliminate germs. Safety signals and

SEVEN STRATEGIES FOR OVERCOMING DISEASE PHOBIA

You are probably familiar with the old saying "If you fall off a horse and become frightened of riding, then the thing to do is to get back on." In other words, we can overcome our phobias by gradually and systematically confronting the things we fear. Easier said than done? Not if you work through the following steps, which are clinically proven ways of overcoming phobias, including excessive fears of contracting a disease. These steps are best accomplished by working with your therapist.

1. **Set a goal.** It is easier to accomplish something if you have a clear goal in mind, something you can work toward. If you have a phobia of hospitals, for example, then your goal might be "To be able to visit a friend in hospital without feeling terrified."

2. **Write out the small steps needed to accomplish your goal.** Remember, baby steps are best. What are the small, manageable steps that you can take to accomplish your goal? You might decide to develop a hierarchy, starting with a task that creates only mild anxiety (e.g., walking past a hospital). Once you are comfortable with that task, then you can move on to a somewhat more challenging task (e.g., going into an empty hospital waiting area). And once you become comfortable at that task, you can move on to something even more challenging (e.g., going to the waiting area of a very busy hospital, in which there are many sick people).

3. **Give up your "crutches."** People with phobias often rely on a number of things to make them feel less anxious. A person with a phobia of getting HIV might check his or her body each day and constantly seek reassurance from his or her doctor. A person with a phobia of getting cancer might carry a lucky rabbit's foot to ward off danger. Excessive checking, reassurance seeking, and reliance on lucky charms are all crutches—they prevent you from overcoming your fears. Try to gradually discontinue relying on them.

4. **Schedule time to practice.** The more you practice going into feared situations, the less distressing they become. Regular, daily practice is often best. For example, you might attempt 20–30 minutes each day until your goal is accomplished.

5. **Keep track of your progress.** Use the monitoring form provided by your therapist.

(continued)

6. **Don't let setbacks get you down.** Sometimes overcoming a phobia is smooth sailing, where you steadily becomes less and less frightened. More often, however, progress consists of two steps forward and one step back. You might become gradually more comfortable in a feared situation, but periodically experience mini-increases in fear. For example, you might be less anxious around sick people but then one day you might, for some reason, feel a little more anxious. Don't worry about these minor setbacks. Persistent practice is what counts.

7. **Reward your efforts.** Remember your good reasons for overcoming your phobia. And take time to reward yourself for your efforts at overcoming your phobia. After all, working on phobias can require some effort. Reward yourself for accomplishing each of the small steps (e.g., congratulate yourself, treat yourself to something you enjoy).

safety behaviors can prevent dysfunctional (e.g., catastrophic) beliefs from being disconfirmed. Safety signals and behaviors are, therefore, important to eliminate from all kinds of exposure therapy. Thus, situational exposure is usually combined with some form of response prevention, such as the gradual discontinuation of using safety signals and safety behaviors. The following are ways of eliminating safety signals and safety behaviors during exposure and response prevention:

- *Identify obvious and subtle safety signals and behaviors.* Observe patients during exposure exercises and ask them whether they did anything to cope with the situation or to prevent something bad from happening. Different safety signals or safety behaviors may be used in different situations or on different occasions in the same situation, so the therapist needs to assess in detail what patients do during their exposure assignments.
- *Show patients the effects of safety signals and safety behaviors* by comparing what happens when they use versus don't use them.
- *Encourage patients to drop safety behaviors altogether*, and not to seek out or carry safety signals with them. Safety signals and safety behaviors can be gradually faded out over successive exposure trials.
- *Enlist, with the patient's permission, the assistance of significant others.* This involves reducing family reassurance giving (e.g., "Doctor's orders are that I don't give you reassurance. Let's change the topic and talk about something else"). It is often appropriate to discourage all health-related discussions between patient and family members because such discussions are often used for reassurance seeking.

To illustrate exposure plus response prevention, let's suppose that a person with a fear of contracting rabies is asked to handle puppies in a pet store without engaging in reassurance seeking from the store clerk about the health of the puppies, and without engaging afterward in bodily checking for "signs" of rabies. Guidelines about handwashing after handling the puppies would also be specified (e.g., washing only with soap and water for 1 minute).

The following cases illustrate exposure therapy defined primarily by the *withdrawal* of safety signals. For one patient with a phobia of contracting germs, exposure exercises involved her traveling increasingly greater distances from the "safety" of a hospital (to test, e.g., the idea that the patient is especially vulnerable to medical emergencies, such as a burst appendix). For other patients, exposure exercises involve them giving up or traveling without their portable safety signals. One medically healthy but health-anxious person wouldn't travel without his cellular telephone, which he carried "just in case" he had a medical emergency requiring ambulance assistance. Treatment involved traveling increasingly further distances from home without his telephone.

A Graded Approach

Exposure and response prevention typically proceeds up a hierarchy, beginning with the least fear-evoking stimulus. This is achieved by generating a list of fear stimuli and then rating the likely distress level that the patient would experience when exposed to them. Table 10.3 gives an example and shows how safety signals (i.e., protective gloves and a surgical mask) were used to create a fear hierarchy. Anxiety levels tend to be lower when safety signals are present. Accordingly, these can be gradually faded out over the course of exposure therapy as the patient works up the hierarchy. The goal is to eventually have the patient experience the phobic stimuli without relying on safety signals or safety behaviors.

    Successful therapy is indicated by reductions in anxiety within treatment sessions and between sessions (Foa & Kozak, 1986). When planning exposure plus response prevention exercises, the patient and the therapist should con-

TABLE 10.3. Exposure Hierarchy for Cancer Phobia, Introducing Situational Exposure (Cancer Stimuli) While Fading Safety Signals (Protective Gloves and Surgical Mask)

Exercise	Anxiety level (0 = none, 100 = extreme)
1. Looking at an illustrated medical article on cancer	15
2. Touching photos in the article, without wearing protective gloves	25
3. Sitting in the hospital waiting area, where cancer patients have been, while wearing protective gloves and a surgical mask	30
4. Touching the seats in the waiting area, without wearing gloves or a mask	40
5. Walking down a corridor in a cancer ward, while wearing gloves and a mask	45
6. Walking down the corridor with gloves but without a mask	50
7. Walking down the corridor without gloves and mask	55
8. Walking down the corridor and touching the signs on the doors (e.g., "Chemotherapy Clinic" sign), while wearing gloves (without mask)	65
9. Touching the signs without gloves or mask	70
10. Walking into the cancer ward, while wearing gloves and mask	75
11. Walking into the ward, with gloves but without the mask	78
12. Walking into the ward, without gloves and mask	82
13. Talking to a cancer patient on the ward, without gloves and mask	85
14. Touching a cancer patient on the hand, with gloves but no mask	90
15. Touching a cancer patient on the hand, without gloves or mask	100

sider the activities that can be performed in place of checking or reassurance seeking. What can the patient do instead? Diverting, practical activities are often best. Tania L. had an intense fear of contracting parasites, particularly scabies. She avoided busy downtown areas for fear that someone with scabies might brush up against her. Her exposure assignments involved traveling to these feared (but objectively harmless) locations, and then refraining from checking her body for lesions when she returned home. Tania and her therapist generated a list of activities that she could perform instead of checking. These included watching favorite TV programs, walking her dog, and talking on the telephone with friends. Tania found that these activities helped distract her from the urge to check. As she performed a number of exposure and response prevention exercises, she gradually became less anxious and more convinced that she was unlikely to contract scabies. Her urge to check her body correspondingly declined, to the point that she no longer needed to perform the substitute activities to help her "ride out" her urges to check.

To further help Tania resist urges to check her body, she was given strategies for managing itchy skin. Tania often focused on her skin sensations. She noticed itches, which she feared to be indication of scabies infestation. She scratched her skin so much that it became inflamed, which, in turn, worsened her itchiness. Tania was instructed to pat rather than scratch itchy skin areas so that inflammation would not occur (Salkovskis & Warwick, 1986). This intervention lessened her troublesome itchiness and also provided her with evidence that the skin sensations where largely a result of inflammation due to excessive scratching, rather than parasitic infestation (i.e., patting the skin would be of no help if the itching sensations were caused by parasites).

Graded Exposure versus Flooding

The advantage of using graded situational exposure is that it teaches patients a skill they can continue to use after finishing a course of CBT. That is, the use of a hierarchy teaches patients a structured, step-by-step method for overcoming seemingly insurmountable fears. After the formal course of treatment ends, patients can continue to devise hierarchies themselves for overcoming any remaining fears.

A disadvantage of graded situational exposure is that it can be time-consuming. If time is of the essence, then intensive exposure (i.e., "flooding") plus response prevention can be attempted. This involves situational exposure to stimuli at the very top of the patient's hierarchy (or hierarchies). Although quicker than graded exposure, intensive exposure does not teach patients a skill that they can readily use on their own. Patients often find it too distressing to put themselves through a self-directed program of flooding. A further concern is that patients may be more likely to refuse or to drop out of very intensive programs compared to less demanding programs.

Troubleshooting

If the patient finds situational exposure exercises to be too distressing, then this form of exposure can be preceded by any of a number of interventions. Cognitive restructuring (see Chapter 9) can be implemented beforehand to weaken patient beliefs about the dangerousness of the fear stimuli. Imaginal exposure (discussed below) also can be used to prepare the patient for exposure to real-life stimuli. Finally, relaxation training (see Chapter 11) can be used to reduce pre-exposure arousal, thereby making it easier for patients to complete situational exposure assignments.

If distress levels do not abate with exposure, then an assessment should be conducted to identify the source of the problem. One patient with cancer phobia performed a therapist-assisted exposure assignment in which she repeatedly walked along the corridor of a cancer ward. Her distress abated somewhat over trials within treatment sessions, but not between sessions. The therapist discovered that the patient was engaging in a number of subtle avoidance behaviors during exposure, such as holding her breath while walking down the corridor, so as not to inhale "cancer germs," and imagining herself wearing an invisible protective suit. Exposure trials were repeated, this time without the avoidance behaviors. This resulted in more complete exposure to the feared stimulus, and was associated with gradual reduction in patient distress within and between sessions.

Well-meaning but misguided efforts from people in the patient's life can also interfere with situational exposure. The spouse of a person with disease phobia might convey the message, "You'd better not do the exposure assignments; your health isn't strong enough." A well-meaning primary care physician might persist in reassuring the patient, even though exposure assignments require the fading of undue reassurance giving. These problems can be addressed by raising them with the patient. Then, with the patient's permission and involvement, the concerns can be discussed with all the relevant others. The latter can usually be persuaded to allow the patient to attempt a course of situational exposure (without reassurance), at least on a trial basis.

INTEROCEPTIVE EXPOSURE

Guidelines

Interoceptive exposure exercises, as illustrated in Table 10.4, are designed to induce feared bodily sensations. Exercises that induce a given sensation (e.g., palpitations) are used to test beliefs about that sensation (e.g., "a racing heart will bring on a stroke"). As the table suggests, interoceptive exposure exercises tend to be quite short, usually requiring a few minutes each. The

TABLE 10.4. Examples of Interoceptive Exposure Exercises

Exercise	Learning objective: The following sensations have no harmful consequences
Hyperventilate (1 minute)	Dizziness, dry mouth
Breathe through a narrow straw (2 minutes)	Shortness of breath
Hold breath for 30 seconds, exhaling beforehand	Chest tightness, shortness of breath
Breathe with chest muscles rather than diaphragm	Chest tightness
Swallow and then hold one's throat in "midswallow" (10 seconds)	Throat tightness, lump in throat
Swallow five times in quick succession	Throat tightness, lump in throat
Clear throat five times quickly	Sore throat
Place head between knees for 30 seconds and then lift head rapidly to an upright position	Lightheadedness
Drink hot coffee	Palpitations, sweating, hot flushes
Tense all muscles while sitting in a chair (1 minute)	Tension, trembling
Jog on the spot (2 minutes)	Palpitations, fatigue
Take aerobics class (30 minutes)	Palpitations, fatigue, sweating

exercises are usually practiced repeatedly in the therapy session and repeated as homework until corrective learning takes place. A patient might perform, for example, three trials of two of these exercises in a 60-minute treatment session (six trials in all), and then practice the six trials four times in the following week.

Commonplace but avoided physical activities can be used as naturalistic interoceptive exposure exercises. The patient might be encouraged to take part in an exercise program, such as cycling, jogging, aerobics, weight training, dancing classes, swimming classes, or water aerobics. These activities induce a variety of bodily sensations, such as palpitations and dyspnea. Water aerobics is useful for patients whose physical condition (e.g., joint diseases, lower back pain, severe obesity) prevents them from participating in other exercise programs. Exercise programs not only disconfirm catastrophic beliefs (e.g., "My lungs are weak"), but also are very useful for testing the noncatastrophic alternative that the feared sensations are due to a lack of physical fitness (e.g., "I'm short of breath because I'm out of shape"). As the patient's fear of bodily sensations abates, her or his preoccupation with these sensations should also diminish. In other words, the patient becomes less likely to notice the sensations. This is a beneficial side effect for patients who regard their heightened awareness of sensations as evidence that there is something seriously wrong with them.

The distinction between naturalistic interoceptive exposure and situational exposure is arbitrary but clinically useful. Both entail some degree of exposure to bodily sensations. They differ in the intent of the exercise and, to some degree, in the nature of the experience. *Interoceptive exposure* is designed to induce intense bodily sensations. *Situational exposure* emphasizes encounters with situations that are feared and avoided, regardless of whether the situations induce intense sensations. The distinction between the two types of exposure is useful to underscore the fact that it is important to reduce patient's fear and avoidance of situations and bodily sensations.

The choice of exercise depends on which sensations are feared the most. The following is a protocol for conducting interoceptive exposure exercises:

- Identify a dysfunctional (e.g., catastrophic) belief that appears to contribute to the patient's health anxiety.
- In collaboration with the patient, generate an alternative belief statement that is plausible and noncatastrophic.
- Rate the strength of the dysfunctional and alternative beliefs on a 0–100 scale, ranging from 0 = do not believe that _____ is true, to 100 = completely believe that _____ is true.
- The therapist and the patient select an interoceptive exercise (e.g., from Table 10.4) that will test predictions arising from the dysfunctional belief and its noncatastrophic alternative.
- Two predictions are set up. One prediction, based on the patient's dysfunctional belief, is that there will be a catastrophic outcome (e.g., physical collapse). The other prediction, based on the noncatastrophic alternative, is that the outcome will be harmless.
- The chosen exercise is initially performed in the therapist's office. The duration of the exercise is determined, in part, on what the patient thinks she or he is able to do. Ask the patient to rate her or his confidence about performing the task for the required duration (0 = not at all confident, 100 = completely confident). To ensure the task is performed, select a duration that has an 80 or higher confidence rating.
- The therapist demonstrates (i.e., models) the task and describes what sensations were experienced. This shows the patient that he or she is safe. As a rationale, the therapist might tell the patient, "I wouldn't ask you to do something that I wouldn't do myself, so I'm going to show you how this exercise is done."
- The patient performs the task, attempting to make the sensations as intense as possible.
- The therapist and the patient discuss whether the exercise induced the

feared sensations, and then they review whether the outcome supported the prediction from the dysfunctional belief or its noncatastrophic alternative. Ratings of belief strength are also obtained. If the strength of the dysfunctional belief remains high, and if the patient believes the exercise didn't represent a strong test, then the patient and the therapist review why this was so. The therapist should look for safety signals and safety behaviors that might have undermined the exercise.

- Repeat the exposure exercises as often as needed, increasing the "difficulty" level with each successive trial. Difficulty can be raised by increasing the duration or intensity of the exercise, and by successively eliminating safety signals and safety behaviors.
- Assign the exposure exercise or a similar task as homework.
- Look for opportunities for introducing naturalistic interoceptive exposures that test the same beliefs (i.e., build in generalization).
- Encourage patients to chart their progress in terms of tasks completed and reactions to those tasks. Review these records with the patient during therapy sessions.

To illustrate interoceptive exposure, let's suppose that a patient named Rose B. worried that she had throat cancer. She attempted to check for "tumors" by repeatedly swallowing to see whether her throat was constricted. This induced globus (i.e., the sensation of a lump in the throat), which she took as evidence of cancer. The therapist and Rose contrasted two beliefs: "The lump in my throat is evidence of cancer" and "The lump in my throat is due to excessive checking [i.e., swallowing]." Rose was then asked to swallow repeatedly, thereby inducing the frightening lump in her throat. This sensation abated shortly after she stopped the exercise. Rose realized that she was inducing the feared sensation, rather than it being caused by cancer. By repeatedly inducing globus she also gradually became less distressed by throat sensations and thus experienced less of a need to check her throat.

Troubleshooting

Patients sometimes refuse to perform interoceptive exposure exercises or distract themselves during the exercises. Other avoidance behaviors involve limiting the intensity or duration of exposure. For example, a patient might avoid deep, rapid breathing during a hyperventilation exercise, and may stop the task as soon as any sensations are noticed. The best strategy for dealing with adherence problems is to limit the chances that they will occur. Ensure that patients know why the exercises are being performed, and periodically check their understanding. Ensure that the patient understands that the selection of exercises is a collaborative venture, negotiated between therapist and patient.

The exercises can be readily modified in such a way that the patient can perform them. If the patient is too frightened to hyperventilate for 1 minute, for example, then a shorter duration can be used. Adherence can be maintained at an adequate level if the patient is sufficiently motivated to complete the various treatment exercises. To sustain motivation, the therapist can reinforce (e.g., verbally praise) the patient for her or his efforts in completing each therapy assignment, and encourage the patient to self-reinforce for these efforts (e.g., praising oneself or using other incentives). Initially, reinforcement from the therapist may occur frequently. As therapy progresses, reinforcement from the therapist can be faded out as the patient continues to use self-reinforcement.

If patient adherence continues to be poor, then consider whether the exercises are credible tests of the patient's beliefs. If not, then the patient may regard the tasks as pointless. Is the timing right for interoceptive exposure? More sessions may need to be spent on developing a trusting therapeutic relationship. Also, more time may be needed for cognitive restructuring to address beliefs about the exercises and beliefs about the sensations they induce. If the patient is using safety signals or safety behaviors, then a hierarchy can be constructed, where the sources of safety are gradually faded out.

Interoceptive exposure exercises provide the patient with particularly powerful disconfirmatory evidence when the exercises are used to bring on the things the patient fears—for example, jogging on the spot to test the patient's belief that palpitations will lead to a heart attack, voluntary hyperventilation to test the patient's belief that dizziness will lead to physical collapse, or weight training to test the patient's idea that muscle "overuse" will lead to physical degeneration. In some cases, however, it is difficult to devise interoceptive exercises that disprove the patient's dysfunctional beliefs. If this problem arises, then therapy can focus primarily on collecting evidence to support an innocuous interpretation of the feared bodily changes or sensations (Wells, 1997). This process might entail collecting information for the roles of stress, selective attention, and bodily checking.

IMAGINAL EXPOSURE

Guidelines

In the previous chapter we discussed how imaginal methods are used to facilitate cognitive restructuring. Imaginal interventions can also be used for the purpose of exposure, to reduce disease-related fears. Imaginal exposure can be used to treat fears of stimuli that cannot be readily procured (e.g., imaginal exposure to people with leprosy for someone with a phobia of this disease). Imaginal exposure also plays an important role in treating death-related fears (e.g., imaginal exposure to death scenarios).

Imaginal exposure can be conducted in a variety of ways. The patient could narrate a detailed description of the feared stimulus into a tape recorder, and repeatedly listen to the recording until it no longer evokes anxiety. Alternatively, the patient could produce a detailed written description of the feared stimulus, and then read the description over and over until it is no longer upsetting. Such descriptions are more effective if written by hand, rather than typed, because patients can be distracted from the fear-evoking content by the mechanics of typing (e.g., selecting font size, spell-checking, formatting). Written descriptions should be produced without concern for spelling or grammar.

The patient should try to imagine all the components of the feared situation as vividly as possible, including visual, auditory, olfactory, and somatic stimuli, and the thoughts, behaviors, and feelings imagined to occur in the situation. As with other forms of exposure, 0–100 anxiety ratings can be obtained to assess whether the exposure is evoking distress, and whether within- and between-session habituation is occurring.

Imaginal exposure scripts can be constructed hierarchically, beginning with mildly distressing scenarios and progressing to more upsetting ones. Understanding the most distressing aspects of the fear stimulus can facilitate imaginal exposure. People with fears of contracting disease are often frightened of consulting their primary care physician because of concern that their worst fears might be confirmed (e.g., "He'll tell me that I have cancer"). Imaginal exposure is most comprehensive when all the fears are addressed. Therefore, we encourage patients to imagine the worst possible consequences of the feared disease.

Medical texts can be used to develop sufficiently vivid material for imaginal exposure scripts. Tania L., whom we met earlier in this chapter, had a fear of being infested with parasites, particularly scabies. After her fear of scabies was reduced by situational exposure, her other parasitic fears were addressed, beginning with her fear of consuming parasite-infested meat. Imaginal exposure was used to expose her to the scenario of actually being infested. Tania was asked to read the following description from a medical dictionary:

Trichinosis: The disease induced by larvae of the trichina worm, *Trichinella spiralis*, usually acquired through ingestion of raw or insufficiently cooked meat, especially pork, infected with the worm. It is divided into three phases corresponding to periods in the life cycle of the worm. The intestinal phase occupies the time of growth and maturation of the larvae from the initial infection, and is marked by intestinal disturbance, nausea, pain, and diarrhea. The blood-migratory and muscle-penetration phase, during the migration of larvae from the next generation of worms, is characterized by fever, sweating, malaise, high eosinophilia, intense muscle pain, and rheumatic aches, usually preceded by puffiness around the eyes. Death from toxemia, respiratory distress, or other effect may occur during this phase." (Churchill Livingstone Inc., 1989, p. 1986)

This information was used to develop a detailed imaginal exposure script. Tania read, into a tape recorder, a description of becoming infected herself with the trichina worm. Her narration included all the symptoms, along with descriptions of the larvae growing inside her, leading to sickness and death. She listened to the narrative on several occasions until her fear subsided. Situational exposure (eating pork, properly cooked) was used to supplement imaginal exposure.

Death-Related Fears

Imaginal exposure can reduce death-related fears (Peal, Handal, & Gilner, 1985). The goal is not to be happy about death, but to be able to face it without excessive fear—to enjoy one's life rather than squandering it on worry. The therapist conveys the expectation that most people are able to come to terms with the inevitability of their own demise (Furer & Walker, 2000). Imaginal exposure can involve images of death, the process of dying, and whatever aftermath the patient fears. Imaginal exposure is commonly combined with situational exposure (e.g., Furer & Walker, 2000; Kalish, 1985). A treatment package of imaginal and situational exposure, for example, could involve the following exercises:

- Write a detailed description of your death, including the process of dying and whatever aftermath you fear.
- Read the obituary section of a local newspaper.
- Imagine that yesterday you died. Write your obituary for a newspaper.
- Prepare a will.
- Obtain information about the type, availability, and cost of funeral services; this will involve visits to funeral homes.
- Visit cemeteries and read inscriptions on the headstones.
- Visit an art gallery or museum to observe all the ways that death and dying are depicted.

Some patients may object that they are already confronting their fears of death because they are "constantly" worrying about their demise. Worry differs from therapeutic exposure because worry episodes tend to be brief, interspersed with efforts at distraction, and coupled with checking and reassurance seeking. Worries can be converted into therapeutic exposure by increasing the uninterrupted duration of worry (e.g., to 20–30 minutes) and by eliminating safety behaviors such as reassurance seeking.

Troubleshooting

For imaginal exposure to be effective the patient must be able to imagine the feared stimuli with sufficient vividness for some degree of anxiety to be evoked. If the patient reports that the image is not vivid, then a more evocative script can be developed, one that contains vivid descriptions of the sensory and other elements of the feared stimuli. Vividness may also be improved by changing the modality of exposure. Patients who have trouble imagining stimuli in one modality (e.g., listening to a narrated tape recording) may do better with another modality (e.g., reading a written description).

If imagery abilities are sufficient but the image does not evoke much distress, then the therapist might ask the patient to imagine an exaggerated version of the feared consequence. This approach, known as *implosion*, has proved successful in several studies (O'Donnell, 1978; Tearnan et al., 1985), and is worth considering when lesser approaches prove unsuccessful. Implosion can lead patients to conclude that their fears are exaggerated. O'Donnell's (1978) case study of the treatment of cancer phobia illustrates this type of imaginal exposure:

> A 30-minute implosive segment . . . began by suggesting the subjective sensations of tumor-like growths developing throughout critical bodily areas of fearful concern. Each growth was graphically described and presented in terms of a loathsome appearance, smell, texture, and taste. A process of bodily deterioration and a gradual transformation from a person into one large, massive tumor was vividly described. All throughout her miserable ordeal, the client was told to envision family physicians, and friends, shrinking away in horror at her monstrous grotesqueness. Everyone refused to attend to her in her misery, and she was "abandoned by everyone for months-on-end to die a long, drawn-out, excruciatingly painful, and lonely death." Even death itself brought no relief however; and she was "forced to go through an eternity as a pulsating, writhing mass of detestable putrescence." (p. 10)

ADDING COGNITIVE INTERVENTIONS TO BEHAVIORAL EXERCISES

Cognitive interventions (see Chapter 9) can be used before, during, and after all types of behavioral exercises. When used for preparatory purposes, cognitive interventions are used (1) to help the patient make specific predictions for the forthcoming exposure, and (2) to help manage anticipatory anxiety (e.g., "This exposure exercise is short-term pain for long-term gain").

When implemented during exposure, cognitive interventions can be used in the form of coping statements or self-instructions (e.g., "Just let the fear happen, don't try to fight it"). Patients often have difficulty thinking clearly when distressed, so the coping statements or instructions should be written down. If coping statements distract the patient from the task at hand, then she or he should simply observe the fear-evoking stimuli, without resorting to coping statements or self-instructions. However, an important exception is when the patient is on the brink of fleeing from the feared situation. The point of escape can be used as a cue for using self-instructions to help the patient remain in the situation (e.g., "If I'm about to leave I must be predicting something awful will occur. I'll stay here for another minute to see what happens").

When used after a behavioral exercise, cognitive interventions can help patients objectively examine the outcome of the exercise. The patient might take a belief such as "I failed at the assignment" and reframe it in a more adaptive fashion: "I didn't stay in the graveyard for as long as we planned, but at least I tried. I can learn from this experience so I can do better next time." Postexposure cognitive interventions also can help patients review the evidence for and against their dysfunctional beliefs and the noncatastrophic alternatives, and can be used for planning future exposure assignments (e.g., "What do you think would have happened if you'd stayed in the graveyard longer?"). If the patient attributed the absence of catastrophe to a "lucky escape" from some health threat (e.g., germs), then a more rigorous exposure exercise could be devised.

SUMMARY AND CONCLUSIONS

There are several related forms of behavioral exercises, including behavioral experiments, situational exposure, interoceptive exposure, and imaginal exposure. All are methods for changing dysfunctional beliefs. Behavioral methods are used in treating fears of acquiring diseases and fears that one actually has a disease. Behavioral exercises can be fruitfully combined with one another, as in the case where imaginal exposure is used to prepare patients for situational exposure. Behavioral methods also can be integrated with cognitive interventions. This combination forms, in our view, the key ingredients for treating health anxiety disorders.

11

Stress Management

WHY STRESS MANAGEMENT?

Stress can be defined as the process of dealing with things that make demands on the person's coping ability (Lazarus, 1966). Stress reactions include emotional distress and the various bodily reactions listed in Handout 11.1 (Davis, Eshelman, & McKay, 2000; Hambly & Muir, 1997). Stress reactions occur when the demands placed on the person tax or exceed his or her resources for dealing with those demands. In this chapter we describe the stress management procedures that are useful for reducing health anxiety: psychoeducation for stress management, applied relaxation training, breathing retraining, a general approach to problem solving, and time management techniques.

Although there are many books on stress management, we devote a chapter to this topic so as to provide the reader with a complete set of resources, within a single volume, for treating health anxiety. Our approach to stress management is based on, but expanded from, Clark et al.'s (1998) behavioral stress management program. Unlike Clark's research protocol, our approach integrates stress management with cognition-behavioral therapy (CBT) for health anxiety, where stress management plays an adjunctive role.

Stress management techniques can supplement cognitive restructuring exercises by helping health-anxious patients learn about whether their feared bodily changes or sensations are stress reactions. Stress management can also reduce the person's anxious arousal, and can thereby make it easier for people with disease-related fears to complete behavioral assignments in which they are exposed to distressing disease cues. Some stress management methods, such as problem–solving strategies, can be used to help patients plan how they can work on and overcome disease fears and other facets of health anxiety.

COMMON STRESS-RELATED BODILY REACTIONS

Stressors, big and small, can produce bodily reactions. Sometimes these reactions happen while you are experiencing a stressful event, and sometimes they occur later on. The following is a list of some of the common stress-related bodily reactions. Not all of these sensations occur together; people typically experience one or two (or sometimes more) of these sensations during times of stress. Circle the ones that you have experienced in the past week.

Muscle spasms	Stomach cramps
Chest pain	Nausea
Feeling restless or fidgety	Indigestion
Fatigue	Stomach churning
Headache	Diarrhea
Neck pain	Frequent need to urinate
Chest tightness	Difficulty swallowing
Leg cramps	Weight gain
Back ache	Weight loss
Aches and pains	Heart thumping
Trembling	Heart racing
Difficulty taking a deep breath	Heart skipping a beat
Tingling in the feet or hands	Dry mouth
Muscle twitches	Dizziness
Hot flashes	Feeling light-headed
Sweating	Insomnia

The focus of stress management differs in an important way from the foci of the cognitive and behavioral methods discussed in previous chapters. Stress management is aimed at reducing emotional distress and concomitant bodily reactions, including many of the bodily changes and sensations feared by health-anxious people. Changes in health-related beliefs are secondary consequences. In comparison to stress management, the cognitive and behavioral methods described in Chapters 9 and 10 are aimed primarily at weakening or eliminating dysfunctional beliefs and strengthening adaptive beliefs. Reduction in bodily reactions is not the primary aim of the cognitive and behavioral methods, although the frequency of stress-related bodily changes or sensations typically declines as the person becomes less anxious about her or his health.

Stress management methods can be useful as a treatment engagement strategy for patients who are willing to accept the notion that some of their troublesome bodily sensations are stress-related. Some health-anxious people may recognize that they have emotional distress that merits stress management—while insisting that it bears no causal relation to their somatic complaints—whereas other health-anxious people will accept stress management because they believe that stress adversely affects their health (Barsky, 2001).

Stress management also can be helpful in simultaneously treating health anxiety and comorbid disorders, such as comorbid generalized anxiety disorder, panic disorder, chronic headaches, or irritable bowel syndrome (IBS). This is because stress management interventions such as applied relaxation are broad in their effects, influencing health anxiety and other anxiety- or arousal-related phenomena.

CAVEATS

Stress management methods should be implemented with care when treating health anxiety disorders. If improperly applied, patients may use these methods as ways of avoiding frightening bodily changes or sensations. A person with concerns about his heart would be misusing relaxation exercises if he were using the exercise to avoid rapid heart beat. A person with tension headaches would be misusing time management strategies if she was using these interventions to avoid "nerve damage" that she believed to be caused by the headaches. In these cases the stress management methods are misused as ways of avoiding feared bodily sensations, and so they do not help the person learn that the sensations are not indications of danger to one's health. If stress management methods are used with health-anxious patients, the therapist should emphasize that the methods are intended to reduce unpleasant but harmless bodily reactions. If a patient persistently worries about the harmful effects of stress on the body, then cognitive restructuring may be needed before any stress management exercises are implemented. Restructuring would focus on the patient's beliefs about the dangerousness of stress. The patient might be asked to consider whether it is helpful to continually worry about the effects of stress. Patients can typically recognize that worrying about stress makes them feel more distressed and is therefore self-defeating.

SELECTION AND TIMING OF INTERVENTIONS

The choice of stress management method depends on the principal sources of stress in the patient's life. If poor time management appears to be the main source of difficulties, then time management skills would be implemented. If the person is especially reactive to stressors, as indicated by readily induced bodily reactions to even minor stressors, then cognitive restructuring could be used (aimed at beliefs about the stressors) or applied relaxation could be implemented.

There are a variety of ways in which stress management interventions can be combined with other interventions for health anxiety. One can begin with a course of, say, 12 sessions of CBT for health anxiety followed, as necessary, by several sessions of stress management. This sequential approach has two advantages. First, the initial focus on reducing health anxiety beliefs helps underscore the message that the feared bodily changes or sensations are due to some major disease. Second, CBT for health anxiety often reduces the frequency and intensity of arousal-related bodily reactions, thereby obviating the need for stress management.

An alternative approach is that stress management can be introduced in the same sessions in which other health anxiety interventions are used. The first half of a session could be devoted to relaxation training, for example, and the later half could involve some form of exposure exercise. This integrated approach can be especially useful for people with comorbid disorders. A person with a fear of contracting cancer and comorbid IBS, for instance, might have difficulty with cancer-related exposure exercises because these exercises are distressing and therefore can exacerbate IBS. Relaxation exercises, implemented prior to exposures (so as to reduce anticipatory anxiety) can reduce this problem, and more generally can alleviate symptoms of IBS (Blanchard, 2001).

PSYCHOEDUCATION FOR STRESS MANAGEMENT

Psychoeducation about stressors and stress reactions is an extension of the psychoeducational strategies discussed in earlier chapters. Patients are given Handout 11.1, which illustrates common stress-related bodily reactions, and asked to circle those they have experienced in the past week. It is not uncommon for health-anxious people, particularly those with full-blown hypochondriasis, to resist the idea that their bodily complaints are due to stress. And the bodily reactions listed in the handout can be caused by things other than stress. Monitoring the occurrence of stressors and bodily reactions can be used to collect information on which reactions are likely to be stress-related. The therapist can underscore the value of examining the notion that stress is an important cause.

PATIENT: I don't see how my digestion troubles could be due to stress. My friend had the same problems and it turned out to be stomach cancer.

THERAPIST: It sounds like you're reluctant to accept the idea that stress could be a source of your troubles. Are you saying that it's impossible that stress could be involved?

PATIENT: Well, I wouldn't go that far.

THERAPIST: OK. Then imagine for a moment that your stomach problems are due to stress and not stomach cancer. How would that make you feel?

PATIENT: It wouldn't be as bad. Stomach cancer is deadly.

THERAPIST: So maybe we can collect some information to see if stress is relevant. And if it is, then stress management could help you deal with your problems.

It is not unusual for people to overlook the many stressors in their lives, and thereby to underestimate the role of stressors in producing unwanted bodily changes or sensations. To educate patients about stressors, they can be asked to read Handout 11.2, and to circle the stressors that they had experienced in the past week. The handout lists many minor stressors (also known as "hassles") that are common sources of bodily reactions (DeLongis, Folkman, & Lazarus, 1988). The list of stressors has been compiled from a number of sources (Hambly & Muir, 1997; Lazarus & Folkman, 1989; Seaward, 1997; Zalaquett & Wood, 1997). Once the patient completes Handouts 11.1 and 11.2, he or she can be asked to consider whether there are any links between stressors and bodily reactions.

To further help the patient and the therapist to examine the effects of stress, the patient can be asked to keep a daily record of stressors and bodily reactions, using Handout 11.3. The records can be completed for 2 or more weeks to see whether stressors and bodily reactions are correlated. Bodily reactions can occur during the stressor (e.g., trembling and nausea during a

COMMON STRESSORS

Stress is a fact of life, although people commonly fail to recognize how it affects them. This is because stressors are often minor irritants or hassles. When hassles do occur, people often experience stress-related bodily reactions. This is especially likely when many stressors occur at the same time or in succession. The following are some common stressors. Circle the ones that you experienced in the past week.

Household
  Difficulty arranging child care
  Too many household chores
  Shopping problems
  Crowded living space
  Difficulties with home maintenance
  Misplacing or losing things
  Conflicts with partner or children
  Divorce or separation
  Car trouble

Social
  Too few friends
  Feeling isolated
  Friends or relatives living too far away
  Arguments with friends
  Dating problems
  Unwanted social obligations

Neighborhood and environment
  Weather (e.g., too hot, too cold, too humid)
  Things that you are allergic to
  Pollution
  Crime
  Traffic
  Commuting
  Noise
  Waiting lines
  Neighborhood crowding
  Troublesome neighbors
  Inconsiderate smokers
  Parking problems
  Problems with other drivers

(continued)

Neighborhood and environment (cont.)
   Discrimination or harassment
   Disturbing news stories

Work
   Difficult duties
   Inadequate training
   Lack of a clear job description
   Lack of appreciation
   No avenue to voice concerns
   Insufficient resources
   Boring job
   Doing job below level of competence
   Concerns about shift work
   Insufficient backup
   Long work hours
   A lot of responsibility with little or no authority
   Unrealistic deadlines or expectations
   Conflict with coworkers
   Incompetent colleagues
   Hassles from boss
   Problems with supervisees
   Staff shortages
   Difficult clients
   Computer problems (hardware or software)
   Difficulty keeping up with technological developments
   Poor promotional prospects
   Unpleasant working conditions (e.g., noisy, dirty, no privacy, cramped)
   Too much travel (e.g., to meetings)
   Lack of work boundaries (i.e., being contacted after hours by e-mail, phone, or pager)
   Corporate downsizing, restructuring, or job relocation
   Workplace violence
   Lack of job security
   Unemployment

School or university
   Conflicts with roommates
   Conflicts with other students or instructors
   Academic deadlines
   Difficult or boring courses
   Too much schoolwork
   Concerns about career path
   Financial problems (e.g., problems with student loans)
   Budgeting problems

(continued)

Finances
  Debts
  Credit problems
  Lack of money to pay bills
  Insufficient money for recreational activities (e.g., movies)
  Problems with taxes
  Retirement concerns
  Auto payments

Time pressures
  Too much to do
  Too little to do
  Too many interruptions
  Insufficient time for recreation
  Too many meetings
  Too many responsibilities

Health
  Physical illness
  Physical disability
  Concerns with medical treatment
  Treatment side effects
  Concerns about physical appearance
  Overweight
  Underweight
  Sexual problems

Inner concerns
  Inability to express oneself
  Conflicts about life choices (e.g., career, choice of dating partner)
  Too much time on one's hands
  Concerns about the meaning of life
  Too little sleep

Legal
  Parking tickets
  Speeding fines
  Other legal problems

Other stressors in your life (please list)

_____

_____

_____

_____

_____

_____

HANDOUT 11.3. Form for Monitoring Stressors and Bodily Reactions

STRESS AND BODILY REACTIONS DIARY

Instructions: Record any stressful experiences, even minor ones, that you experience, and also record any bodily reactions that you notice. The sensations need not occur at the same time as the stressors.

EXAMPLE:

Date	Time	Stressful event	Bodily reactions
2/20/04	Morning Afternoon Evening	Fight with spouse Caught in traffic jam	Flushed face, rapid heartbeat Upset stomach, headache

YOUR DIARY:

Date	Time	Stressful event	Bodily reactions
	Morning Afternoon Evening		
	Morning Afternoon Evening		
	Morning Afternoon Evening		
	Morning Afternoon Evening		
	Morning Afternoon Evening		

stressful business meeting) or some time afterward (e.g., headaches after a difficult day of child care).

> Robert G. has been preoccupied with his bodily temperature for several months, after a bout of influenza had spread through his office complex. Since then, Robert worried constantly about feeling "feverish." He often felt hot, flushed, and sweaty during the day, which he interpreted as indications of viral infection. Self-monitoring, however, revealed that he was most likely to experience the unwelcome sensations at times of stress, such as when he was working on projects with tight deadlines. The sensations were unlikely to occur when the work pace had lessened, such as on "casual Fridays," or when he was relaxing after work. This pattern was inconsistent with a viral infection. The results of the monitoring helped Robert realize that he was periodically stressed rather than "feverish."

The effects of stressors can be cumulative, with a succession of minor irritants gradually giving rise to unpleasant bodily reactions. Cathy B. was late for a morning meeting because she was stuck in traffic, and then had to rush to the school to take her ill son to the doctor. Parking was difficult to find and she had to wait for 45 minutes in the doctor's waiting room with her sick, complaining child. As a result of the day's stressors, Cathy's heart was racing, her face was hot and flushed, and her chest felt tight by the time she got home.

Once the patient understands the relationship between stressors and bodily reactions, the therapist can provide information about the types of stress management interventions that may be useful. The interventions fall into four main classes, depending on the nature of the problem:

1. Modifying the stressor, if possible—for example, through training in time management to better deal with workload requirements.
2. Changing how the person appraises the stressor, using cognitive restructuring. This would be used if dysfunctional beliefs appear to be playing a role in the person's reaction to stress (e.g., misinterpreting minor stressors as catastrophes).
3. Buffering the effects of stress with exercises aimed at directly reducing arousal and related bodily sensations (e.g., relaxation training, breathing retraining).
4. Reducing or eliminating the use of self-defeating stress management strategies, such as overeating or excessive use of alcohol to reduce distress. These strategies can reduce stress-related arousal in the short term, but create problems in the longer term.

APPLIED RELAXATION

Applied relaxation (Öst, 1987) consists of exercises to help the patient rapidly relax in a variety of situations, particularly stressful circumstances. It is among the most effective and versatile relaxation programs (Öst, 1987; Taylor, 2000). It typically requires several weeks of practice for patients to become proficient at all the components of the program. The full package consists of six exercises:

1. Progressive muscle relaxation (tense–release relaxation).
2. Release-only relaxation.
3. Cue-controlled relaxation (pairing the word "relax" with a state of relaxation).
4. Differential relaxation (relaxing some muscle groups while others remain tensed—e.g., standing up while relaxing all muscles except those required to remain upright).
5. Rapid relaxation (a brief exercise for quickly relaxing, practiced in calm settings).
6. Application training (practicing rapid relaxation in stressful situations).

Abbreviated forms of applied relaxation are often used (e.g., Davis et al., 2000), in which applied relaxation is taught along with other stress management strategies, in as few as three weekly sessions (along with several weeks of homework practice). Our abbreviated protocol involves combining some of the steps. Steps 2 and 3 are combined by using the cue word "relax" throughout release-only relaxation. Steps 4–6 are also combined. That is, patients practice rapid relaxation in the therapist's office under increasingly more active conditions. Patients initially practice a few trials of rapid relaxation while sitting in a comfortable chair, then practice while standing up, and then while walking about, and so on. Homework exercises involve practicing rapid relaxation in both calm and stressful situations. In summary, our version of applied relaxation consists of three exercises: tense–release relaxation, release-only relaxation, and rapid relaxation.

Applied relaxation begins by educating patients that its purpose is to teach a coping skill to enable them to recognize the early signs of arousal, and then to relax rapidly in order to reduce harmless but unpleasant stress-related bodily reactions. The goal is to relax within 20–30 seconds. The protocol is summarized in Handout 11.4. The handout is supplemented by an audiotape, recorded by the therapist specifically for a given patient, in which the therapist goes through each of the exercises.

The patient listens to the tape as a homework assignment. The audiotape is particularly useful in guiding the patient through the early stages of practic-

APPLIED RELAXATION

1. What Is Applied Relaxation?

Applied relaxation (AR) is a portable skill that helps you recognize and overcome the effects of stress, including tension, pain, and a host of other bodily reactions (please see the handout "Common Stress-Related Bodily Reactions" [Handout 11.1]). Just like any other skill, such as learning to play the piano or drive a car, AR requires practice in order to become good at implementing the relaxation exercises. Your therapist will help you by making a relaxation tape for you to listen to. With sufficient practice, you will be able to implement the AR exercises rapidly in practically any situation. The goal is to be able to relax in 20–30 seconds. To achieve this goal, follow these steps:

- *Tense–release relaxation*: Practice tensing and relaxing various muscle groups. Each muscle group is tensed for a brief period and then relaxed. The purpose is to increase your awareness of muscle tension, and to enhance relaxation from the inertia built up by tensing then releasing. The entire exercise takes about 15 minutes. After that, we will begin to shorten the procedure to develop more portable relaxation skills. We do this by working through the following exercises:
- *Release-only relaxation*: This is the same as the above but without tensing the muscles first. This takes 10 minutes. During this exercise we teach you to connect the self-instruction "relax" to the bodily state of relaxation.
- *Rapid relaxation*: You will be asked to practice a quick relaxation exercise many times each day in nonstressful situations. This also involves practicing relaxation while doing various activities, such as walking. You will then be asked to practice rapid relaxation in daily stressful situations.

Please be aware that when you first begin to use AR, you probably won't become very relaxed. Don't give up! With practice you will get better and better at relaxing.

2. Tense–Release Relaxation

Duration: 15 minutes

Instructions: (1) Sit in a comfortable position, free from distractions. (2) Close your eyes and scan your body, looking for areas of muscle tension. Attempt to "let go" of any tension. (3) Work through each of the following muscle groups, tensing them for 5 seconds and then relaxing for 10–15 seconds. Work through each muscle group twice. This will be easier to do if you follow the relaxation tape recorded by your therapist.

(continued)

Muscle group	Activity
Fingers and hands	Clench each hand into a fist, one hand at a time
Wrists and forearms	Bend wrists back toward forearms
Biceps	Tense both biceps ("Strong Man" act)
Shoulders	Hunch shoulders
Forehead	Raise eyebrows and then frown
Eyes	Squint eyes
Jaw	Jut lower jaw outward
Tongue	Push tongue against roof of mouth
Throat	Yawn
Neck	Gently rotate neck left, right, back, and then forward
Chest	Take a deep breath and then slowly exhale
Chest and upper back	Pull shoulders back and push chest outward
Abdomen	Push out stomach and then suck it all the way in
Lower back	Arch lower back
Thighs and legs - I	Knees locked, feet pointing upward
Thighs and legs - II	Knees locked, feet pointing down
Toes and feet - I	Toes curled down
Toes and feet - II	Toes curled upward

3. Release-Only Relaxation

Duration: 10 minutes, twice per day.

Instructions: (1) Sit in a comfortable position, free from distractions. (2) Close your eyes and scan your body, looking for areas of muscle tension. Attempt to "let go" of any tension. (3) Go over each of your muscle groups and focus on relaxing them—your face, chest, arms, hands, stomach, legs, feet—while continuing to say "relax" each time you breathe out. Do this for about 5 minutes. (4) Say to yourself, under your breath, the word "inhale" each time you breathe in, and the word "relax" each time you breathe out. Continue this for about 5 minutes.

4. Rapid Relaxation

Duration: 20–30 seconds, about 20 times each day.

Instructions: (1) Take three slow, deep breaths, thinking to yourself "inhale" as you breathe in and "relax" as you breathe out. Remember to breathe in slowly, and let the air out slowly. (2) As you do this, let go of as much muscle tension as you can. (3) Practice doing activities, such as standing or walking, while letting go of all the muscle tension that is not involved in these activities. For example if you are standing, you can relax the muscles in your face, shoulders, and stomach. (4) Practice relaxing in your daily life, initially in calm situations and then in increasingly more challenging circumstances (e.g., while taking a stressful phone call). Use reminders to prompt yourself to practice Rapid Relaxation. For example, a Post-it note on the dash of your car or on your computer monitor at work might contain the message "Practice RR every 30 minutes." Similarly, you could place a colored dot on your wristwatch or telephone. Every time you used the phone or looked at your watch, the dot would remind you to practice Rapid Relaxation.

ing tense–release and release-only relaxation. The tape is eventually faded out in order to encourage the patient to implement self-directed relaxation, without having to rely on an audiotape. Clinically, we have found that applied relaxation can be taught in three weekly sessions. Patients then practice the exercises for several weeks until they become proficient at relaxing. Then the exercises are used as needed. Details of the relaxation procedures are described in the following sections.

Tense–Release Relaxation

This exercise involves working through various muscle groups, as described in Handout 11.4. The exercise can be practiced in a comfortable chair. Each muscle group is tensed for 5 seconds and then relaxed for 5–15 seconds. Muscle tensing and releasing is used to deepen relaxation and to sharpen the patient's ability to identify the difference between tension and relaxation. The better the ability to detect tension, the greater the chances of implementing relaxation when tension develops. Otherwise, tension may build up, undetected, until it become so intense that it produces headaches, muscle cramps, or related problems.

The goal of the tense–release relaxation is not to tense the muscles until they hurt. If pain or cramps occur—or if the patient has a history of some sort of recurrent pain (e.g., low back pain)—then the afflicted muscles should be weakly tensed or not tensed at all. People wearing contact lenses should be instructed not to tightly squint their eyes.

Tense–release relaxation begins by having the patient work through all the muscle groups (Handout 11.4) during the therapy session and as homework. Then the patient practices by relaxing more rapidly by using fewer and fewer muscle groups. The assumption is that relaxation will spread to the remaining groups.

Homework consists of practicing for 15–30 minutes, twice per day, for at least 2 weeks. As with other relaxation methods, the exercises can be audiotaped to facilitate homework practice. The audiotape is then faded out as the patient learns to relax without the tape. The importance of regular practice is emphasized.

Release-Only Relaxation

The next step is to repeat the protocol for tense–release relaxation, but this time omitting the tensing portion of the exercise. Patients are simply asked to focus on releasing tension from the various muscle groups, starting at the top of the head and working down to the toes. If patients notice tension in a particular muscle group, then they can briefly tense and release those muscles. As before, the exercise is practiced in the session and as homework. The latter should be done twice per day for at least a week. The protocol can be audiotaped to facilitate practice, and then the tape is faded out. The following is a sample script of release-only relaxation, which the therapist uses to guide the patient through the exercise. This script pairs the cue "relax" with the relaxation of each muscle group.

> "Breathe with calm, regular breaths and feel how you relax more and more with every breath. . . . Just let go. . . . And as you relax, say to yourself, under your breath, the word 'relax' each time you breathe out. . . . Imagining the word 'relax' each time you breathe out. . . . Relax your forehead . . . eyebrows . . . eyelids . . . jaws . . . tongue and throat . . . lips . . . your entire face. . . . Imagining the word 'relax' each time you breathe out. . . . Relax your neck . . . shoulders . . . arms . . . hands . . . and all the way out to your fingertips. . . . Imagining the word 'relax' each time you breathe out. . . . Breathe calmly and regularly with your stomach all the time. . . . Let the relaxation spread to your stomach . . . waist and back. . . . Relax the lower part of your body, your behind . . . thighs . . . knees . . . calves . . . feet . . . and all the way down to the tips of your toes. . . . Imagining the word 'relax' each time you breathe out. . . . Breathe calmly and regularly and feel how you relax more and more by each breath. . . . Take a deep breath and hold your breath a couple of seconds . . . and let the air out slowly . . . slowly. . . . Notice how you relax more and more."

Rapid Relaxation

Rapid relaxation is used to teach patients to relax in everyday situations and to further reduce the time it takes to relax. The goal is to relax within 20–30 seconds. Rapid relaxation consists of (1) taking one to three deep breaths and slowly exhaling, (2) thinking "relax" before each exhalation, and (3) scanning one's body for tension and trying to relax as much as possible as one breathes out. The exercise is initially practiced in nonstressful situations, such as in the therapist's office, and then practiced 15–20 times per day in everyday situations. Colored dots or other salient stimuli are used as cues or reminders to practice relaxation. To illustrate, a blue dot might be stuck on a patient's cell phone as a reminder to use the relaxation exercise. Cues are changed periodically (e.g., blue dots are replaced with red dots) to prevent habituation to the reminders.

In-session practice begins with a few trials of relaxation in a comfortable chair. Then the patient practices relaxing under increasingly more active circumstances. Patients are asked to perform a series of exercises during which only the essential muscles are tensed. Examples include (1) opening one's eyes and looking around while relaxing all the muscles except those required to sit upright and look about; (2) lifting one arm, and then the other, lifting one foot, one leg, and then the other, while relaxing all the muscles that are not needed for those activities; and (3) tensing the biceps while keeping the hands relaxed. Patients then practice relaxing under increasingly more active circumstances, such as walking about while relaxing all the muscles except those required for ambulation. For homework, the exercises are practiced in various settings at least 20 times per day.

Indications and Caveats

Applied relaxation exercises can be used to calm the patient down if she or he is too anxious to concentrate on whatever other interventions are being used in the therapy session. Relaxation also can be used if the patient feels too anxious to undertake in-session exposure assignments. Similarly, relaxation exercises can be used to facilitate homework exposure assignments, particularly when anticipatory anxiety is so high that it interferes with the patient's willingness to attempt the assignments. In these applications, a short (e.g., 10-minute) relaxation exercise can be used, such as release-only relaxation, and then the exposure exercise is attempted.

Relaxation training can sometimes lead patients to see that bodily sensations are harmless. This may happen because relaxation exercises can convince some patients that the feared sensations are simply the harmless by-products of tension—that is, sensations that can be simply "switched off" if desired. However, sometimes patients misuse relaxation methods as safety behaviors, where they strive to reduce arousal because they fear its consequences.

If relaxation training is used, it is important to check whether or not the relaxation exercises interfere with the reduction in erroneous beliefs about the dangerousness of stress. If interference occurs, then the patient can be asked to periodically refrain from using the relaxation exercises in order to prove to him- or herself that stress does not have catastrophic consequences. It is also important to inform patients that some degree of anxiety is normal and adaptive. By allowing themselves to periodically experience anxiety—in full—patients are reminded that this emotion is harmless.

BREATHING RETRAINING

Indications

Clinical observations suggest that hyperventilation, such as stress-induced overbreathing, can cause some of the bodily sensations that trouble people with hypochondriasis (Kaplan, 2002). Accordingly, breathing retraining may be of some value. Breathing retraining instructs patients in slow diaphragmatic breathing. It is used to alleviate unpleasant but harmless sensations, including those due to hyperventilation (e.g., dizziness, dyspnea) and those due to chest breathing (e.g., chest pain). Breathing retraining can also abort panic attacks (Taylor, 2000), and so could be used to treat panicking, health-anxious people. With repeated practice, slow diaphragmatic breathing becomes habitual. Acute hyperventilators can be taught to identify stimuli that trigger hyperventilation (e.g., stressful events) and to implement slow, diaphragmatic breathing at these times.

There are several ways of assessing whether the patient tends to hyperventilate. One is to ask patients to demonstrate how they breathe when they are feeling stressed or anxious. Another is to ask patients to hyperventilate for 1–2 minutes and then to assess their emotional reactions and the similarity of the resulting sensations to sensations of naturally occurring bodily sensations. A third approach is to ask patients if they often feel short of breath (even when not panicking), and whether they tend to yawn or sigh a lot, or take in gulps of air.

Caveats

An important caveat in using breathing retraining is that breathing exercises can become safety behaviors. That is, patients may use them to avoid or escape feared sensations, and thereby fail to learn that the sensations are harmless. Related safety behaviors include procedures to abort hyperventilation, such as breathing into a paper bag or through cupped hands. If breathing retraining is used, it is important that the patient learn that the feared sensations are harmless (Taylor, 2001).

Breathing Retraining Procedures

Diaphragmatic breathing consists of a number of simple exercises that can be taught in a couple of sessions. Details are as follows:

- In the first session of breathing retraining, patients are educated about the distinction between "chest breathing" and "diaphragm breathing." Patients are informed about how chest breathing can produce harmless but uncomfortable sensations such as chest tightness or pain, and is associated with hyperventilation. The therapist should emphasize that hyperventilation is harmless, but can cause unpleasant sensations, such as dizziness or shortness of breath. An overview of breathing retraining is presented.
- The therapist demonstrates the two types of breathing and shows how to best observe the difference between the two. Placing one hand on

his or her chest and the other on his or her stomach (in order to notice differences in movement), the therapist demonstrates how the ribcage moves upward and outward during chest breathing. Then the therapist demonstrates how the stomach but not the chest moves in and out during diaphragmatic breathing. Patients then place their own hands over their own chest and stomach, practicing the two types of breathing and observing the differences.

- Patients are then asked to practice diaphragmatic breathing for 10 minutes in the therapist's office. Respiration should be at a comfortable rate, breathing through the nose rather than the mouth. The goal is to achieve a slow, smooth, shallow pattern of breathing.

- Patients can practice diaphragmatic breathing either by sitting in a chair or by lying in a supine position.

- The patient should observe the abdomen rising and falling with each breath, while breathing with the diaphragm and keeping the chest still. Patients are instructed to notice the cool air slowly coming in through the nostrils as they inhale, then pause for 1–2 seconds, and then notice the warm air slowly flowing out as they exhale. Initially, the target respiration rate is about 12 breaths per minute (i.e., inhaling for 2 seconds, pausing for 1 second, and exhaling for 2 second).

- For homework, the patient is requested to sit or lie down in a quiet place at home, free from distractions, and practice the diaphragmatic breathing two to three times per day for 10 minutes each time. Breathing should be at a comfortable rate. Patients are instructed to use a monitoring form to record the duration of each practice period. The importance of regular practice is emphasized.

- A 5-minute pacing tape can be recorded during the session to be used as a homework aid to help the patient breathe at the desired rate (Clark, 1989). The pacing on the tape is at the patient's usual rate of respiration or, if possible, a little slower. The patient follows the tape for 5 minutes, and then for the next 5 minutes practices without the tape. Such tapes typically consist of the therapist saying "in" for 2 seconds, pausing for 1 second, and then "out" for 2 seconds (12 breaths per minute). Pacing can be faster if this is too slow for the patient. By prolonging the articulation of "in" and "out," gentle and extended inspirations and expirations are achieved, in contrast to the sharp gasps that characterize hyperventilation.

- Application training usually commences in the second treatment session. To train patients to abort episodes of hyperventilation, they are asked to hyperventilate for 1–2 minutes and then to practice controlling their respiration by implementing slow diaphragmatic breathing. This is practiced several times during the therapy session. Patients should be advised that their breathing rate should always feel comfortable. If they are engaging in some physical activity, then their respiratory rate should increase to match the body's oxygen requirements.

- For homework, the patient continues practicing slow diaphragmatic breathing while sitting at home for 10 minutes two to three times per day. The respiration rate can be slowed down to 8–10 breaths per minute. A slower pacing tape can be recorded for use on alternate days for the following week, and then the tape is discontinued.
- Patients are also asked to complete application training homework. This consists of practicing slow diaphragmatic breathing in a variety of everyday situations: while watching TV, waiting in lines in stores, sitting in the car at traffic lights, sitting in crowded cinemas, and so forth. Patients gradually practice in increasingly challenging situations. Various stimuli can be used as cues or reminders to practice a breathing exercise, including particular situations (e.g., stressful circumstances) and sensations (e.g., dizziness, chest tightness, or other sensations suggesting that respiration may have increased).

PROBLEM SOLVING

Problem-solving interventions provide brief, structured approaches to solving life difficulties, and can thereby reduce emotional distress and stress-related bodily reactions (D'Zurilla, 1986; Hawton & Kirk, 1989). One approach is illustrated in Handout 11.5. This begins by encouraging patients to define their problems, to develop goals, and to identify and implement the steps for attaining those goals. Obstacles to goal attainment are identified, such as practical constraints (e.g., a lack of necessary skills or resources) and cognitive obstacles (e.g., distorted beliefs about one's ability to solve the problem). The patient and the therapist can work through the worksheet during a problem-solving session, starting with an easy problem to illustrate the process, and then the patient can work on problem solving as a homework assignment.

Problem solving might involve working on health anxiety. For example, the person might devise a series of steps for overcoming a disease fear, such as developing an exposure hierarchy (see Chapter 10). The patient and the therapist can work together to ensure that goals are realistic and are specified sufficiently clearly so that one knows when the goal has been attained. If a health-anxious person specifies a goal of "being healthy," the therapist can encourage the patient to define this goal more clearly and realistically (e.g., having a clean bill of health during an annual physical exam, while accepting that 100% certainty is impossible). Cognitive restructuring methods (see Chapter 9) can be used in such cases to facilitate problem solving.

TWELVE STEPS TO SOLVING PROBLEMS

There are solutions to most of life's problems. The odds of solving problems depends on the approach you take. The following steps increase the chances of solving important problems in your life.

1. **Pick a problem** that you would like to work on. It could be a big, urgent problem that may take some effort to solve, or it might be a little one. Successfully tackling small problems can increase your confidence of solving bigger problems. List your problem as specifically as possible:

_____

_____

2. **State your goal**. Please be as specific as possible. What is the outcome that you are hoping to attain? For example, if you are an unemployed accountant, your goal might be to find a full-time accounting position.

_____

_____

3. **Is your goal realistic?** If not, list another, more attainable goal.

_____

_____

4. **What are your resources for attaining your goal?** This would include material resources (e.g., money, transportation) and social resources (e.g., people who could help you or offer support).

_____

_____

_____

_____

5. **Brainstorm!** List all the possible ways of attaining your goal that you can think of. List these possibilities regardless of whether they're plausible or not. Use an extra sheet if necessary.

_____

_____

_____

_____

(continued)

6. **Refine your solutions.** Look through your list of solutions and see if you can think of ways of improving your solutions. If you think of extra solutions while doing this, then write them down as well.

_____

_____

_____

_____

7. **Evaluate.** List the pros and cons of each solution. Which one looks the best?

_____

_____

_____

_____

8. **Baby steps.** Can you break your goal up into subgoals? For example, if your goal was to find a dating partner, your subgoals might be the following: (1) Put yourself in situations in which you will meet people that you might like to date (e.g., join a sporting club or enroll in a course at a community center). (2) Get to know people—make friends. Even if you don't find a dating partner, at least you'll have friends. (3) If you find someone attractive, arrange to have coffee with him or her . . . and so on.

_____

_____

_____

_____

_____

9. **Identify obstacles.** What are the things that might get in the way of solving your problems? These might be behavioral obstacles (e.g., lack of job skills) or thinking obstacles (e.g., negative thoughts like "Nobody would ever hire me"). List your obstacles here.

_____

_____

_____

_____

_____

(continued)

10. **Overcome your roadblocks.** List ways of overcoming the obstacles. This might involve improving your skills or challenging your negative thoughts.

_____

_____

_____

_____

_____

_____

11. **Make a commitment** to solving your problems. Plan to do something each day.

12. **Track your progress** toward achieving your goals. Are you making steady progress? If so, good. If not, then identify the roadblocks and try to come up with solutions. Sometimes it helps to reward yourself for your efforts in overcoming problems, especially big problems. Treat yourself to something nice.

TIME MANAGEMENT

Poor time management can be a source of significant distress, leading the person to feel overwhelmed with responsibilities. Time management is likely to be a problem if the patient feels that she or he is (1) often rushing from one activity to another, (2) frequently late, (3) low in productivity, or (4) having difficulty finishing important tasks (Davis et al., 2000). Training in time management skills can be used to improve coping at work, at home, and in other areas of the person's life. Time management builds on the problem-solving skills described in the previous section—for example, setting realistic goals and deadlines, and specifying the steps for achieving goals. There are three fundamental strategies for good time management (Seaward, 1997):

- *Prioritizing.* Listing one's current responsibilities and ranking their order of importance. Tasks that are unimportant can be discarded, leaving more time to focus on essential tasks. Self-defeating activities (e.g., excessive bodily checking or undue reassurance seeking) can be omitted. Prioritizing involves planning ahead and setting realistic goals. Dysfunctional beliefs about performing tasks (e.g., believing that you should never say "no" to requests) can be examined and modified in order to set realistic priorities.
- *Scheduling.* Patients can be encouraged to make lists or keep a day planner to specify when they will perform specific tasks. Scheduling an "appointment" for a given task increases the likelihood that it will get done. Where possible, things can be done to reduce distractions while tasks are performed (e.g., taking the telephone off the hook until you have completed an important assignment).
- *Execution.* When possible, finish a task or an important component of a task rather than jumping from task to task. To increase efficiency, tasks can be delegated, where possible.

Handout 11.6 provides a simple but informative summary of these time management methods. This handout has been adapted from several sources (Conduit, 1995; Ellis & Knaus, 1977; Davis et al., 2000; Morgenstern, 2000; Seaward, 1997), which readers should consult for a more extensive discussion of time management methods.

Good time management involves keeping the health-anxious person productively occupied with things that bring a sense of mastery or enjoyment, rather than squandering his or her time on maladaptive behaviors such as checking medical textbooks and doctor shopping. The following vignette illustrates how training in time management can be used in treating health-anxious patients:

TIME MANAGEMENT

Are you constantly late? Always rushing from one task to the next? Feel like you get little accomplished during your day? Does your "to-do" list keep growing? If you answered yes to any of these questions, then you might have a problem with time management. The following methods may help you better manage your time:

- **List your goals**. Write down the tasks you want to accomplish this week. Create a "to-do" list. This encourages you to plan ahead.
- **Set priorities**. Rate the priority of each task: high, medium, or low.
- **How long?** Estimate the amount of time required to do each task.
- **Make a schedule.** Use a day planner to schedule when you'll do each task. Assign realistic deadlines.
- **Match the task to your energy level.** For example, are you a "morning person"? If so, then schedule your challenging tasks for the morning. Don't wait until the afternoon or evening, when you're too tired.
- **Too many tasks?** Then try one or more of the following:
  - Delegate. Assign some of your tasks to other people.
  - Streamline. Is there a way of doing things more efficiently? Things rarely need to be perfect.
  - Discard. Some tasks can be omitted.
  - Reduce disruptions to improve efficiency. If you need a block of time to complete something important, for example, then shut your office door and forward your phone calls.
- **Is procrastination a problem?** Then try one or more of the following:
  - Examine your beliefs. Are you telling yourself that the task is too difficult? That it needs to be done perfectly? That you're not good enough to do it? Are these beliefs realistic? People often procrastinate because they overestimate the task's difficulty and underestimate their competence.
  - Motivate yourself. Think of motivating self-statements like "Doing gets it done" or "Just do it!" Then reward yourself for finishing the task.
  - Make a date with destiny. Using your day planner, set aside a specific time for doing the task.
  - The 5-minute rule. Tell yourself you'll work on that difficult task for 5 minutes and then see if you feel like continuing. Chances are that once you get started, you'll want to continue.

Jill K., a student in a demanding graduate program, learned in therapy that her chest pain was stress-related and not due to a heart condition. This greatly alleviated her health anxiety, but Jill continued to have recurrent episodes of pain, particularly when she was rushing to complete course essays before their deadline. Time management strategies were used to reduce the pain and to reinforce the message that the pain was stress-related. Instead of procrastinating and then frantically working all night to complete her essays, Jill learned to devise a less stressful schedule. Using a day planner, she scheduled times to complete various aspects of each essay (e.g., doing a literature review, compiling an essay outline, working on each section of the essay), and planned to complete each component over a period of 2 weeks before the due date. Jill also learned to avoid time-wasting distractions while working on her essays. For example, during a 1-hour block of "essay time" she refrained from checking her e-mail until she had worked on the essay for the allotted hour. As a result of using these strategies, Jill less frequently experienced episodes of chest pain and became further convinced that the pain was a result of stress.

When training patients in time management, it is important for the clinician to consider whether time management is a realistic option. Sometimes workers are overwhelmed with tasks that they simply don't have the time and resources to perform. In such cases restructuring or changing jobs may be the most viable options. Patients also should be encouraged to lead a balanced lifestyle, allocating time to all the important spheres of life (e.g., work, family activities, personal recreation).

OTHER METHODS OF STRESS MANAGEMENT

A number of other stress management interventions can be used, depending on the nature of the problem. If distorted beliefs appear to play a role in the person's stress reactions, then cognitive approaches can be used, in a manner similar to that described in Chapter 9 and elsewhere (Beck, 1993; Davis et al., 2000; Meichenbaum, 1993). If the person's stress reactions arise from assertiveness or social skills deficits, then interpersonal skills training can be used (e.g., Paterson, 2000). If the person's stress reactions arise from a competitive, time-pressured, and hostile personality style (Type A behavior pattern), then Friedman's (1996) protocol can be used. Motivational interviewing methods (see Chapter 8) can be used to reduce self-defeating ways of coping with stress, such as overeating or excessive use of alcohol (e.g., see Miller & Rollnick, 2002).

Work-related stress can also be managed by improving one's job skills and by setting boundaries between work and home, thereby allowing the person to separate "job time" from "leisure time" (Conduit, 1995). Boundaries can be made salient by changing clothes on return from work and confining weighty correspondence (including e-mail) to the work environment and office hours. Other lifestyle changes can also be implemented to reduce stress reactions, such as cutting down one's caffeine consumption, getting regular exercise, scheduling leisure or recreational time, and eating a well-balanced diet.

SUMMARY AND CONCLUSIONS

Stress management interventions can be useful adjuncts to the CBT methods described in previous chapters. However, the therapist must ensure that the patient is not using stress management methods as ways of avoiding feared but harmless bodily reactions. This misuse can perpetuate health anxiety. Stress management can be fruitfully used either (1) to reduce unpleasant bodily reactions, once the patient accepts that the sensations are not signs of dire disease; or (2) as ways of showing patients that their bodily changes or sensations are due to stress, rather than a result of disease.

12

Extending and Maintaining Treatment Gains

In this chapter we consider the issues and interventions used toward the end of, and after, a formal course of cognitive-behavioral therapy (CBT) for health anxiety disorders. Most patients will have experienced at least some reduction in health anxiety after, for example, 12–16 sessions of CBT (with or without stress management). The final sessions can fruitfully address the following:

- Extending treatment gains to other areas of the patient's life—in particular, enhancing the person's quality of life. This includes improving a person's health habits (e.g., diet, exercise). Despite their bodily concerns, health-anxious people often have no better health habits than other people (APA, 2000). The decision of whether to extend treatment into these areas depends on the patient's goals.
- Developing a maintenance program to increase the chances that treatment gains will be maintained after the end of the formal course of CBT. This involves relapse prevention strategies.
- Coming up with treatment options for patients who have not benefited sufficiently from CBT.

Throughout this chapter we consider the principles for extending and maintaining treatment gains for health anxiety disorders in general. We also consider principles that apply to specific forms of health anxiety, such as disease phobia and delusional disorder (somatic type).

Little has been written on these topics in the treatment of health anxiety. In developing the ideas for this chapter, we drew on the small literature on the topic (e.g., Clark et al., 1998; Salkovskis, 1989; Wells, 1997), along with our own clinical experiences. We also drew on the literature on maintaining gains for other disorders. There is a small but growing body of research on treatment maintenance for obsessive–compulsive disorder (Espie, 1986; Hiss, Foa, & Kozak, 1994; McKay, Todero, Neziroglu, & Yaryura-Tobias, 1996) and body dysmorphic disorder (McKay, 1999), both of which bear phenomenological similarities to hypochondriasis (e.g., both are characterized by fears and repeated checking). We also drew on the literature on maintaining gains for phobias and panic disorder (Öst, 1989; Taylor, 2000) because this work can be applied to health anxiety in which phobic avoidance and fear are prominent (e.g., disease phobia). Regardless of disorder, most maintenance programs are based on the work on relapse prevention for alcohol and substance-use disorder (Marlatt & Gordon, 1985), which we have also drawn upon to develop relapse prevention strategies for health anxiety disorders.

TOWARD THE END OF THERAPY

Patients with health anxiety as their primary (i.e., most severe) problem would typically be treated first for this condition, and then treated for any remaining disorders. A patient might enter treatment with severe hypochondriasis and a less severe mood disorder. Once the former has been treated, the latter may still require clinical attention, which could be treated with CBT for depression (Beck et al., 1979). Other specific CBT protocols could be implemented for other remaining disorders (e.g., Beck, Freeman, & Associates, 2003; Beck & Emery, 1985; Hawton, Salkovskis, Kirk, & Clark, 1989; Taylor, 2000).

Enhancing Quality of Life

The absence of psychopathology does not ensure the presence of happiness. Patients can benefit from a few sessions devoted to improving their quality of life. The latter is the person's appraisal of the degree to which his or her most important needs, goals, and wishes have been fulfilled (Frisch, Cornell, Villaneuva, & Retzlaff, 1992). Thus, quality of life entails life satisfaction and subjective well-being. Quality of life issues can be addressed at any point in therapy. In fact, some methods that improve quality of life, such as physical exercise for improving one's health, can be used during CBT as behavioral experiments, to test patients' beliefs about their health (e.g., "My body is too frail to take any physical exertion"; see Chapter 10). Even so, quality of life issues tend to be more important toward the end of therapy. Once the patient's health concerns have abated, other issues may come to the fore, such as concerns about employment or marital satisfaction. Patients tend to have more free time once they are devoting less time to bodily checking, reassurance seeking, and related behaviors. Quality of life issues emerge when they begin thinking about how to productively fill this time.

CBT for health anxiety does not target all areas of a person's life relevant for improving well-being and life satisfaction. The therapist may need to implement strategies from Frisch's (2003) cognitive-behavioral quality of life therapy. This contains specific treatment strategies for each of 16 domains of quality of life: health, self-esteem, goals and values, money, work, play, learning, creativity, helping others, love, friends, children, relatives, home, neighborhood, and community. The therapy also offers several general strategies that can be used for boosting satisfaction in any of these domains. General strategies include the following, which can be summarized by the acronym CASIO (Frisch, 2003).

- *Circumstances*. Changing the objective circumstances of a life domain (e.g., increasing one's circle of friends, changing where one lives or works).
- *Attitude*. Changing one's attitude about life domains (e.g., learning to be satisfied with one's current job).
- *Standards*. Examining one's goals and standards for fulfillment. This involves setting realistic goals and lowering excessive standards (e.g., "Do I have to drive a Porsche Boxster in order to be happy?").
- *Importance*. Examining the importance placed on each domain for one's overall happiness. Priorities may be revised to emphasize those domains the person can change. If one's job is unsatisfying and other employment opportunities are limited, for example, the person could increasingly cultivate other life domains, such as friends, family, and recreational pursuits.
- *Other*. Cultivating interests in other areas not considered before, such as hobbies and other pleasant activities, even while continuing to work on improving other life domains. This could include areas that divert the patient's attention away from the issue of physical health and disease.

To commence work on quality of life issues, the patient can be asked to generate a list of goals associated with each valued area of life (e.g., family, work). The goals are then prioritized and translated into manageable subgoals and strategies. For example, the quality of relationships with one's children can be improved by training in parenting skills (e.g., Christophersen &

Mortweet, 2003). Vocational training may be useful for patients who have long avoided work situations.

Pleasant event scheduling, based on Beck's cognitive therapy for depression (Beck et al., 1979), is another simple but very useful method for improving quality of life. Patients can be asked to complete a checklist like the one in Handout 12.1 which incorporates elements from MacPhillamy and Lewinsohn (1982) and from Linehan (1993). The patient indicates which of the activities she or he did in the past week. The patient and the therapist can then review the checklist to see if there are other enjoyable activities that the patient has not been doing. The patient can then be encouraged to attempt these activities in order to improve her or his quality of life. Activity scheduling such as this can also reduce depressive symptoms (Beck et al., 1979; Jacobson et al., 1996), which are commonly associated with health anxiety disorders (see Chapter 1). Activities that confer a sense of mastery (e.g., returning to employment, even on a part-time basis) are also useful in improving quality of life and reducing depression. Such activities can be identified by reviewing, with the patient, the areas that he or she would like to improve, and then devising a step-by-step approach for achieving these goals (see Beck et al., 1979, for further details). Ideally, these are pleasant or productive activities that direct attention away from the body.

Quality of life can be improved by implementing strategies for a healthy lifestyle (e.g., regular exercise, a balanced diet, sufficient sleep, reduction in smoking and alcohol consumption), along with other stress management strategies (see Chapter 11). A useful effect of these strategies is that they can strengthen the patient's view of him- or herself as a person who is healthy and resilient, instead of someone who is especially vulnerable to disease. For patients choosing to improve their physical health, therapists should check that they are not compulsively pursuing a healthy lifestyle—by physical exercise, dieting, or taking dietary supplements—as safety behaviors to ward off dreaded diseases.

Treatment Tapering

According to clinical wisdom, as the formal course of CBT draws to an end, the treatment sessions should be spaced increasingly further apart, so as to fade out reliance on the therapist and encourage the patient him- or herself to take an increasingly active role in extending and maintaining treatment gains. The final four treatment sessions might be successively spaced 2, 4, 8, and 12 weeks apart.

Remarkably, there has been very little research on the wisdom of this approach. Craske and colleagues have examined the effects of uniform versus increasingly spaced sessions in the treatment of various sorts of fears and phobias,

ACTIVITIES FOR ENHANCING YOUR QUALITY OF LIFE

Instructions: Enjoyable activities are essential to one's quality of life. But sometimes people neglect these activities when they are preoccupied or worried about their health. Please look through the following checklist of activities. Did you do any of them in the past week? If so, did you enjoy the activity? Are there any activities that you haven't done but would like to do? This list of activities might help you think about ways of improving your quality of life. Some of these activities might distract you from your health worries, while others can improve your health and fitness.

Please note: This checklist is concerned with enjoyable activities that enhance your quality of life (e.g., watching a romantic movie), not activities to do with health and disease (e.g., not phoning friends to discuss your health).

Activities unrelated to health worries	Indicate (√) which of these activities you did in the past week.	For the activities you indicated, were they enjoyable? (yes/no)	Indicate (√) which of these activities you didn't do but would like to do.
Creative activities			
Doing artwork or crafts			
Knitting, needlework, sewing			
Taking a course in something creative (e.g., cooking, photography)			
Decorating or redecorating your house or apartment			
Woodwork, carpentry, or furniture restoration			
Repairing things			
Mechanical hobbies (e.g., fixing gadgets)			
Photography			
Creative writing or doing a journal			
Musical hobbies (e.g., singing, dancing, playing an instrument)			
Games and entertainments			
Watching TV, videos, or DVDs			
Playing videogames			
Listening to music or radio programs			
Going to the cinema			

(continued)

Going to a play, concert, opera, or ballet	_____	_____	_____
Going to a museum, art gallery, or exhibition	_____	_____	_____
Going to a sporting event	_____	_____	_____
Educational activities that *do not* have to do with gathering information about health and disease			
Reading books, magazines, or newspapers	_____	_____	_____
Going to a lecture on a topic that interests you	_____	_____	_____
Learning a foreign language	_____	_____	_____
Surfing the Internet	_____	_____	_____
Learning about computers (e.g., learning to make a web page).	_____	_____	_____
Going to the library	_____	_____	_____
Physical activities			
Playing tennis, squash, or racquetball	_____	_____	_____
Playing golf or lawn sports such as bowls	_____	_____	_____
Ten-pin bowling	_____	_____	_____
Water activities (e.g., swimming, sailing, canoeing)	_____	_____	_____
Walking or hiking	_____	_____	_____
Jogging, aerobics classes, or working out at a fitness center	_____	_____	_____
Snow sports (skiing, skating, snow boarding)	_____	_____	_____
Bike riding	_____	_____	_____
Horse riding	_____	_____	_____
Playing team sports (e.g., volleyball, hockey, basketball)	_____	_____	_____
Fishing or hunting	_____	_____	_____
Playing snooker or pool	_____	_____	_____
Social and community activities that *do not* involve discussing health and disease			
Writing, telephoning, or e-mailing friends	_____	_____	_____
Visiting a friend or inviting a friend to your place	_____	_____	_____
Going out to lunch or dinner with a friend	_____	_____	_____
Giving a party or going to a party	_____	_____	_____
Going on a date	_____	_____	_____
Joining a club (e.g., a book club or social club)	_____	_____	_____

(continued)

228

Going to a bar or restaurant	_____	_____	_____
Involvement in community or political activities	_____	_____	_____
Involvement in religious or church activities	_____	_____	_____
Other			
Sitting in the sun	_____	_____	_____
Going for a scenic drive	_____	_____	_____
Gardening, caring for houseplants, or arranging flowers	_____	_____	_____
Visiting fun or interesting places (e.g., park, beach, zoo)	_____	_____	_____
Caring for, or being with pets	_____	_____	_____
Planning or going on a holiday	_____	_____	_____
Going to a sauna	_____	_____	_____
Soaking in the bathtub	_____	_____	_____
Doing yoga or meditation	_____	_____	_____
Buying yourself something special	_____	_____	_____
Hobbies (e.g., stamp collecting, model building, flying a kite)	_____	_____	_____
List your favorite activities here, if they are not listed above: _____ _____ _____	_____ _____ _____	_____ _____ _____	_____ _____ _____

Adapted from MacPhillamy and Lewinsohn (1982) and Linehan (1993).

although they have not studied health anxiety disorders. The results of their research have been mixed, although there is some evidence that the likelihood of relapse may be reduced by increasingly spacing sessions (Lang & Craske, 2000; Rowe & Craske, 1998; Tsao & Craske, 2000). The same may apply to health anxiety disorders.

When such treatment tapering is used, the CBT practitioner and the patient should work together to ensure that there is no increase in self-defeating compensatory behavior. As a patient with hypochondriasis is tapered off CBT, for instance, he or she might increase the frequency of his or her consultations with the primary care physician in order to seek reassurance. This is particularly likely to happen if the CBT practitioner is seen by the patient as a source of safety ("I'm safe as long as I'm seeing my therapist, who won't let anything bad happen to me"). To prevent this from happening, the CBT practitioner can examine the patient's beliefs about ending CBT. Dysfunctional beliefs can be addressed by cognitive restructuring.

THERAPIST: How do you feel about our sessions coming to an end?

PATIENT: I'm worried about how I will cope on my own.

THERAPIST: What are your particular concerns?

PATIENT: I've never been without a doctor that I can depend on. I feel safe knowing that someone is looking out for my health.

THERAPIST: What would it be like if you could rely more on yourself?

PATIENT: I suppose I wouldn't feel so vulnerable.

THERAPIST: That would be good. I'm wondering what you could do to feel more confident about relying on yourself?

PATIENT: I don't know.

THERAPIST: Hmmm. Let's think for a moment. Is there anything in your life that you're confident about? For example, are you confident in your job as a certified general accountant?

PATIENT: Yes, I suppose I am.

THERAPIST: How did you develop that confidence?

PATIENT: At first it wasn't easy. I was always asking my supervisor to check things, but then she retired and I had to fend for myself.

THERAPIST: Did that make you nervous?

PATIENT: Yes, it was a stressful time.

THERAPIST: So, how long were you nervous?

PATIENT: For a few weeks, and then I got used to managing on my own.

THERAPIST: Do you think the same thing could happen here, in developing confidence in handling your health anxiety?

PATIENT: I guess so.

THERAPIST: And maybe your confidence would be improved if we develop a plan for coping by yourself, something that we call a maintenance program.

PATIENT: That sounds like a good idea.

MAINTAINING TREATMENT GAINS

Developing a Maintenance Program

The final few sessions of a course of CBT can focus on developing plans for maintaining and furthering treatment gains. For some patients this involves plans for further reducing health anxiety, while for others it involves plans for preventing relapse. The general elements of a maintenance program are listed in Table 12.1. Therapy is presented as a continuing process that continues after a course of CBT has ended.

In the final sessions it is useful for the patient and the therapist to review the gains made during treatment and the extent to which the therapy goals were met. A graph of the treatment gains, such as a chart (or other self-monitoring data) showing reductions in the percentage of each day spent worrying about one's health, can be used to illustrate treatment gains, thereby encouraging patients to continue using, as needed, the exercises they learned in CBT. This approach can be effective for patients who fail to appreciate that reductions in health anxiety were due to their own efforts during therapy. Such patients often forget how severe their problems were at the beginning of treatment.

Patients should consider what they did to produce the treatment gains. Which interventions were most helpful for them? One can ask patients to produce a written description of what they learned during treatment so that the CBT exercises can be used again in the future, if needed. This would involve generating a list of specific interventions, the steps involved in their implementation, and the rationale for each intervention. Interventions should be described in specific, concrete terms. This is done in a collaborative fashion, with the therapist using careful questioning to help the patient come up with most of the information.

Checking the patient's understanding of the rationale (during and at the end of treatment) is important to prevent an intervention from being misused. For example, one patient might use exposure exercises to remind him- or

TABLE 12.1. General Elements of a Maintenance Program

Review of treatment progress
- What problems have diminished over the course of treatment? What problems remain to be addressed?
- What interventions were most useful?

Establish appropriate expectations for posttreatment functioning
- Some ongoing practice of some treatment exercises may be required to address outstanding problems
- Setbacks may occur
- Coping strategies can overcome setbacks

Written maintenance plan
- Ongoing interventions
- Appropriate medical consultations
- Remind patients to retain the handouts they received during therapy

Relapse prevention
- Distinguish between "setback" and "relapse"
- Discuss "abstinence violation effect"
- Identify high-risk situations
- Develop plans for coping with setbacks

Arrange for periodic check-in with CBT practitioner
- Booster sessions, if needed
- Telephone or e-mail consultations

herself that bodily sensations are harmless. That would be an appropriate use of the intervention. In contrast, another patient might use exposure exercises to reduce anxiety because she believes that anxiety is harmful. This would be an inappropriate use of the intervention because it would prevent the patient from learning that anxiety is harmless. When misconceptions are identified, the therapist can correct them by using cognitive restructuring (see Chapter 9).

As part of the review of treatment progress, the patient is reminded of strategies for helping him or her determine when he or she is simply suffering from health anxiety ("When am I worrying excessively?"). Patients can be asked to generate a list of reasons why he or she would want to continue using the exercises (as needed) in the future, and to identify and develop plans for overcoming anticipated obstacles for implementing the interventions.

By the end of treatment, the strength of dysfunctional disease-related beliefs may be substantially reduced, but not to the point that the patient confidently regards the beliefs as false. To identify any lingering doubts the therapist can ask the patient to generate a list of evidence *for* their dysfunctional beliefs and *against* the alternative, noncatastrophic beliefs. If the patient is able to generate such a list, then the dysfunctional beliefs have not been completely eradicated. If so, then cognitive and exposure interventions can be set as tasks to be performed during the maintenance program. Patients could be asked to conduct further tests of their beliefs.

For patients with remaining problems at the end of CBT, the therapist and the patient can generate a written list of the problems, ranked in order of importance. Plans, based on the skills learned in CBT, can then be developed for each problem. The patient can be encouraged to work through each problem, beginning with the most pressing concern. Of course, if these problems are severe, then the patient and the therapist may decide to extend the course of therapy.

Relapse Prevention

A relapse prevention plan is an essential feature of any maintenance program. Even when health anxiety disorders are successfully treated, health anxiety may reoccur at some point in the future. The important issue is not whether the problems return, but how the patient deals with them. In order to successfully maintain treatment gains, it is important that a *setback* or *lapse*—defined as a transient increase in symptoms of a health anxiety disorder—does not progress into a relapse of the disorder. The maintenance program should provide the patients with relapse prevention strategies. These should be written down so patients can consult them in the future, if necessary. The points to convey are described below and can be supplemented by a written handout or worksheet such as that shown in Handout 12.2.

- Unrealistic patient expectations, such as expectations that she or he will never experience another bout of health anxiety, should be identified and challenged. Patients are likely to have anxiety about their health in the future. Sometimes this will be a normal reaction to health problems, while at other times the anxiety reactions may be disproportionate. The important point is for patients to expect and prepare to deal with anxiety in the future.
- A lapse (setback) is not a relapse. A future occurrence of excessive health anxiety does not mean that the patient has lost all the gains that he or she made during treatment. It simply means that it's time to practice the exercises learned in therapy.
- Lapses can be framed as *opportunities* for continuing to practice the skills learned during treatment. Patients can be asked to write out a plan of what CBT strategies they would implement if they had another epi-

HEALTH ANXIETY RELAPSE PREVENTION (HARP)

Everyone experiences anxiety about their health at some time or other. You too will probably have a bout of health anxiety in the future. It is important to cope with these episodes when they occur. This is important for preventing a minor *setback* or lapse (i.e., some return of health anxiety) from turning into a major *relapse* (the full return of health anxiety). This handout is intended to help you design a relapse prevention program for your particular problems so that you can cope with setbacks in the future. Let us begin by considering some examples of how two people coped poorly with their setbacks:

Examples of Poor Coping

Allen had a long history of excessive health anxiety that had been successfully treated with therapy. But one morning he woke up with a dry cough, and began to worry that it could be something serious. "Maybe I have tuberculosis" he thought. Soon Allen had worked himself up into an extremely anxious state. Allen realized that he had become very anxious, just like he was before he went into therapy. Allen thought, "Therapy hasn't helped me! I'm back at square 1." As a result of his thoughts, Allen didn't use the coping skills he learned in therapy, and so his health anxiety continued to worsen.

Mary had a phobia of developing cancer that had been successfully treated in therapy. However, her cancer fear started to return when a close friend was diagnosed with breast cancer. Mary didn't notice that her fear had returned until it had become severe. By that stage she avoided everything that reminded her about cancer, including her friend. She forgot about the things she had learned in therapy and so she felt helpless to deal with the return of her cancer phobia.

Good Coping

Write down three things that Allen could have done to better cope with his worries about tuberculosis.

(*Hint*: How might Allen's thoughts influence his health anxiety? Is there any evidence to support his thoughts about tuberculosis? What might he say to himself to feel less anxious? What sorts of things might Allen be doing to make his health anxiety worse? What could he do differently? Does his lapse really mean that he's back at "square 1"?)

1. _____

_____

_____

2. _____

_____

_____

(continued)

3. _____

_____

_____

Now write down three things that Mary could have done to better cope with her cancer phobia.

(*Hint*: Does avoidance help her overcome her phobia? What sorts of things could she do in a step-by-step fashion to tackle her phobia? Should she visit her friend?)

1. _____

_____

_____

2. _____

_____

_____

3. _____

_____

_____

DEVELOPING YOUR OWN PERSONALIZED HARP PROGRAM: PREPARATION FOR COPING WITH SETBACKS

Preventing relapse consists of several steps. The first step comes *before* you have experienced any setbacks:

1. Write down all the things you have learned about the *causes* of your health anxiety. Use additional pages if necessary.

_____

_____

_____

_____

2. Write down the things that might help you in the short term, but make your health anxiety *worse* in the longer term.

_____

_____

3. What sorts of things have you learned that help you cope with, or even overcome, your health anxiety?

(*Hint*: These could have to do with the way you think about things or the way you do things, or they might involve practicing particular exercises.)

_____

_____

(continued)

YOUR HARP PROGRAM (CONT.): ADMINISTERING EMOTIONAL FIRST AID IN THE EVENT OF A SETBACK

Now let us develop some strategies for coping with setbacks when they occur. If you begin to experience problems with health anxiety, then complete the following:

1. *Is the setback a catastrophe?* Write out your reasons.

(*Hint*: Have you had a full relapse or was it just a temporary failure to cope? If you have had a full relapse, is it a catastrophe? Why, or why not?)

_____

_____

_____

_____

2. *Analyze the situation.* Try to learn why the setback occurred. Write out the frightening thoughts you had during the period of health anxiety, including thoughts of what you feared might happen. You might have had frightening thoughts, for example, about the significance of bodily sensations (e.g., "My chest pain means I have heart disease").

_____

_____

_____

_____

3. Now *review the evidence* for and against your frightening thoughts. Can you think of any alternative explanations for your troublesome bodily sensations (e.g., "My chest pain is due to increased tension in the muscles in my chest, which had nothing to do with my heart").

_____

_____

_____

_____

4. *Practice other exercises you learned in therapy*, such as (a) other methods for examining the validity of your beliefs, (b) exposure and response prevention exercises, or (c) stress management exercises. Write down the exercises that you used to cope with your current episode of health anxiety. What was the outcome?

_____

_____

_____

_____

(continued)

5. *Restrict the setback.* Refrain from doing things that make health anxiety worse, such as seeking reassurance, checking your body, and avoiding fear-evoking things. Please list the things that you are trying to refrain from doing (e.g., "I am avoiding searching medical web sites in order to control my health worry").

_____

_____

_____

_____

6. *Return to any situations that you are starting to avoid.* Do this as soon as possible. Develop a step-by-step plan for returning to these situations. If an avoided situation is too anxiety-provoking to enter, then try an easier, related situation and then gradually work up to more difficult situations. Example: Mary could begin to overcome her cancer phobia by, first, looking at magazine articles about survivors of cancer, and then gradually working up to more anxiety-provoking situations such as having coffee with her friend who had been diagnosed with cancer.

Write down the situations that you are avoiding because of excessive fear. Then list the steps for gradually exposing yourself to these situations, in order to overcome the fear.

_____

_____

_____

_____

7. If these methods haven't helped you, then *call your therapist* to discuss the problem or to arrange for further therapy sessions.

Therapist name: _____

Therapist telephone number: _____

Note. Parts of the HARP adapted from Öst (1989).

sode of health anxiety. As part of this exercise, the patient can write out and challenge any dysfunctional beliefs she or he has about the recurrence of his or her problems (e.g., "If my problems return then that will mean the effects of therapy have worn off"). It is important that patients realize that, as a result of therapy, they have acquired effective skills for dealing with setbacks.

- To prepare to deal with setbacks, the patient and the therapist can compile a list of "high–risk" situations. These are events or circumstances most likely to lead to the return of health anxiety. To identify these situations, the therapist can review the case formulation, including circumstances in which the patient's problems initially developed. This provides clues about what might contribute to lapses. Common high–risk situations include stressful life events (which induce bodily reactions), episodes of personal disease, and serious disease or death in significant others or acquaintances (which can heighten one's sense of mortality). Patients can be trained to anticipate and prepare for such events.
- To inoculate against the future development of catastrophic beliefs, one should review body sensations that patients might not have experienced before. The therapist might ask, for example, "Suppose that one day you noticed that you had difficulty breathing. What would you think was happening?" Socratic dialogue can be used to elicit dysfunctional interpretations of the new sensations, and to discuss ways of testing the interpretations.
- If a setback does occur, then the patient should attempt to analyze the situation to identify any dysfunctional beliefs. Once identified, the patient can use cognitive and exposure strategies learned in therapy to evaluate these beliefs. Patients are encouraged to restrict the lapse before it gets worse, using the approach described in Handout 12.2.
- If the patient is unable to manage the setback, then the therapist should be contacted for one or more telephone contacts or face-to-face booster sessions. Consultations should focus on the cause of the setback and should thereby lead to a plan for correcting the problem.

As part of the maintenance plan, arrangements can be made for the patient to periodically check in with the CBT practitioner in order to review progress and discuss any ongoing problems. This can be done by brief telephone, e-mail, or face-to-face booster sessions. Check-in sessions can be arranged, say, 3, 6, and 12 months after the end of a formal course of, say, 12 CBT sessions. Such contacts are used to assess the maintenance of treatment gains, to reinforce the patient's efforts, to provide assistance in helping the patient deal with any new or enduring problems, and to develop plans for ongoing exposure or other therapeutic exercises. Patients should write down what they learned from these contacts so the information is not forgotten.

Issues in Maintaining Gains for Specific Forms of Health Anxiety

In cases of disease phobia, the patient may need to periodically practice exposure exercises in order to reduce the likelihood of a return of fear. The driver's license analogy is useful in conveying this idea (Öst, 1989). Overcoming fears is like acquiring driving skills. It is insufficient to get your driver's license: one must periodically practice driving in order to maintain one's skills.

For patients with delusional disorder (somatic type), the review of treatment progress is likely to be largely concerned with reviewing the effects of medication on bodily sensations. It can be useful to inquire as to whether the patient's beliefs about the cause of the sensations has changed with treatment. Has there been a time during treatment when she or he has wondered, even momentarily, whether she or he really had a severe medical condition such as parasitic infestation? The patient and the therapist can further explore these thoughts to reinforce the idea that the patient's problems arose from misinterpretation of real, but benign, bodily sensations. Patients with delusional disorder (somatic type) may express the desire to discontinue their medications once their troublesome bodily sensations have subsided. Under these circumstances it would be wise for them to remain in regular consultation with the prescribing physician, so that medication can be reinitiated if relapse occurs.

Ongoing Medical Care

To avoid unnecessary medical evaluations, the patient, the CBT practitioner, and the patient's primary care physician can generate a tailored list of guidelines for when a physician should be consulted. The guidelines should be phrased in simple, unambiguous terms. Consultation with a physician might be indicated when:

- New, painful symptoms develop (e.g., chest pain).
- There are unambiguously abnormal bodily changes or sensations (e.g., blood in the urine, loss of continence, inability to speak).
- Symptoms of chronic, medically established diseases flare up that warrant medical intervention (e.g., a resurgence of ulcerative colitis).
- Annual medical examinations or inoculations are due (e.g., mammography, prostate exam, or influenza shot).

Specific guidelines for seeking medical care will depend on the nature of the patient's physical health, and are best formulated with the input of the patient's primary care physician. For elderly or infirm patients, it may be medically necessary for frequent (e.g., monthly) medical checkups.

TREATMENT DROPOUTS AND FAILURES

Although there are a number of effective methods for reducing health anxiety disorders, there is ample room for improving treatment acceptability and efficacy. Some patients will refuse treatment, others will drop out prematurely, and still more will complete a course of therapy but continue to experience health anxiety. Timing is an important issue for treatment refusal. Before they are willing to accept a course of CBT (or other health anxiety treatment), some health-anxious patients will first need to hear the repeated message, from numerous doctors, that their problem is one of health anxiety. Only then will they be willing to try a nonmedical approach to their problems. Other patients will find that practical problems, such as arranging for child care or time off work, prevent them from entering or completing a course of CBT. Sometimes the patient and the therapist can solve these difficulties but on other occasions it may be necessary to defer CBT until the timing is more appropriate.

What should the therapist do when a patient completes a course of CBT but fails to adequately respond? Ongoing monitoring of health anxiety during the course of treatment should alert the clinician to this problem long before the end of a treatment program. To overcome problems with poor treatment response, the therapist should try to develop a hypothesis or formulation of the problem. Then the therapist, in collaboration with the patient, may be able to develop a plan for overcoming the difficulties. There are several reasons for incomplete or poor responses to treatment:

- *Misunderstanding the patient's problems.* In formulating the origins of the problem, the therapist should consider whether the formulation of the patient's health anxiety needs to be revised. In some cases the problem may be one of misdiagnosis. The therapist might assume a patient is suffering from hypochondriasis when, in fact, the patient is expressing appropriate worry about symptoms of a serious, undiagnosed disease such as multiple sclerosis.
- *Failing to establish a sound therapeutic relationship.* Treatment nonadherence may occur if the patient feels that his or her therapist is not listening or not taking his or her problems seriously. Such patients may respond by incessantly talking about their somatic concerns, without

listening to the therapist. This problem can be addressed by the therapist making greater use of empathic, reflective listening, to demonstrate that the therapist is listening and taking the problem seriously. The patient's beliefs about the need to provide a complete, detailed description of his or her "symptoms" can also be explored (see Chapter 9).

- *Noncompletion of homework assignments.* Patients who fail to complete homework assignments are unlikely to fully benefit from CBT. The reasons for nonadherence should be explored in order to find a solution to the problem. Sometimes the problem is one of logistics (e.g., finding sufficient time to complete assignments). At other times the problem is one of therapy timing and pacing (e.g., assigning too many assignments in quick succession, or assignments that are too anxiety-provoking).

- *Environmental contingencies.* Reinforcement contingencies can also interfere with treatment progress, such as significant others in the patient's life who encourage somatic focus (by continually fussing over the patient's health), or significant others who continually criticize patients for not progressing fast enough in overcoming their health anxiety (thereby leading to demoralization and helplessness). Involving the significant other in treatment can be useful in overcoming these obstacles. In cases in which the significant other actively sabotages treatment, couple therapy may be warranted to overcome this interpersonal problem.

- *Overvalued ideation.* Strong disease conviction can be difficult to treat with CBT, and may warrant the addition of antipsychotic medication, particularly in cases of somatic delusions.

- *Interference due to comorbid psychopathology.* Comorbid disorders, such as coexisting personality disorders or substance-use disorders, can sometimes interfere with the treatment of health anxiety. Comorbid benzodiazepine abuse, for example, would interfere with treatment if the patient were taking such high doses that he or she was too sedated to undertake homework assignments or to appreciate what was learned in these assignments. Sometimes comorbid disorders need to be treated before progress can be made in reducing health anxiety.

If the patient has failed to respond to CBT, and if the therapist is unable to identify reasons for the failure, then one might consider extending the duration of CBT, replacing CBT with medication, combining CBT with medication, or referring the patient to another practitioner. These strategies are empirically driven because they are based on a "try it and see" approach, rather than on a case formulation. Although such treatment approaches are not conceptually elegant, they are pragmatic, and are sometimes the best we can do to help our health-anxious patients.

SUMMARY AND CONCLUSIONS

For many people with health anxiety disorders, therapy is an ongoing process, extending beyond the formal course of CBT. Treatment would ideally do more than reduce symptoms; it would enhance the patient's quality of life. The latter can be addressed in the final stages of a formal course of CBT. To foster autonomous functioning, treatment sessions are gradually tapered and the patient is educated in ways of maintaining treatment gains. Relapse prevention strategies are an important element in any maintenance program. Printed handouts and worksheets can facilitate treatment maintenance. For patients who fail to respond to treatment, it is important for the clinician to do a thorough evaluation to identify the reasons for the problem. The treatments outlined in this book are generally effective, although not all patients will benefit from them. There is ample room for improving treatment outcome. In the coming years there will likely be many new developments in treatments for health anxiety disorders, both cognitive-behavioral and pharmacological. We expect that treatment advances will arise from a combination of accumulating research, refined models of health anxiety disorders, and from carefully listening to, and learning from, our health-anxious patients.

APPENDICES
Instruments for Assessing Health Anxiety

I. PROBE QUESTIONS

1. Do you have a lot of medical problems?   Yes   No
2. Do you have symptoms that bother you?   Yes   No
3. Are you concerned about your health?   Yes   No
4. Is your health on your mind a lot?   Yes   No
5. Do you think your body is malfunctioning?   Yes   No

Note: If respondent answers *No* to all questions, discontinue interview.

II. HYPOCHONDRIASIS

i. DSM-IV CRITERION A   Preoccupation with fears of having, or the idea that one has, a serious disease based on the person's misinterpretation of bodily symptoms.

(A1) Disease Fear or Conviction

1. Are you concerned that you might have a serious   Yes   No
   disease that doctors have not been able to find?
2. Do you worry a lot about getting sick or being sick?   Yes   No

(A2) Symptom Misinterpretation

3. What are your symptoms and why do you think they indicate disease?

         Possible symptom misinterpretation   Yes   No

             CRIT MET   NOT MET

Note: If respondent fails to meet Hypochondriasis Criterion A, skip to Section III. Disease Phobia. If the person exhibits an extraordinary conviction or the disease concerns and symptoms seem impossible with regard to content, then consider Delusional Disorder (Somatic Type) (Section IV).

ii. DSM-IV CRITERION B   The preoccupation persists despite appropriate medical evaluation and reassurance.

(B1) Appropriate Medical Evaluation

1. Have you seen a doctor for these symptoms?   Yes   No
2. What types of test did the doctor perform?
   Appropriate medical evaluation   Yes   No

(B2) Reassurance

1. Has your doctor tried to reassure you about your symptoms? Yes   No
2. Did the doctor make you feel better?   Yes   No

             CRIT MET   NOT MET

(continued)

iii. DSM-IV CRITERION D   The preoccupation causes clinically significant distress or impairment in social, occupational, or other important areas of functioning.

  1. Have your symptoms caused you problems   Yes   No
in your home, leisure, or work activities?

                    CRIT MET NOT MET

iv. DSM-IV CRITERION E   The duration of the disturbance is at least 6 months.

  1. How long has your health been giving   > 6 mo.   < 6 mo.
you trouble like this?

                    CRIT MET NOT MET

v. SPECIFIER

(Specifier) With Poor Insight

  1. Do you think you worry more about these symptoms   Yes   No
than is warranted?

Note: If the above criteria are all met, ensure that exclusionary criteria are ruled out.

vi. DSM-IV Criteria C and F

Are symptoms:

(C) better accounted for by Delusional Disorder or restricted to concerns about appearance

1.	Delusional Disorder (Somatic Type)	No	Yes
2.	Body Dysmorphic Disorder	No	Yes

(D) better accounted for by Axis I Disorders

1.	Generalized Anxiety Disorder	No	Yes
2.	Obsessive–Compulsive Disorder	No	Yes
3.	Panic Disorder	No	Yes
4.	Major Depressive Disorder	No	Yes
5.	Separation Anxiety	No	Yes
6.	Other Somatoform Disorder	No	Yes

                    CRIT MET NOT MET

III. DISEASE PHOBIA

i. DSM-IV CRITERION A   Marked and persistent fear of contracting a disease that is excessive or unreasonable.

  1. Are you concerned that you might contract   Yes   No
a serious disease or illness?   CRIT MET NOT MET

Note: If respondent fails to meet Disease Phobia Criterion A, skip to Section IV. Delusional Disorder (Somatic Type).

(continued)

    ii. DSM-IV CRITERION B   Exposure to disease-related stimuli invariably provokes an immediate anxiety response.

    1.   Do you get anxious or panicky whenever you see   Yes   No
or hear about disease-related things (e.g., sick people,
hospitals, medical news)?   CRIT MET NOT MET

    iii. DSM-IV CRITERION C   The person recognizes that the fear is excessive or unreasonable.

    1.   Do you feel that you are more fearful of disease-related   Yes   No
things when compared to most people? Do you think
your fear is excessive?   CRIT MET NOT MET

    DSM-IV CRITERION D   Are disease related stimuli avoided *or* endured with intense anxiety or distress?

    1.   Do you avoid things that are associated with disease   Yes   No
(e.g., medical shows on TV, visiting a sick relative in
the hospital, using public restrooms)?

    2.   When you have to be around things that you associate   Yes   No
with disease, do you feel anxious or distressed?

If affirmative response to 1 or 2, then score CRIT MET.   CRIT MET NOT MET

    iv. DSM-IV CRITERION E   The avoidance, anxious anticipation, or distress interferes significantly with normal routine, social, occupational, or other important areas of functioning, *or* is associated with marked distress.

    1.   Have your symptoms caused you problems in   Yes   No
your home, leisure, or work activities?

    2.   Have your symptoms been distressing to you?   Yes   No
        CRIT MET NOT MET

If affirmative response to 1 or 2, then score CRIT MET.

IV. DELUSIONAL DISORDER (SOMATIC TYPE)

    1. Are parts of your body malfunctioning?   Yes   No

    2. Does your body, or parts of your body, smell foul?   Yes   No

    3. Is your skin infested by insects?   Yes   No

    4. Is your body occupied by parasites?   Yes   No

Note. If an affirmative response is provided to any of these probes, a thorough assessment of Delusional Disorder is warranted. In this assessment it is crucial to establish whether delusions are nonbizarre or bizarre. Nonbizarre delusions are those that might conceivably occur in real life, while those that are bizarre are clearly implausible in this context.

(continued)

    i. DSM-IV CRITERION A Non-bizarre delusions have persisted for more than 1 month.

        1. How long has your health been giving you trouble like this?   > 1 mo.   < 1 mo.

                                                                       CRIT MET NOT MET

    ii. DSM-IV CRITERION B and E Criterion A for Schizophrenia has *never* been met. Delusions are *not* due to effects of a substance or general medical condition.

From history or additional assessment, determine whether Criterion A for Schizophrenia has ever been met. If affirmative for history or current Criteria A for Schizophrenia, discontinue interview.

Determine whether delusions are likely due the effects of a substance (e.g., drug abuse, medication) or general medical condition (e.g., Alzheimer's Disease). If affirmative for either, discontinue interview.

    iii. DSM-IV CRITERION C Aside from impact of delusions, functional abilities are *not* markedly impaired and behavior is *not* bizarre.

        1. Have your health concerns caused you serious problems in your home, leisure, or work activities?   No   Yes

        2. Has anyone close to you ever commented that your behavior is unusual or nonsensical? If yes, please explain.   No   Yes

                                                        CRIT MET NOT MET

    iv. DSM-IV CRITERION D Duration of mood changes, if present, have been brief relative to delusions.

        1. Have you or people close to you noticed any significant changes in your mood?   Yes   No

        2. When did these changes first become apparent?   Brief   Lengthy

        3. Has this mood been fairly constant for the past while?   No   Yes

                                                         CRIT MET NOT MET

V. CURRENT CIRCUMSTANCES

    1. Tell me a little bit more about your home and work environments. Who do you live with? Do you have a group of close friends that you do things with on a regular basis? Do you interact with your coworkers? How do your family, friends, and coworkers respond to you when you express your concerns about health or disease to them?

(continued)

2. Do you exercise or participate in a regular physical activity? What kind of activity and how often?

3. How often have you seen your family physician over the past 6 months? What about specialists?

4. What has your doctor told you about the purpose of you coming to see me?

VI. HISTORY AND DEVELOPMENT OF HEALTH ANXIETY

1. When did you start to become concerned about your health? What happened? What else was happening in your life at the time?

2. What was your physical health like when you were a child?

3. How did your parents (or caregivers) react when you got sick when you were a child?

4. Were your parents (or caregivers) worried about their own health? What about your siblings or close relatives? Can you give me some examples?

5. Has anything else occurred in your life that's influenced the way you think about health and disease? For example, did anything happen to family or friends that made you worried about getting sick?

APPENDIX 2a. Whiteley Index

Here are some questions about your health. Circle either YES or NO to indicate your answer to each question.

1. Do you often worry about the possibility that you have got a serious illness?　　YES　　NO

2. Are you bothered by many pains and aches?　　YES　　NO

3. Do you find that you are often aware of various things happening in your body?　　YES　　NO

4. Do you worry a lot about your health?　　YES　　NO

5. Do you often have the symptoms of very serious illness?　　YES　　NO

6. If a disease is brought to you attention (through the radio, television, newspapers, or someone you know) do you worry about getting it yourself?　　YES　　NO

7. If you feel ill and someone tells you that you are looking better, do you become annoyed?　　YES　　NO

8. Do you find that you are bothered by many different symptoms?　　YES　　NO

9. Is it easy for you to forget about yourself, and think about all sorts of other things?　　YES　　NO

10. Is it hard for you to believe the doctor when he or she tells you there is nothing for you to worry about?　　YES　　NO

11. Do you get the feeling that people are not taking your illness seriously enough?　　YES　　NO

12. Do you think that you worry about your health more than most people?　　YES　　NO

13. Do you think there is something seriously wrong with your body?　　YES　　NO

14. Are you afraid of illness?　　YES　　NO

Note. Wording "or she" has been added to item 10. Reprinted with kind permission from Professor Issy Pilowsky. User manual available by contacting Ms. Sue Sullivan, Department of Psychiatry (RAH), University of Adelaide, South Australia 5001, Australia.

APPENDIX 2b. Scoring Sheet for the Whiteley Index

Name:

ID number:

Date:

Scoring instructions: Give 1 point for each affirmative response. Item 9 is reverse scored—that is, 1 point is given for a negative response.

Index	Items	Score
WI total score	Sum all 14 items*	
Disease fear	6 + 9* + 12 + 14	
Disease conviction	7 + 11 + 13	
Bodily preoccupation	2 + 3 + 8	

Note. Barsky et al. (1992) introduced a modification to the scoring by changing to a 5-point Likert scale ranging from 1 ("Not at all") to 5 ("A great deal"). Total and subscale scores are calculated as above.
*Item 9 is reverse scored (i.e., 1 point given for negative response)
Subscale scores are based on factors derived in Pilowsky (1967) and do not contain all WI items.

APPENDIX 3a. Illness Behavior Questionnaire for Clinical Setting

Here are some questions about your illness. Circle YES or NO to indicate your answer to each question.

1. Do you worry a lot about your health? — Yes No
2. Do you think there is something seriously wrong with your body? — Yes No
3. Does your illness interfere with your life a great deal? — Yes No
4. Are you easy to get on with when you are ill? — Yes No
5. Does your family have a history of illness? — Yes No
6. Do you think you are more liable to illness than other people? — Yes No
7. If the doctor told you that he could find nothing wrong with you would you believe him? — Yes No
8. Is it easy for you to forget about yourself and think about all sorts of other things? — Yes No
9. If you feel ill and someone tells you that you are looking better, do you become annoyed? — Yes No
10. Do you find that you are often aware of various things happening in your body? — Yes No
11. Do you ever think of your illness as a punishment for something you have done wrong in the past? — Yes No
12. Do you ever have trouble with your nerves? — Yes No
13. If you feel ill or worried, can you be easily cheered up by the doctor? — Yes No
14. Do you think that other people realize what it is like to be sick? — Yes No
15. Does it upset you to talk to the doctor about your illness? — Yes No
16. Are you bothered by many pains and aches? — Yes No
17. Does your illness affect the way you get on with your family or friends a great deal? — Yes No
18. Do you find that you get anxious easily? — Yes No
19. Do you know anybody who has had the same illness as you? — Yes No
20. Are you more sensitive to pain than other people? — Yes No
21. Are you afraid of illness? — Yes No
22. Can you express your personal feelings easily to other people? — Yes No
23. Do you feel sorry for you when you are ill? — Yes No
24. Do you think that you worry about your health more than most people? — Yes No
25. Do you find that your illness affects your sexual relations? — Yes No
26. Do you experience a lot of pain with your illness? — Yes No
27. Except for your illness, do you have any problems in your life? — Yes No
28. Do you care whether or not people realize you are sick? — Yes No
29. Do you find that you get jealous of other people's good health? — Yes No
30. Do you ever have silly thoughts about your health which you can't get out of your mind, no matter how hard you try? — Yes No

(continued)

31.	Do you have any financial problems?	Yes	No
32.	Are you upset by the way people take your illness?	Yes	No
33.	Is it hard for you to believe the doctor when he or she tells you there is nothing for you to worry about?	Yes	No
34.	Do you often worry about the possibility that you have got a serious illness?	Yes	No
35.	Are you sleeping well?	Yes	No
36.	When you are angry, do you tend to bottle up your feelings?	Yes	No
37.	Do you often think that you might suddenly fall ill?	Yes	No
38.	If a disease is brought to your attention (through the radio, television, newspapers, or someone you know) do you worry about getting it yourself?	Yes	No
39.	Do you get the feeling that people are not taking your illness seriously enough?	Yes	No
40.	Are you upset by the appearance of your face or body?	Yes	No
41.	Do you find that you are bothered by many different symptoms?	Yes	No
42.	Do you frequently try to explain to others how you are feeling?	Yes	No
43.	Do you have any family problems?	Yes	No
44.	Do you think there is something the matter with your mind?	Yes	No
45.	Are you eating well?	Yes	No
46.	Is you bad health the biggest difficulty in your life?	Yes	No
47.	Do you find that you get sad easily?	Yes	No
48.	Do you fuss over small details that seem unimportant to others?	Yes	No
49.	Are you always a cooperative patient?	Yes	No
50.	Do you often have the symptoms of a very serious disease?	Yes	No
51.	Do you find that you get angry easily?	Yes	No
52.	Do you have any work problems?	Yes	No
53.	Do you prefer to keep your feelings to yourself?	Yes	No
54.	Do you often that you get depressed?	Yes	No
55.	Would all your worries be over if you were physically healthy?	Yes	No
56.	Are you more irritable toward other people?	Yes	No
57.	Do you think that your symptoms may be caused by worry?	Yes	No
58.	Is it easy for you to let people know when you are cross with them?	Yes	No
59.	Is it hard for you to relax?	Yes	No
60.	Do you have personal worries which are not caused by physical illness?	Yes	No
61.	Do you often find that you lose patience with other people?	Yes	No
62.	Is it hard for you to show people your personal feelings?	Yes	No

Note. Wording "or she" has been added to item 33. Reprinted with kind permission from Professor Issy Pilowsky. User manual available by contacting Ms. Sue Sullivan, Department of Psychiatry (RAH), University of Adelaide, South Australia 5001, Australia.

APPENDIX 3b. Scoring Sheet for the Illness Behavior Questionnaire

Name:

ID number:

Date:

Scoring instructions: Give 1 point for each response scored as indicated in the key below. Note that not all items contribute to subscale scores.

Index	Items	Score
General hypochondriasis	9 + 20 + 21 + 24 + 29 + 30 + 32 + 37 + 38	
Disease conviction	2 + 3 + 7R + 10 + 35R + 41	
Psychological versus somatic concern	11 + 16R + 44 + 46R + 57	
Affective inhibition	22R + 36 + 53 + 58R + 62	
Affective disturbance	12 + 18 +47 + 54 + 59	
Denial	27R + 31R + 43R + 55 + 60R	
Irritability	4R + 17 + 51 + 56 + 61	
Whiteley Index	1 + 2 + 8R + 9 + 10 + 16 + 21 + 24 + 33 + 34 + 38 + 39 + 41 + 50	

Note. "R" indicates items to be reverse scored (i.e., 1 point given for negative response).

APPENDIX 4a. Illness Attitude Scales

Please circle your answers to all questions with the exception of the few questions that require a few words or sentences. Do not think long before answering. Work quickly!

1. Do you worry about your health?	No Rarely Sometimes Often Most of the time
2. Are you worried that you may get a serious illness in the future?	No Rarely Sometimes Often Most of the time
3. Does the thought of a serious illness scare you?	No Rarely Sometimes Often Most of the time
4. If you have pain, do you worry that it may be caused by a serious illness?	No Rarely Sometimes Often Most of the time
5. If a pain lasts for a week or more, do you see a physician?	No Rarely Sometimes Often Most of the time
6. If a pain lasts a week or more, do you believe that you have a serious illness?	No Rarely Sometimes Often Most of the time
7. Do you avoid habits that may be harmful to you such as smoking?	No Rarely Sometimes Often Most of the time
8. Do you avoid foods that may not be healthy?	No Rarely Sometimes Often Most of the time
9. Do you examine your body to find whether there is something wrong?	No Rarely Sometimes Often Most of the time
10. Do you believe that you have a physical disease but the doctors have not diagnosed it?	No Rarely Sometimes Often Most of the time
11. When your doctor tells you that you have no physical disease, do you refuse to believe it?	No Rarely Sometimes Often Most of the time
12. When you have been told by a doctor what he or she found, do you soon begin to believe that you may have developed the illness?	No Rarely Sometimes Often Most of the time
13. Are you afraid of news that reminds you of death (such as funerals, obituary notices)?	No Rarely Sometimes Often Most of the time
14. Does the thought of death scare you?	No Rarely Sometimes Often Most of the time
15. Are you afraid that you may die soon?	No Rarely Sometimes Often Most of the time
16. Are you afraid that you may have cancer?	No Rarely Sometimes Often Most of the time
17. Are you afraid that you may have heart disease?	No Rarely Sometimes Often Most of the time
18. Are you afraid that you may have another serious illness?	No Rarely Sometimes Often Most of the time

(continued)

Which illness? _____

19. When you read or hear about an illness, do you get symptoms similar to those of the illness?
    No Rarely Sometimes Often Most of the time

20. When you notice a sensation in your body, do you find it difficult to think of something else?
    No Rarely Sometimes Often Most of the time

21. When you feel a sensation in your body, do you worry about it?
    No Rarely Sometimes Often Most of the time

22. Has your doctor told you that you have an illness now?
    If yes, what illness? _____

23. How often do you see a doctor?

Almost never	Only very rarely
About 4 times a year	About once a month
About once a week	

24. How many different doctors, chiropractors, or other healers have you seen in the past year?

None	1
2 or 3	4 or 5
6 or more	

25. How often have you been treated in the last year (e.g., drugs, change of drugs, surgery, etc.)?

Not at all	Once
2 or 3 times	4 or 5 times
6 or more times	

26. If yes, what were the treatments?
    _____
    _____

The next three questions concern your bodily symptoms (e.g., pain, aches, pressure in your body, breathing difficulties, tiredness, etc.).

27. Do your bodily symptoms stop you from working?
    No Rarely Sometimes Often Most of the time

28. Do your bodily symptoms stop you from concentrating on what you are doing?
    No Rarely Sometimes Often Most of the time

29. Do your bodily symptoms stop you from enjoying yourself?
    No Rarely Sometimes Often Most of the time

Note. Reprinted with kind permission of the University of New Mexico. User manual available by contacting Mrs. Tina Lujan, Department of Psychiatry, University of New Mexico, School of Medicine, 2400 Tucker NE, Albuquerque, NM 87131.

APPENDIX 4b. Scoring Sheet for the Illness Attitude Scales

Name:

ID number:

Date:

Scoring instructions: Sum item responses (0 = no; 1 = rarely; 2 = sometimes; 3 = often; 4 = most of the time) as indicated in the key below.

Index	Items	Score
IAS total score	Sum all items, excluding item 22 and item 26	
Worry about illness	1+ 2 + 3	
Concerns about pain	4 + 5 + 6	
Health habits	7 + 8 + 9	
Hypochondriacal beliefs	10 + 11 + 12	
Thanatophobia	13 + 14 + 15	
Disease phobia	16 + 17 + 18	
Bodily preoccupation	19 + 20 + 21	
Treatment experience	23 + 24 + 25	
Effects of symptoms	27 + 28 + 29	

Note. This scoring method is based on Kellner's (1987) original nine-subscale conceptualization of the IAS. Items 22 and 26 are not used in scoring.

APPENDIX 4c. Alternative Method Scoring Sheet for the Illness Attitude Scales

Name:

ID number:

Date:

Scoring instructions: Sum item responses (0 = no; 1 = rarely; 2 = sometimes; 3 = often; 4 = most of the time) as indicated in the key below.

Index	Items	Score
IAS total score	Sum all items, excluding item 22 and item 26	
Fear of illness, disease, pain, and death	2 + 3 + 4 + 13 + 14 + 15 + 16 + 17 + 18	
Symptoms interference with lifestyle	20 + 27 + 28 + 29	
Treatment experience	5 + 23 + 24 + 25	
Disease conviction	10 + 11 + 12 + 18	

Note. This scoring method is based on Hadjistavropoulos, Frombach, and Asmundson's (1999) four-subscale conceptualization of the IAS. Items 1, 6, 7, 8, 9, 21, 22 and 26 are not used in subscale scoring.

APPENDIX 5a. Health Anxiety Questionnaire

This questionnaire is concerned with people's attitudes about their health. Some of the questions concern your bodily symptoms and feelings which can mean pains, aches, sickness, dizziness, breathing difficulties, tiredness, etc. Read each question and circle the answer that best applies to you.

1. Do you ever worry about your health? Not at all or rarely   Sometimes   Often   Most of the time

2. Are you ever worried that you may get a serious illness in the future?   Not at all or rarely   Sometimes   Often   Most of the time

3. Does the thought of a serious illness ever scare you?   Not at all or rarely   Sometimes   Often   Most of the time

4. When you notice an unpleasant feeling in your body, do you tend to find it difficult to think of anything else?   Not at all or rarely   Sometimes   Often   Most of the time

5. Do you ever examine your body to find whether there is something wrong?   Not at all or rarely   Sometimes   Often   Most of the time

6. If you have an ache or pain do you worry that it may be caused by a serious illness?   Not at all or rarely   Sometimes   Often   Most of the time

7. Do you ever find it difficult to keep worries about your health out of your mind?   Not at all or rarely   Sometimes   Often   Most of the time

8. When you notice an unpleasant feeling in your body, do you ever worry about it?   Not at all or rarely   Sometimes   Often   Most of the time

9. When you wake up in the morning do you find you very soon begin to worry about your health?   Not at all or rarely   Sometimes   Often   Most of the time

10. When you hear of a serious illness or the death of someone you know, does it ever make you more concerned about your own health?   Not at all or rarely   Sometimes   Often   Most of the time

11. When you read or hear about an illness on TV or radio, does it ever make you think you may be suffering from that illness?   Not at all or rarely   Sometimes   Often   Most of the time

12. When you experience unpleasant feelings in your body do you tend to ask friends or family about them?   Not at all or rarely   Sometimes   Often   Most of the time

13. Do you tend to read up about illness and diseases to see if you may be suffering from one?   Not at all or rarely   Sometimes   Often   Most of the time

(continued)

14. Do you ever feel afraid of news that reminds you of death (such as funerals, obituary notices)?   Not at all or rarely   Sometimes   Often   Most of the time

15. Do you ever feel afraid that you may die soon?   Not at all or rarely   Sometimes   Often   Most of the time

16. Do you ever feel afraid that you may have cancer?   Not at all or rarely   Sometimes   Often   Most of the time

17 Do you ever feel afraid you might have heart disease?   Not at all or rarely   Sometimes   Often   Most of the time

18. Do you ever feel afraid that you may have any other serious illness? Which illness? _____   Not at all or rarely   Sometimes   Often   Most of the time

19. Have your bodily symptoms stopped you from working during the past 6 months or so?   Not at all or rarely   Sometimes   Often   Most of the time

20. Do your bodily symptoms stop you from concentrating on what you are doing?   Not at all or rarely   Sometimes   Often   Most of the time

21. Do your bodily symptoms stop you from enjoying yourself?   Not at all or rarely   Sometimes   Often   Most of the time

Note. Reprinted with kind permission from Professor Stephen Morley and Dr. Michael Lucock as well as the British Psychological Society. Original work appears in Lucock, M. P., & Morley, S. (1996). The Health Anxiety Questionnaire. *British Journal of Health Psychology, 1,* 137–150.

APPENDIX 5b. Scoring Sheet for the Health Anxiety Questionnaire

Name:

ID number:

Date:

Scoring instructions: Sum item responses (not at all or rarely = 0; sometimes = 1; often = 2; most of the time = 3) as indicated in the key below.

Index	Items	Score
HAQ total score	Sum scores for all 21 items	
Health worry and preoccupation	1 + 4 + 6 + 7 + 8 + 9 + 11 + 18	
Fear of illness and death	2 + 3 + 10 + 14 + 15 + 16 + 17	
Reassurance-seeking behavior	5 + 12 +1 3	
Interference with life	19 + 20 + 21	

APPENDIX 6a. Reassurance Questionnaire

These questions concern the extent to which you feel reassured by your physician about your symptoms. Please answer by circling the best answer.

0 = No
1 = Rarely
2 = Sometimes
3 = Often
4 = Usually

1.	If you initially feel reassured by a visit to your physician, does your anxiety return later on?	0	1	2	3	4
2.	Do you keep worrying as long as it is not possible to rule out a serious illness?	0	1	2	3	4
3.	Do you keep worrying as long as you do not know the origins of your symptoms?	0	1	2	3	4
4.	Do you think the diagnosis made by your physician is incorrect?	0	1	2	3	4
5.	Do you ask for a referral to a consultant, even if your physician does not think this is necessary?	0	1	2	3	4
6.	Do you think your physician is keeping something from you?	0	1	2	3	4
7.	Do you think your physician has not examined you properly?	0	1	2	3	4
8.	Do you think that your symptoms should be investigated more extensively (laboratory tests, x-rays, etc.)?	0	1	2	3	4

Note. Reprinted with kind permission from Dr. Anne Speckens and Cambridge University Press. Original work appears in Speckens, A. E. M., Spinhoven, P., van Hamert, A. M., & Bolk, J. H. (2000). The Reassurance Questionnaire (RQ): Psychometric properties of a self-report questionnaire to assess reassurability. *Psychological Medicine, 30*, 841–847.

APPENDIX 6b. Scoring Sheet for the Reassurance Questionnaire

Name:

ID number:

Date:

Scoring instructions: Sum all item responses to obtain a total scale score (0 = no; 1 = rarely; 2 = sometimes; 3 = often; 4 = usually).

Total RQ score: _____

APPENDIX 7a. Somatosensory Amplification Scale

Please indicate the degree to which each of the following statements are true of you in general. Circle your answer.

1 = Not at all true
2 = A little bit true
3 = Moderately true
4 = Quite a bit true
5 = Extremely true

1.	I can't stand smoke, smog, or pollutants in the air.	1	2	3	4	5
2.	I am often aware of various things happening within my body.	1	2	3	4	5
3.	When I bruise myself, it stays noticeable for a long time.	1	2	3	4	5
4.	I sometimes can feel the blood flowing in my body.	1	2	3	4	5
5.	Sudden loud noises really bother me.	1	2	3	4	5
6.	I can sometimes hear my pulse or my heartbeat throbbing in my ear.	1	2	3	4	5
7.	I hate to be too hot or too cold.	1	2	3	4	5
8.	I am quick to sense the hunger contractions in my stomach.	1	2	3	4	5
9.	Even something minor, like an insect bite or a splinter, really bothers me.	1	2	3	4	5
10.	I can't stand pain.	1	2	3	4	5

Note. Reprinted with kind permission from Dr. Arthur Barsky.

APPENDIX 7b. Scoring Sheet for the Somatosensory Amplification Scale

Name:

ID number:

Date:

Scoring instructions: Sum all item responses to obtain a total scale score (1 = not at all true; 2 = a little bit true; 3 = moderately true; 4 = quite a bit true; 5 = extremely true).

Total SSAS score: _____

APPENDIX 8. Daily Diary

Name: _____ Day and date: _____

Instructions: Please complete this diary at the end of each day, so that we can obtain detailed information about your health concerns.

1. Today, did you worry that you *might have* a physical illness, or that you have a physical illness that's getting worse?	YES / NO
2. Which illness?	
3. Was there anything in particular that caused you to worry, such as a particular bodily sensation or symptom, or a newspaper article?	
4. How long were you worried?	
5. How severe was your anxiety when your worry was at its worst? Use a 0 to 10 scale, where 0 = no anxiety and 10 = severe anxiety.	
6. What did you do to try to deal with your worries? For example, did you see your doctor, seek reassurance from a family memory, or take some sort of medication?	
7. Today, did you avoid anything (e.g., people, places, activities) because you were frightened that you *might catch* an illness?	YES / NO
8. What did you avoid?	
9. Which illness were you frightened of catching?	

References

Agras, S., Sylvester, D., & Oliveau, D. (1969). The epidemiology of common fears and phobias. *Comprehensive Psychiatry, 10,* 151–156.

Airola, P. O. (1977). *Hypoglycemia: A better approach.* Phoenix, AZ: Health Plus.

Altamura, A. C., Carta, M. G., Tacchini, G., Musazzi, A., & Pioli, M. R. (1998). Prevalence of somatoform disorders in a psychiatric population: An Italian nationwide survey. *European Archives of Psychiatry and Clinical Neuroscience, 248,* 267–271.

American Psychiatric Association. (1995). Practice guideline for psychiatric evaluation of adults. *American Journal of Psychiatry, 152,* 63–80.

American Psychiatric Association. (2000). *Diagnostic and statistical manual of mental disorders* (4th ed., text rev.). Washington, DC: Author.

Amsterdam, E. A. (1990). Emotions, cardiac arrhythmias, and sudden death. In D. G. Byrne & R. H. Rosenman (Eds.), *Anxiety and the heart* (pp. 251–258). New York: Hemisphere.

Anderson, J. R. (1990). *Cognitive psychology and its implications* (3rd ed.). New York: Freeman.

Andrews, E., Bellard, J., & Walter-Ryan, W. G. (1986). Monosymptomatic hypochondriacal psychosis manifesting as delusions of infestation: Case studies of treatment with haloperidol. *Journal of Clinical Psychiatry, 47,* 188–190.

Asmundson, G. J. G., Taylor, S., & Cox, B. J. (2001). *Health anxiety: Clinical and research perspectives on hypochondriasis and related disorders.* New York: Wiley.

Atmaca, M., Kuloglu, M., Tezcan, E., & Unal, A. (2002). "Detergent is circulating in my blood": A case report. *International Journal of Psychiatry in Clinical Practice, 6,* 117–120.

Avia, M. D., Ruiz, M. A., Olivares, M. E., Crespo, M., Guisado, A. B., Sanchez, A., & Varela, A. (1996). The meaning of psychological symptoms: Effectiveness of a group intervention with hypochondriacal patients. *Behaviour Research and Therapy, 34,* 23–31.

Bagby, R. M., Taylor, G. J., & Ryan, D. (1986). Toronto Alexithymia Scale: Relationship with personality and psychopathology measures. *Psychotherapy and Psychosomatics, 45,* 207–215.

Baker, B., & Merskey, H. (1982). Parental representations of hypochondriacal patients from a psychiatric hospital. *British Journal of Psychiatry, 141,* 233–238.

Balint, M. (1964). *The doctor, his patient and the illness* (2nd ed.). New York: International Universities Press.

Bankier, B., Aigner, M., & Bach, M. (2001). Alexithymia in DSM-IV disorders: Comparative evaluation of somatoform disorders, panic disorder, obsessive–compulsive disorder, and depression. *Psychosomatics, 42,* 235–240.

Barsky, A. J. (1992). Amplification, somatization, and the somatoform disorders. *Psychosomatics, 33,* 28–34.

Barsky, A. J. (1996). Hypochondriasis: Medical management and psychiatric treatment. *Psychosomatics, 37,* 48–56.

Barsky, A. J. (2000). The validity of bodily symptoms in medical outpatients. In A. A. Stone, J. S. Turkkan, C. A. Bachrach, J. B. Jobe, H. S. Kurtzman, & V. S. Cain (Eds.), *The science of self-report: Implications for research and practice* (pp. 339–361). Mahwah, NJ: Erlbaum.

Barsky, A. J. (2001). The patient with hypochondriasis. *New England Journal of Medicine, 345,* 1395–1399.

Barsky, A. J., Ahern, D. K., Bailey, E. D., & Delamater, B. A. (1996). Predictors of persistent palpitations and continued medical utilization. *Journal of Family Practice, 42,* 465–472.

Barsky, A. J., Barnett, M. C., & Cleary, P. D. (1994a). Hypochondriasis and panic disorder: Boundary and overlap. *Archives of General Psychiatry, 51,* 918–925.

Barsky, A. J., Brener, J., Coeytaux, R. R., & Cleary, P. D. (1995a). Accurate awareness of heartbeat in hypochondriacal and non-hypochondriacal patients. *Journal of Psychosomatic Research, 39,* 489–497.

Barsky, A. J., Cleary, P. D., Coeytaux, R. R., & Ruskin, J. N. (1995b). The clinical course of palpitations in medical outpatients. *Archives of Internal Medicine, 155,* 1782–1788.

Barsky, A. J., Cleary, P. D., Sarnie, M. K., & Klerman, G. L. (1993a). The course of transient hypochondriasis. *American Journal of Psychiatry, 150,* 484–488.

Barsky, A. J., Cleary, P. D., Wyshak, G., Spitzer, R. L., Williams, J. B. W., & Klerman, G. L. (1992). A structured diagnostic interview for hypochondriasis: A proposed criterion standard. *Journal of Nervous and Mental Disease, 180,* 20–27.

Barsky, A. J., Coeytaux, R. R., Sarnie, M. K., & Cleary, P. D. (1993b). Hypochondriacal patients' beliefs about good health. *American Journal of Psychiatry, 150,* 1085–1089.

Barsky, A. J., Ettner, S. L., Horsky, J., & Bates, D. W. (2001). Resource utilization of patients with hypochondriacal health anxiety and somatization. *Medical Care, 39,* 705–715.

Barsky, A. J., Fama, J. M., Bailey, E. D., & Ahern, D. K. (1998b). A prospective 4- to 5-year study of DSM-III-R hypochondriasis. *Archives of General Psychiatry, 55,* 737–744.

Barsky, A. J., Frank, C. B., Cleary, P. D., Wyshak, G., & Klerman, G. L. (1991). The relation between hypochondriasis and age. *American Journal of Psychiatry, 148,* 923–928.

Barsky, A. J., Geringer, E., & Wool, C. A. (1988a). A cognitive-educational treatment for hypochondriasis. *General Hospital Psychiatry, 10,* 322–327.

Barsky, A. J., Goodson, J. D., Lane, R. S., & Cleary, P. D. (1988b). The amplification of somatic symptoms. *Psychosomatic Medicine, 50,* 510–519.

Barsky, A. J., & Klerman, G. L. (1983). Overview: Hypochondriasis, bodily complaints, and somatic styles. *American Journal of Psychiatry, 140,* 273–283.

Barsky, A. J., Orav, E. J., Ahern, D. K., Rogers, M. P., Gruen, S. D., & Liang, M. H. (1999). Somatic style and symptom reporting in rheumatoid arthritis. *Psychosomatics, 40,* 396–403.

Barsky, A. J., Orav, E. J., Delamater, B. A., Clancy, S. A., & Hartley, L. H. (1998a). Cardiorespiratory symptoms in response to physiological arousal. *Psychosomatic Medicine, 60,* 604–609.

Barsky, A. J., Saintforth, R., Rogers, M. P., & Borus, J. F. (2002). Nonspecific medication side effects and the nocebo phenomenon. *Journal of the American Medical Association, 287,* 622–627.

Barsky, A. J., Wool, C., Barnett, M. C., & Cleary, P. D. (1994b). Histories of childhood trauma in adult hypochondriacal patients. *American Journal of Psychiatry, 151,* 397–401.

Barsky, A. J., & Wyshak, G. (1989). Hypochondriasis and related health attitudes. *Psychosomatics, 30,* 412–420.

Barsky, A. J., & Wyshak, G. (1990). Hypochondriasis and somatosensory amplification. *British Journal of Psychiatry, 157,* 404–409.

Barsky, A. J., Wyshak, G., & Klerman, G. L. (1986). Hypochondriasis: An evaluation of the DSM-III criteria in medical outpatients. *Archives of General Psychiatry, 43,* 493–500.

Barsky, A. J., Wyshak, G., & Klerman, G. L. (1990a). The somatosensory amplification scale and its relationship to hypochondriasis. *Journal of Psychiatric Research, 24,* 323–334.

Barsky, A. J., Wyshak, G., & Klerman, G. L. (1990b). Transient hypochondriasis. *Archives of General Psychiatry, 47,* 746–752.

Barsky, A. J., Wyshak, G., Klerman, G. L., & Latham, K. S. (1990c). The prevalence of hypochondriasis in medical outpatients. *Social Psychiatry and Psychiatric Epidemiology, 25,* 89–94.

Bartholomew, R. E., & Wessely, S. (2002). Protean nature of mass sociogenic illness: From possessed nuns to chemical and biological terrorism fears. *British Journal of Psychiatry, 180,* 300–306.

Baumann, L. J., Cameron, L. D., Zimmerman, R. S., & Leventhal, H. (1989). Illness representations and matching labels with symptoms. *Health Psychology, 8,* 449–469.

Beck, A. T. (1976). *Cognitive therapy and the emotional disorders.* New York: International Universities Press.

Beck, A. T. (1993). Cognitive approaches to stress. In P. M. Lehrer & R. L. Woolfolk (Eds.), *Principles and practice of stress management* (pp. 333–372). New York: Guilford Press.

Beck, A. T., & Emery, G. (1985). *Anxiety disorders and phobias: A cognitive perspective.* New York: Basic Books.

Beck, A. T., Freeman, A., & Associates. (2003). *Cognitive therapy of personality disorders* (2nd ed.). New York: Guilford Press.

Beck, A. T., Rush, A. J., Shaw, B. F., & Emery, G. (1979). *Cognitive therapy of depression.* New York: Guilford Press.

Ben-Tovim, D. I., & Esterman, A. (1998). Zero progress with hypochondriasis. *Lancet, 352,* 1798–1799.

Bernstein, I. C., Callahan, W. A., & Jaranson, J. M. (1975). Lobotomy in private practice: Long-term follow-up. *Archives of General Psychiatry, 32,* 1041–1047.

Bianchi, G. N. (1971). Origins of disease phobia. *Australian and New Zealand Journal of Psychiatry, 5,* 241–257.

Black, D. W. (1996). Iatrogenic (physician-induced) hypochondriasis: Four patient examples of "chemical sensitivity." *Psychosomatics, 37,* 390–393.

Blanchard, E. B. (2001). *Irritable bowel syndrome: Psychosocial assessment and treatment.* Washington, DC: American Psychological Association.

Bond, M. R. (1971). The relation of pain to the Eysenck Personality Inventory, Cornell Medical Index and Whitely Index of Hypochondriasis. *British Journal of Psychiatry, 119,* 671–678.

Borkovec, T. D., Wilkinson, L., Folensbee, R., & Lerman, C. (1983). Stimulus control applications to the treatment of worry. *Behaviour Research and Therapy, 21,* 247–251.

Bouman, T. K. (2002). A community-based psychoeducational group approach to hypochondriasis. *Psychotherapy and Psychosomatics, 71,* 326–332.

Bouman, T. K., & Meijer, K. J. (1999). A preliminary study of worry and metacognitions in hypochondriasis. *Clinical Psychology and Psychotherapy, 6,* 96–101.

Bouman, T. K., & Visser, S. (1998). Cognitive and behavioural treatment of hypochondriasis. *Psychotherapy and Psychosomatics, 67,* 214–221.

Bouton, M. E. (2000). A learning theory perspective on lapse, relapse, and the maintenance of behavior change. *Health Psychology, 19*(Suppl.), 57–63.

Brehm, J. W. (1962). *A theory of psychological reactance.* New York: Academic Press.

Brodal, A. (1969). *Neurological anatomy in relation to clinical medicine* (2nd ed.). New York: Oxford University Press.

Brotman, A. W., & Jenike, M. A. (1984). Monosymptomatic hypochondriasis treated with tricyclic antidepressants. *American Journal of Psychiatry, 141,* 1608–1609.

Brown, H. D., Kosslyn, S. M., Delamater, B., Fama, J., & Barsky, A. J. (1999). Perceptual and memory biases for health-related information in hypochondriacal individuals. *Journal of Psychosomatic Research, 47,* 67–78.

Brown, H. N., & Valliant, G. E. (1981). Hypochondriasis. *Archives of Internal Medicine, 141,* 723–726.

Burns, D. D. (1980). *Feeling good: The new mood therapy.* New York: Morrow.

Burton, R. (1927). *The anatomy of melancholy* (F. Dell & P. Jordan-Smith, Ed. and Trans.). New York: Tudor. (Original work published 1651)

Canadian Pharmacists Association. (2002). *Compendium of pharmaceuticals and specialties* (37th ed.). Toronto: Webcom.

Carpenter, M. B. (1976). *Human neuroanatomy* (7th ed.). Baltimore: Williams & Wilkins.

Cedro, A., Kokoszka, A., Popiel, A., & Narkiewicz, J. W. (2001). Alexithymia in schizophrenia: An exploratory study. *Psychological Reports, 89,* 95–98.

Cetin, M., Ebrinc, S., Agargun, N. Y., & Yigit, S. (1999). Respiridone for the treatment of monosymptomatic hypochondriacal psychosis. *Journal of Clinical Psychiatry, 60,* 554.

Chadda, R. K., & Ahuja, N. (1990). Dhat syndrome: A sex neurosis of the Indian subcontinent. *British Journal of Psychiatry, 156,* 577–579.

Chadwick, P., Birchwood, M., & Trower, P. (1996). *Cognitive therapy for delusions, voices and paranoia.* New York: Wiley.

Chaplin, E. W., & Levine, B. A. (1981). The effects of total exposure duration and interrupted versus continued exposure in flooding therapy. *Behavior Therapy, 12,* 360–368.

Chobanian, A. V. (1982). Orthostatic hypotension. In H. R. Brunner & H. Gavras (Eds.), *Clinical hypertension and hypotension* (pp. 435–454). New York: Marcel Dekker.

Christophersen, E. R., & Mortweet, S. L. (2003). *Parenting that works: Building skills that last a lifetime.* Washington, DC: American Psychological Association.

Churchill Livingstone Inc. (1989). *Churchill's medical dictionary.* New York: Author.

Cioffi, D. (1991). Asymmetry of doubt in medical self-diagnosis: The ambiguity of "uncertain wellness." *Journal of Personality and Social Psychology, 61,* 969–980.

Clark, D. M. (1986). A cognitive approach to panic. *Behaviour Research and Therapy, 24,* 461–470.

Clark, D. M. (1989). Anxiety states: Panic and generalized anxiety. In K. Hawton, P. M. Salkovskis, J. Kirk, & D. M. Clark (Eds.), *Cognitive behaviour therapy for psychiatric problems: A practical guide* (pp. 52–96). Oxford, UK: Oxford University Press.

Clark, D. M. (1999). Anxiety disorders: Why they persist and how to treat them. *Behaviour Research and Therapy, 37,* S5–S27.

Clark, D. M., Salkovskis, P. M., Hackmann, A., Wells, A., Fennell, M., Ludgate, J., Ahmad, S., Richards, H. C., & Gelder, M. (1998). Two psychological treatments for hypochondriasis: A randomized controlled trial. *British Journal of Psychiatry, 173,* 218–225.

Clifft, M. A. (1986). Writing about psychiatric patients: Guidelines for disguising case material. *Bulletin of the Menninger Clinic, 50,* 511–524.

Cloninger, C. R., Sigvardsson, S., von Knorring, A.-L., & Bohman, M. (1984). An adoption study of somatoform disorders: II. Identification of two discrete somatoform disorders. *Archives of General Psychiatry, 41,* 863–871.

Cohen, J. (1988). *Statistical power analysis for the behavioral sciences* (2nd ed.). Hillsdale, NJ: Erlbaum.

Conduit, E. (1995). *The body under stress: Developing skills for keeping healthy.* Hillsdale, NJ: Erlbaum.

Côté, G., O'Leary, T., Barlow, D. H., Strain, J. J., Salkovskis, P. M., Warwick, H. M. C., Clark, D. M., Rapee, R., & Rasmussen, S. A. (1996). Hypochondriasis. In T. A. Widiger, A. J. Frances, H. A. Pincus, R. Ross, M. B. First, & W. W. Davis

(Eds.), *DSM-IV sourcebook* (Vol. 2, pp. 933–947). Washington, DC: American Psychiatric Association.

Cox, B. J., Borger, S. C., Asmundson, G. J. G., & Taylor, S. (2000). Dimensions of hypochondriasis and the five-factor model of personality. *Personality and Individual Differences, 29,* 99–180.

Craig, T. K. J., Boardman, A. P., Mills, K., Daly-Jones, O., & Drake, H. (1993). The south London somatisation study: I. Longitudinal course and the influence of early life experiences. *British Journal of Psychiatry, 163,* 579–588.

Croyle, R. T., & Sande, G. N. (1998). Denial and confirmatory search: Paradoxical consequences of medical diagnoses. *Journal of Applied Social Psychology, 18,* 473–490.

Davis, M., Eshelman, E. R., & McKay, M. (2000). *The relaxation and stress reduction workbook* (5th ed.). Oakland, CA: New Harbinger.

Deiker, T., & Counts, D. K. (1980). Hypnotic paradigm-substitution therapy in a case of hypochondriasis. *American Journal of Clinical Hypnosis, 23,* 122–127.

de Jong, P. J., Haenen, M. A., Schmidt, A., & Mayer, B. (1998). Hypochondriasis: The role of fear-confirming reasoning. *Behaviour Research and Therapy, 36,* 65–74.

de Leon, A. C., & Cheng, T. O. (1986). History and physical examination. In J. W. Hurst (Ed.), *The heart: Arteries and veins* (6th ed., pp. 22–46). New York: McGraw-Hill.

DeLongis, A., Folkman, S., & Lazarus, R. S. (1988). The impact of daily stress on health and mood: Psychological and social resources as mediators. *Journal of Personality and Social Psychology, 54,* 485–495.

Devine, E. C. (1992). Effects of psychoeducational care for adult surgical patients: A meta-analysis of 191 studies. *Patient Education and Counselling, 19,* 129–142.

DiLalla, D. L., Carey, G., Gottesman, I. I., & Bouchard, T. J. (1996). Heritability of MMPI personality indicators of psychopathology in twins reared apart. *Journal of Abnormal Psychology, 105,* 491–499.

Ditto, P. H., Jemmott, J. B., & Darley, J. M. (1988). Appraising the threat of illness: A mental representational approach. *Health Psychology, 7,* 183–201.

Dorfman, W. (1968). Hypochondriasis as a defense against depression. *Psychosomatics, 9,* 248–251.

Drossman, D. A. (1978). The problem patient: Evaluation and care of medical patients with psychosocial disturbances. *Annals of Internal Medicine, 88,* 366–372.

Durso, F. T., Reardon, R. S., Shore, W. J., & Delys, S. M. (1991). Memory processes and hypochondriacal tendencies. *Journal of Nervous and Mental Disease, 179,* 279–283.

D'Zurilla, T. J. (1986). *Problem solving therapy.* New York: Springer.

Easterling, D. V., & Leventhal, H. (1989). Contribution of concrete cognition to emotion: Neutral symptoms as elicitors of worry about cancer. *Journal of Applied Psychology, 74,* 787–796.

Ellis, A., & Knaus, W. J. (1977). *Overcoming procrastination.* New York: Signet.

Elmer, K. B., George R. M., & Peterson, K. (2000). Use of risperidone for the treatment of monosymptomatic hypochondriacal psychosis. *Journal of the American Academy of Dermatology, 43,* 683–686.

Emmons, K. M., & Rollnick, S. (2001). Motivational interviewing in health care settings: Opportunities and limitations. *American Journal of Preventive Medicine, 20,* 68–74.

Enns, M. W., Kjernisted, K., & Lander, M. (2001). Pharmacological management of hypochondriasis and related disorders. In G. J. G. Asmundson, S. Taylor, & B. J. Cox (Eds.), *Health anxiety: Clinical and research perspectives on hypochondriasis and related conditions* (pp. 193–219). New York: Wiley.

Escobar, J. I. (1995). Transcultural aspects of dissociative and somatoform disorders. *Psychiatric Clinics of North America, 18,* 555–569.

Escobar, J. I., Allen, L. A., Hoyos Nervi, C., & Gara, M. A. (2001). General and cross-cultural considerations in a medical setting for patients presenting with medically unexplained symptoms. In G. J. G. Asmundson, S. Taylor, & B. J. Cox (Eds.), *Health anxiety: Clinical and research perspectives on hypochondriasis and related conditions* (pp. 220–245). New York: Wiley.

Escobar, J. I., Gara, M., Waitzkin, H., Silver, R. C., Holman, A., & Compton, W. (1998). DSM-IV hypochondriasis in primary care. *General Hospital Psychiatry, 20,* 155–159.

Escobar, J. I., Swartz, M., Rubio-Stipec, M., & Manu, P. (1991). Medically unexplained symptoms: Distribution, risk factors, and comorbidity. In L. J. Kirmayer & J. M. Robbins (Eds.), *Current concepts of somatization: Research and clinical perspectives* (pp. 63–78). Washington, DC: American Psychiatric Association.

Espie, C. A. (1986). The group treatment of obsessive–compulsive ritualizers: Behavioural management of identified patterns of relapse. *Behavioural Psychotherapy, 14,* 21–33.

Fabricant, N. D. (1960). *13 famous patients.* Philadelphia: Chilton.

Fahrenberg, J., Frank, M., Bass, U., & Jost, E. (1995). Awareness of blood pressure: Interoception or contextual judgement. *Journal of Psychosomatic Research, 39,* 11–18.

Fallon, B. A. (1999). Somatoform disorders. In R. E. Feinstein & A. A. Brewer (Eds), *Primary care psychiatry and behavioral medicine: Brief office treatment and management pathways* (pp. 146–170). New York: Springer.

Fallon, B. A. (2001). Pharmacologic strategies for hypochondriasis. In V. Starcevic & D. R. Lipsitt (Eds.), *Hypochondriasis: Modern perspectives on an ancient malady* (pp. 329–351). New York: Oxford University Press.

Fallon, B. A., Javitch, J. A., Hollander, E., & Liebowitz, M. R. (1991). Hypochondriasis and obsessive compulsive disorder: Overlaps in diagnosis and treatment. *Journal of Clinical Psychiatry, 52,* 457–460.

Fallon, B. A., Liebowitz, M. R., Salman, E., Schneier, F. R., Insino, C., Hollander, E., & Klein, D. F. (1993). Fluoxetine for hypochondriacal patients without major depression. *Journal of Clinical Psychopharmacology, 13,* 438–441.

Fallon, B. A., Schneier, F. R., Marshall, R., Campeas, R., Vermes, D., Goetz, D., & Liebowitz, M. R. (1996). The pharmacotherapy of hypochondriasis. *Psychopharmacology Bulletin, 32,* 607–611.

Fava, G. A., Grandi, S., Rafanelli, C., Fabbri, S., & Cazzaro, M. (2000). Explanatory therapy in hypochondriasis. *Journal of Clinical Psychiatry, 61,* 317–322.

Fava, G. A., Kellner, R., Zielezny, M., & Grandi, S. (1988). Hypochondriacal fears and beliefs in agoraphobia. *Journal of Affective Disorders, 14,* 239–244.

Fava, M., Bless, E., Otto, M. W., Pava, J. A., & Rosenbaum, J. F. (1994). Dysfunctional attitudes in major depression: Changes with pharmacotherapy. *Journal of Nervous and Mental Disease, 182*, 45–49.

Fawcett, R. G. (2002). Olanzapine for the treatment of monosymptomatic hypochondriacal psychosis. *Journal of Clinical Psychiatry, 63*, 169.

Fedoroff, I. C., & Taylor, S. (2001). Psychological and pharmacological treatments for social phobia: A meta-analysis. *Journal of Clinical Psychopharmacology, 21*, 311–324.

Feld, R., Woodside, D. B., Kaplan, A. S., Olmsted, M. P., & Carter, J. C. (2001). Pretreatment motivational enhancement therapy for eating disorders: A pilot study. *International Journal of Eating Disorders, 29*, 393–400.

Ferguson, E. (1996). Hypochondriacal concerns: The roles of raw and calibrated medical knowledge. *Psychology, Health and Medicine, 1*, 315–318.

Ferguson, E. (1998). Hypochondriacal concerns, symptom reporting and secondary gain mechanisms. *British Journal of Medical Psychology, 71*, 281–295.

Ferguson, R. J., & Ahles, T. A. (1998). Private body consciousness, anxiety and pain symptom reports of chronic pain patients. *Behaviour Research and Therapy, 36*, 527–535.

Fink, P. (1993). Admission patterns of persistent somatization patients. *General Hospital Psychiatry, 15*, 211–218.

First, M. B., Spitzer, R. L., Gibbon, M., & Williams, J. B. W. (1996). *Structured Clinical Interview for DSM-IV*. New York: New York State Psychiatric Institute, Biometrics Research Department.

First, M. B., Spitzer, R. L., Gibbon, M., Williams, J. B. W., & Lorna, B. (1994). *Structured Clinical Interview for DSM-IV Axis II Personality Disorders (SCID-II; Version 2.0)*. New York: New York State Psychiatric Institute, Biometrics Research Department.

Fishbain, D. A., Barsky, S., & Goldberg, M. (1992). Monosymptomatic hypochondriacal psychosis: Belief of contracting rabies. *International Journal of Psychiatry in Medicine, 22*, 3–9.

Fitzpatrick, R. (1996). Telling patients there is nothing wrong. *British Medical Journal, 313*, 311–312.

Foa, E. B., & Kozak, M. J. (1986). Emotional processing of fear: Exposure to corrective information. *Psychological Bulletin, 99*, 20–35.

Foa, E. B., Steketee, G. S., & Milby, J. B. (1980). Differential effects of exposure and response prevention in obsessive compulsive washers. *Journal of Consulting and Clinical Psychology, 48*, 71–79.

Ford, C. V. (1983). *The somatizing disorders: Illness as a way of life*. New York: Elsevier.

Frazier, L. D., & Waid, L. D. (1999). Influences on anxiety in later life: The role of health status, health perceptions, and health locus of control. *Aging and Mental Health, 3*, 213–220.

Friedman, M. (1996). *Type A behavior: Its diagnosis and treatment*. New York: Plenum Press.

Frisch, M. B. (2003). *Quality of life therapy*. New York: Wiley.

Frisch, M. B., Cornell, J., Villanueva, M., & Retzlaff, P. J. (1992). Clinical validation of the Quality of Life Inventory: A measure of life satisfaction for use in treatment planning and outcome assessment. *Psychological Assessment, 4*, 92–101.

Fritz, G. K., & Williams, J. R. (1989). Issues of adolescent development for survivors of childhood cancer. *Journal of the American Academy of Child and Adolescent Psychiatry, 27,* 712–715.

Fukunishi, I., Kikuchi, M., Wogan, J., & Takubo, M. (1997). Secondary alexithymia as a state reaction in panic disorder and social phobia. *Comprehensive Psychiatry, 38,* 166–170.

Furer, P., & Walker, J. R. (2000). *Intense illness worries treatment manual.* Unpublished manuscript, University of Manitoba, Department of Clinical Health Psychology, MB, Canada.

Furer, P., Walker, J. R., & Freeston, M. H. (2001). Integrated approach to cognitive-behavioral therapy for intense illness worries. In G. J. G. Asmundson, S. Taylor, & B. J. Cox (Eds.), *Health anxiety: Clinical and research perspectives on hypochondriasis and related conditions* (pp. 161–192). New York: Wiley.

Furst, J. B., & Cooper, A. (1970). Combined use of imaginal and interoceptive stimuli in desensitizing fear of heart attacks. *Journal of Behavior Therapy and Experimental Psychiatry, 1,* 87–91.

Gallucci, G., & Beard, G. (1995). Risperidone and the treatment of delusions of parasitosis in an elderly patient. *Psychosomatics, 36,* 578–580.

Gelder, M. G., Gath, D., & Mayou, R. A. (1983). *Oxford textbook of psychiatry.* Oxford, UK: Oxford University Press.

Gerdle, B., Brulin, C., Elert, J., Eliasson, P., et al. (1995). Effect of a general fitness program on musculoskeletal symptoms, clinical status, physiological capacity, and perceived work environment among home care service personnel. *Journal of Occupational Rehabilitation, 5,* 1–16.

Gershon, M. D. (1998). *The second brain.* New York: HarperCollins.

Goldberg, R. L., Buongiorno, P. A., & Henkin, R. I. (1985). Delusions of halitosis. *Psychosomatics, 26,* 325–331.

Goldstein, S. E., & Birnbom, F. (1976). Hypochondriasis and the elderly. *Journal of the American Geriatrics Society, 24,* 150–154.

Goodstein, R. K. (1985). Common clinical problems in the elderly: Camouflaged by ageism and atypical presentation. *Psychiatric Annals, 15,* 299–312.

Gottesman, I. I. (1962). Differential inheritance of the psychoneuroses. *Eugenics Quarterly, 9,* 223–227.

Gould, W. M., & Gragg, T. M. (1976). Delusions of parasitosis: An approach to the problem. *Archives of Dermatology, 112,* 1745–1748.

Gramling, S. E., Clawson, E. P., & McDonald, M. K. (1996). Perceptual and cognitive abnormality model of hypochondriasis: Amplification and physiological reactivity. *Psychosomatic Medicine, 58,* 423–431.

Greenblatt, M. (1959). Relation between history, personality and family pattern and behavioral responses after frontal lobe surgery. *American Journal of Psychiatry, 116,* 193–202.

Gureje, O., Üstün, T. B., & Simon, G. E. (1997). The syndrome of hypochondriasis: A cross-national study in primary care. *Psychological Medicine, 27,* 1001–1010.

Hadjistavropoulos, H. D., Frombach, I. K., & Asmundson, G. J. G. (1999). Exploratory and confirmatory factor analytic investigations of the Illness Attitudes Scale in a nonclinical sample. *Behaviour Research and Therapy, 37,* 671–684.

Haenen, M. A., de Jong, P. J., Schmidt, A. J. M., Stevens, S., & Visser, L. (2000). Hypochondriacs' estimation of negative outcomes: Domain-specificity and responsiveness to reassuring and alarming information. *Behaviour Research and Therapy, 38,* 819–833.

Haenen, M. A., Schmidt, A. J. M., Kroeze, S., & van den Hout, M. A. (1996). Hypochondriasis and symptom reporting: The effect of attention versus distraction. *Psychotherapy and Psychosomatics, 65,* 43–48.

Haenen, M. A., Schmidt, A. J. M., Schoenmakers, M., & van den Hout, M. A. (1997a). Suggestibility in hypochondriacal patients and elderly control subjects: An experimental case–control study. *Psychosomatics, 38,* 543–547.

Haenen, M. A., Schmidt, A. J. M., Schoenmakers, M., & van den Hout, M. A. (1997b). Tactual sensitivity in hypochondriasis. *Psychotherapy and Psychosomatics, 66,* 128–132.

Haenen, M. A., Schmidt, A. J. M., Schoenmakers, M., & van den Hout, M. A. (1998). Quantitative and qualitative aspects of cancer knowledge: Comparing hypochondriacal subjects and healthy controls. *Psychology and Health, 13,* 1005–1014.

Hahn, R. A. (1999). Expectations of sickness: Concept and evidence of the nocebo phenomenon. In I. Kirsch (Ed.), *How expectancies shape experience* (pp. 333–356). Washington, DC: American Psychological Association.

Hamann, K., & Avnstorp, C. (1982). Delusions of infestation treated with pimozide: A double-blind crossover clinical study. *Acta Dermato-Venereologica, 62,* 55–58.

Hambly, K., & Muir, A. J. (1997). *Stress management in primary care.* Oxford, UK: Butterworth-Heinemann.

Hanback, J. W., & Revelle, W. (1978). Arousal and perceptual sensitivity in hypochondriasis. *Journal of Abnormal Psychology, 87,* 523–530.

Hankin, J., & Oktay, J. S. (1979). *Mental disorder of primary medical care: An analytical review of the literature* (U.S. DHEW Publication No. 78–661). Washington, DC: U.S. Department of Health, Education, and Welfare.

Hawton, K., & Kirk, J. (1989). Problem-solving. In K. Hawton, P. M. Salkovskis, J. Kirk, & D. M. Clark (Eds.), *Cognitive behaviour therapy for psychiatric problems: A practical guide* (pp. 406–426). Oxford, UK: Oxford University Press.

Hawton, K., Salkovskis, P. M., Kirk, J., & Clark, D. M. (1989). *Cognitive behaviour therapy for psychiatric problems: A practical guide.* Oxford, UK: Oxford University Press.

Hiss, H., Foa, E. B., & Kozak, M. J. (1994). Relapse prevention program for treatment of obsessive–compulsive disorder. *Journal of Consulting and Clinical Psychology, 62,* 801–808.

Hitchcock, P. B., & Mathews, A. (1992). Interpretation of bodily symptoms in hypochondriasis. *Behaviour Research and Therapy, 30,* 223–234.

Hollander, E. (1993). *Obsessive–compulsive related disorders.* Washington, DC: American Psychiatric Press.

Hollifield, M., Paine, S., Tuttle, L., & Kellner, R. (1999). Hypochondriasis, somatization, and perceived health and utilization of health care services. *Psychosomatics, 40,* 380–386.

Honkalampi, K., Hintikka, J., Tanskanen, A., Lehtonen, J., & Viinamaeki, H. (2000). Depression is strongly associated with alexithymia in the general population. *Journal of Psychosomatic Research, 48*, 99–104.

Hotopf, M., Mayou, R., Wadsworth, M., & Wessely, S. (1999). Childhood risk factors for adults with medically unexplained symptoms: Results from a national birth cohort study. *American Journal of Psychiatry, 156*, 1796–1800.

House, A. (1989). Hypochondriasis and related disorders: Assessment and management of patients referred for a psychiatric opinion. *General Hospital Psychiatry, 11*, 156–165.

House, A. (1995). The patient with medically unexplained symptoms: Making the initial psychiatric contact. In R. Mayou, C. Bass, & M. Sharpe (Eds.), *Treatment of functional somatic symptoms* (pp. 89–102). Oxford, UK: Oxford University Press.

Howes, O. D., & Salkovskis, P. M. (1998). Health anxiety in medical students. *Lancet, 351*, 1332.

Humfress, H., Igel, V., Lamont, A., Tanner, M., Morgan, J., & Schmidt, U. (2002). The effect of a brief motivational intervention on community psychiatric patients' attitudes to their care, motivation for change, compliance and outcome: A case control study. *Journal of Mental Health, 11*, 155–166.

Hunter, R. C. A., Lohrenz, J. G., & Schwartzman, A. E. (1964). Nosophobia and hypochondriasis in medical students. *Journal of Nervous and Mental Disease, 139*, 147–152.

Jacobson, N. S., Dobson, K. S., Truax, P. A., Addis, M. E., Koerner, K., Gollan, J. K., Gortner, E., & Prince, S. E. (1996). A component analysis of cognitive-behavioral treatment for depression. *Journal of Consulting and Clinical Psychology, 64*, 295–304.

James, A., & Wells, A. (2002). Death beliefs, superstitious beliefs and health anxiety. *British Journal of Clinical Psychology, 41*, 43–53.

Jibiki, I., & Yamaguchi, N. (1992). A case with delusion of parasitosis as a reactive psychosis following scabies infection. *European Journal of Psychiatry, 6*, 181–183.

Johansson, J., & Öst, L.-G. (1981). Applied relaxation in treatment of "cardiac neurosis": A systematic case study. *Psychological Reports, 48*, 463–468.

Johnson, G. C., & Anton, R. F. (1983). Pimozide in delusions of parasitosis. *Journal of Clinical Psychiatry, 44*, 233.

Jones, T. F. (2000). Mass psychogenic illness: Role of the individual physician. *American Family Physician, 62*, 2649–2653, 2655–2656.

Jones, T. F., Craig, A. S., Hoy, D., Gunter, E. W., Ashley, D. L., Barr, D. B., Brock, J. W., & Schaffner, W. (2000). Mass psychogenic illness attributed to toxic exposure at a high school. *New England Journal of Medicine, 342*, 96–100.

Kalish, R. A. (1985). Coping with death. In R. A. Kalish (Ed.), *The final transition* (pp. 11–23). New York: Baywood.

Kamlana, S. H., & Gray, P. (1988). Fear of AIDS. *British Journal of Psychiatry, 15*, 1291.

Kaplan, N. M. (2002). Hypochondriasis. *New England Journal of Medicine, 346*, 783–784.

Kasteler, J., Kane, R. L., Olsen, D. M., & Thetford, C. (1976). Issues underlying prevalence of "doctor shopping" behavior. *Journal of Health and Social Behavior, 17*, 328–339.

Katz, R. C., Meyers, K., & Walls, J. (1995). Cancer awareness and self-examination practices in young men and women. *Journal of Behavioral Medicine, 18*, 377–384.

Keeley, R., Smith, M., & Miller, J. (2000). Somatoform symptoms and treatment nonadherence in depressed family medicine outpatients. *Archives of Family Medicine, 9*, 46–54.

Kellner, R. (1979). Psychotherapeutic strategies in the treatment of psychophysiologic disorders. *Psychotherapy and Psychosomatics, 32*(Suppl. 4), 91–100.

Kellner, R. (1982). Psychotherapeutic strategies in hypochondriasis: A clinical study. *American Journal of Psychotherapy, 36*, 146–157.

Kellner, R. (1983). Prognosis of treated hypochondriasis: A clinical study. *Acta Psychiatrica Scandinavica, 67*, 69–79.

Kellner, R. (1985). Functional somatic symptoms and hypochondriasis: A survey of empirical studies. *Archives of General Psychiatry, 42*, 821–833.

Kellner, R. (1986). *Somatization and hypochondriasis.* New York: Praeger.

Kellner, R. (1987). *Abridged manual of the Illness Attitudes Scale.* Unpublished manual, University of New Mexico, School of Medicine, Department of Psychiatry, Albuquerque.

Kellner, R. (1991). *Psychosomatic syndromes and somatic symptoms.* Washington, DC: American Psychiatric Press.

Kellner, R. (1992). The treatment of hypochondriasis: To reassure or not to reassure? *International Review of Psychiatry, 4*, 71–75.

Kellner, R., Abbott, P., Winslow, W. W., & Pathak, D. (1987). Fears, beliefs, and attitudes in DSM-III hypochondriasis. *Journal of Nervous and Mental Disease, 175*, 20–25.

Kellner, R., Abbott, P., Winslow, W. W., & Pathak, D. (1989). Anxiety, depression, and somatization in DSM-III hypochondriasis. *Psychosomatics, 30*, 57–64.

Kellner, R., Fava, G. A., Lisansky, J., Perini, G. I., & Zielezny, M. (1986a). Hypochondriacal fears and beliefs in DSM-III melancholia: Changes with treatment. *Journal of Affective Disorders, 10*, 21–26.

Kellner, R., Pathak, D., Romanik, R., & Winslow, W. W. (1983). Life events and hypochondriacal concerns. *Psychiatric Medicine, 1*, 133–141.

Kellner, R., Wiggins, R. G., & Pathak, D. (1986b). Hypochondriacal fears and beliefs in medical and law students. *Archives of General Psychiatry, 43*, 487–489.

Kendler, K. S., Walters, E. E., Neale, M. C., Kessler, R. C., Heath, A. C., & Eaves, L. J. (1995). The structure of the genetic and environmental risk factors for six major psychiatric disorders in women: Phobia, generalized anxiety disorder, panic disorder, bulimia, major depression and alcoholism. *Archives of General Psychiatry, 52*, 374–383.

Kenyon, F. E. (1964). Hypochondriasis: A clinical study. *British Journal of Psychiatry, 110*, 478–488.

Kirmayer, L. J., & Robbins, J. M. (1991). Three forms of somatization in primary care: Prevalence, co-occurrence, and sociodemographic characteristics. *Journal of Nervous and Mental Disease, 179*, 647–655.

Kjernisted, K. D., Enns, M. W., & Lander, M. (2002). An open-label clinical trial of nefazodone in hypochondriasis. *Psychosomatics, 43*, 290–294.

Knight, R. O. (1941). Evaluation of the results of psychoanalytic therapy. *American Journal of Psychiatry, 98*, 434–446.

Koblenzer, C. S. (1997). Psychodermatology of women. *Clinics in Dermatology, 1*, 127–141.

Koo, J., & Lee, C. S. (2001). Delusions of parasitosis: A dermatologist's guide to diagnosis and treatment. *American Journal of Clinical Dermatology, 2*, 285–290.

Kooiman, C. G., Bolk, J. H., Brand, R., Trijsburg, R. W., & Rooijmans, H. G. M. (2000). Is alexithymia a risk factor for unexplained physical symptoms in general medical outpatients? *Psychosomatic Medicine, 62*, 768–778.

Kumar, K., & Wilkinson, J. C. M. (1971). Thought stopping: A useful technique in phobias of internal stimuli. *British Journal of Psychiatry, 119*, 305–307.

Ladee, G. A. (1966). *Hypochondriacal syndromes.* Amsterdam: Elsevier.

Lambert, M., Hatch, D., Kingston, M., & Edwards, B. (1986). Zung, Beck, and Hamilton rating scales as measures of treatment outcome: A meta-analytic comparison. *Journal of Consulting and Clinical Psychology, 54*, 54–59.

Lang, A. J., & Craske, M. G. (2000). Manipulations of exposure-based therapy to reduce return of fear: A replication. *Behaviour Research and Therapy, 38*, 1–12.

Lang. P. J. (1985). The cognitive psychophysiology of emotion: Fear and anxiety. In A. H. Tuma & J. D. Maser (Eds.), *Anxiety and the anxiety disorders* (pp. 131–170). Hillsdale, NJ: Erlbaum.

Lautenbacher, S., Pauli, P., Zaudig, M., & Burbaumer, N. (1998). Attentional control of pain perception: The role of hypochondriasis. *Journal of Psychosomatic Research, 44*, 251–259.

Lazarus, R. S. (1966). *Psychological stress and the coping process.* New York: McGraw-Hill.

Lazarus, R. S., & Folkman, S. (1989). *Manual for the Hassles and Uplifts Scales.* Palo Alto, CA: Consulting Psychologists Press.

Leonhard, K. (1961). On the treatment of ideohypochondriac and sensohypochondriac neuroses. *International Journal of Social Psychiatry, 7*, 123–133.

Lesse, S. (1980). Masked depression—the ubiquitous but unappreciated syndrome. *Psychiatric Journal of the University of Ottawa, 5*, 268–273.

Lidbeck, J. (1997). Group therapy for somatization disorders in general practice: Effectiveness of a short cognitive-behavioural treatment model. *Acta Psychiatrica Scandinavica, 96*, 14–24.

Linehan, M. M. (1993). *Skills training manual for treating borderline personality disorder.* New York: Guilford Press.

Lippert, G. P. (1986). Excessive concern about AIDS in two bisexual men. *Canadian Journal of Psychiatry, 31*, 63–65.

Lishman, W. A. (1987). *Organic psychiatry* (2nd ed.). Oxford, UK: Blackwell Scientific.

Logsdail, S., Lovell, K., Warwick, H., & Marks, I. (1991). Behavioural treatment of AIDS-focused illness phobia. *British Journal of Psychiatry, 159*, 422–425.

Logsdon, C. D., & Hyer, L. (1999). Treating hypochondria in later life: Personality and health factors. In M. Duffy (Ed.), *Handbook of counseling and psychotherapy with older adults* (pp. 414–435). New York: Wiley.

Looper, K. J., & Kirmayer, L. J. (2001). Hypochondriacal concerns in a community population. *Psychological Medicine, 31*, 577–584.

Lucock, M. P., & Morley, S. (1996). The Health Anxiety Questionnaire. *British Journal of Health Psychology, 1,* 137–150.

Lucock, M. P., Morley, S., White, C., & Peake, M. D. (1997). Responses of consecutive patients to reassurance after gastroscopy: Results of self administered questionnaire survey. *British Medical Journal, 315,* 572–575.

Lucock, M. P., White, C., Peake, M. D., & Morley, S. (1998). Biased perception and recall of reassurance in medical patients. *British Journal of Health Psychology, 3,* 237–243.

Lundh, J. G., & Simonsson, S. M. (2001). Alexithymia, emotion, and somatic complaints. *Journal of Personality, 69,* 483–510.

Lyell, A. (1983). Delusions of parasitosis. *British Journal of Dermatology, 108,* 485–499.

Mabe, P. A., Hobson, D. P., Jones, L. R., & Jarvis, R. G. (1988). Hypochondriacal traits in medical inpatients. *General Hospital Psychiatry, 10,* 236–244.

MacLeod, A. K., Haynes, C., & Sensky, T. (1998). Attributions about common bodily sensations: Their associations with hypochondriasis and anxiety. *Psychological Medicine, 28,* 225–228.

MacPhillamy, D., & Lewinsohn, P. M. (1982). The Pleasant Events Schedule: Studies on reliability, validity, and scale intercorrelation. *Journal of Consulting and Clinical Psychology, 50,* 363–380.

Madioni, F., & Mammana, L. A. (2001). Toronto Alexithymia Scale in outpatients with sexual disorders. *Psychopathology, 34,* 95–98.

Malhotra, H. K., & Wig, N. N. (1975). Dhat syndrome: A culture-bound sex neurosis of the Orient. *Archives of Sexual Behavior, 4,* 519–528.

Malis, R. W., Hartz, A. J., Doebbeling, C. C., & Noyes, R. (2002). Specific phobia of illness in the community. *Hospital and Community Psychiatry, 24,* 135–139.

Mandeville, B. (1976). *A treatise of the hypochondiack and hysterick diseases.* New York: Delmar. (Original work published 1730)

Marcus, D. K. (1999). The cognitive-behavioral model of hypochondriasis: Misinformation and triggers. *Journal of Psychosomatic Research, 47,* 79–91.

Marks, I. (1987). *Fears, phobias, and rituals.* New York: Oxford University Press.

Marlatt, G. A., & Gordon, J. R. (1985). *Relapse prevention: Maintenance strategies in the treatment of addictive behaviors.* New York: Guilford Press.

Marshall, W. L. (1985). The effects of variable exposure in flooding therapy. *Behavior Therapy, 16,* 117–135.

Martin, R. L., & Yutzy, S. H. (1994). Somatoform disorders. In R. E. Hales, S. C. Yudofsky, & J. A. Talbott (Eds.), *American Psychiatric Press textbook of psychiatry* (2nd ed., pp. 591–622). Washington, DC: American Psychiatric Press.

Matas, M., & Robinson, C. (1988). Diagnosis and treatment of monosymptomatic hypochondriacal psychosis in chronic renal failure. *Canadian Journal of Psychiatry, 33,* 748–750.

Mayou, R. (1993). Somatization. *Psychotherapy and Psychosomatics, 59,* 69–83.

Mazzeo, S. E., & Espelage, D. L. (2002). Association between childhood physical and emotional abuse and disordered eating behaviors in female undergraduates: An investigation of the mediating role of alexithymia and depression. *Journal of Counseling Psychology, 49,* 86–100.

McCollum, E. E. (1994). "Brief strategic treatment of a male with HIV hypochondria": Comment. *Journal of Family Psychotherapy, 5*, 11–14.

McDonald, I. G., Daly, J., Jelinek, V. M., Panetta, F., & Gutman, J. M. (1996). Opening Pandora's box: The unpredictability of reassurance by a normal test result. *British Medical Journal, 313*, 329–332.

McKay, D. (1999). Two-year follow-up of behavioral treatment and maintenance of body dysmorphic disorder. *Behavior Modification, 23*, 620–629.

McKay, D., Todaro, J. F., Neziroglu, F., & Yaryura-Tobias, J. A. (1996). Evaluation of a naturalistic maintenance program in the treatment of obsessive–compulsive disorder: A preliminary investigation. *Journal of Anxiety Disorders, 10*, 211–217.

McLaren, P. (1992). Psychotherapy by telephone: Experience of patient and therapist. *Journal of Mental Health UK, 1*, 311–313.

McMullin, R. E. (1986). *Handbook of cognitive therapy techniques.* New York: Norton.

Mechanic, D. (1972). Social psychologic factors affecting the presentation of bodily complaints. *New England Journal of Medicine, 286*, 1132–1139.

Mechanic, D. (1978). Effects of psychological distress on perceptions of physical health and use of medical and psychiatric facilities. *Journal of Human Stress, 4*, 26–32.

Mechanic, D. (1980). The experience and reporting of common physical complaints. *Journal of Health and Social Behavior, 21*, 146–155.

Mechanic, D. (1983). Adolescent health and illness behavior: Review of the literature and a new hypothesis for the study of stress. *Journal of Human Stress, 9*, 4–13.

Meichenbaum, D. (1993). Stress inoculation training: A 20–year update. In P. M. Lehrer & R. L. Woolfolk (Eds.), *Principles and practice of stress management* (2nd ed., pp. 373–406). New York: Guilford Press.

Miller, D., Acton, T. M. G., & Hedge, B. (1988). The worried well: Their identification and management. *Journal of the Royal College of Physicians of London, 22*, 158–165.

Miller, L. (1984). Neuropsychological concepts of somatoform disorders. *International Journal of Psychiatry in Medicine, 14*, 31–46.

Miller, M. S., Brody, D. S., & Summerton, J. (1988). Styles of coping with threat: Implications for health. *Journal of Personality and Social Psychology, 54*, 142–148.

Miller, W. R. (1995). *Motivational enhancement therapy with drug users.* Albuquerque, MN: Center on Alcoholism, Substance Abuse, and Addictions, University of New Mexico.

Miller, W. R., & Rollnick, S. (2002). *Motivational interviewing: Preparing people for change* (2nd ed.). New York: Guilford Press.

Morgenstern, J. (2000). *Time management from the inside out.* New York: Holt.

Moss-Morris, R., & Petrie, K. J. (2001). Redefining medical students' disease to reduce morbidity. *Medical Education, 35*, 724–728.

Mountcastle, V. B. (1974). Neural mechanisms in somesthesia. In V. B. Mountcastle (Ed.), *Medical physiology* (13th ed., pp. 307–347). St. Louis: Mosby.

Moyers, T. B., & Rollnick, S. (2002). A motivational interviewing perspective on resistance in psychotherapy. *Journal of Clinical Psychology, 58*, 185–193.

Munro, A., & Chmara, J. (1982). Monosymptomatic hypochondriacal psychosis: A diagnostic checklist based on 50 cases of the disorder. *Canadian Journal of Psychiatry, 27*, 374–376.

Needham, K. (2000, December). Mental insect attacks revisited. *Boreus: Newsletter of the Entomological Society of BC, 20,* 16.

Nemiah, J. C. (1985). Somatoform disorders. In H. I. Kaplan & B. J. Sadock (Eds.), *Comprehensive textbook of psychiatry* (4th ed., pp. 924–942). Baltimore: Williams & Wilkins.

Nemiah, J. C. (1996). Alexithymia: Present, past—and future? *Psychosomatic Medicine, 58,* 217–218.

Nemiah, J. C., & Sifneos, P. E. (1970). Affect and fantasy in patients with psychosomatic disorders. In O. W. Hill (Ed.), *Modern trends in psychosomatic medicine* (Vol. 2, pp. 26–34). London: Butterworths.

Noyes, R. (2001). Hypochondriasis: Boundaries and comorbidities. In G. J. G. Asmundson, S. Taylor, & B. J. Cox (Eds.), *Health anxiety: Clinical and research perspectives on hypochondriasis and related conditions* (pp. 132–160). New York: Wiley.

Noyes, R., Kathol, R. G., Fisher, M. M., Phillips, B. M., Suelzer, M., & Woodman, C. L. (1994a). One-year follow-up of medical outpatients with hypochondriasis. *Psychosomatics, 35,* 533–545.

Noyes, R., Kathol, R. G., Fisher, M. M., Phillips, B. M., Suelzer, M., & Woodman, C. L. (1994b). Psychiatric comorbidity among patients with hypochondriasis. *General Hospital Psychiatry, 16,* 78–87.

Noyes, R., Reich, J., Clancy, J., & O'Gorman, T. W. (1986). Reduction of hypochondriasis with treatment of panic disorder. *British Journal of Psychiatry, 149,* 631–635.

Noyes, R., Roger, G., Fisher, M. M., Phillips, B. M., Suelzer, M. T., & Holt, C. S. (1993). The validity of DSM-III-R hypochondriasis. *Archives of General Psychiatry, 50,* 961–970.

Noyes, R., Stuart, S., Longley, S. L., Langbehn, D. R., & Happel, R. L. (2002). Hypochondriasis and fear of death. *Journal of Nervous and Mental Disease, 190,* 503–509.

O'Donnell, J. M. (1978). Implosive therapy with hypnosis in the treatment of cancer phobia: A case report. *Psychotherapy: Theory, Research and Practice, 15,* 8–12.

Oltmanns, T. F., Emery, R. E., & Taylor, S. (2002). *Abnormal psychology.* Toronto: Prentice-Hall.

Oosterbaan, D. B., van Balkom, A. J. L. M., van Boeijen, C. A., de Meij, T. G. J., & van Dyck, R. (2001). An open study of paroxetine in hypochondriasis. *Progress in Neuro-Psychopharmacology and Biological Psychiatry, 25,* 1023–1033.

Opler, L. A., & Feinberg, S. S. (1991). Pimozide in clinical psychiatry. *Journal of Clinical Psychiatry, 52,* 515–516.

Öst, L.-G. (1987). Applied relaxation: Description of a coping technique and review of controlled studies. *Behaviour Research and Therapy, 25,* 397–409.

Öst, L.-G. (1989). A maintenance program for behavioral treatment of anxiety disorders. *Behaviour Research and Therapy, 27,* 123–130.

Owens, K. M. B., Asmundson, G. J. G., Hadjistavropoulos, T., & Owens, T. J. (2001). *Attentional bias toward illness threat in individuals with elevated health anxiety.* Unpublished manuscript, University of Regina, SK, Canada.

Pålsson, N. (1988). Functional somatic symptoms and hypochondriasis among general practice patients: A pilot study. *Acta Psychiatrica Scandinavica, 78,* 191–197.

Papageorgiou, C., & Wells, A. (1998). Effects of attention training on hypochondriasis: A brief case series. *Psychological Medicine, 28,* 193–200.

Paris, J. (1998). Does childhood trauma cause personality disorder in adults? *Canadian Journal of Psychiatry, 43,* 148–153.

Parker, G., & Lipscombe, P. (1980). The relevance of early parental experiences to adult dependency, hypochondriasis and utilization of primary physicians. *British Journal of Medical Psychology, 53,* 355–363.

Parsons, T. (1951). *The social system.* Glencoe, IL: Free Press.

Paterson, R. J. (2000). *The assertiveness workbook.* Oakland, CA: New Harbinger.

Pauli, P., & Alpers, G. W. (2002). Memory bias in patients with hypochondriasis and somatoform pain disorder. *Journal of Psychosomatic Research, 52,* 45–53.

Pauli, P., Schwenzer, M., Brody, S., Rau, H., & Birbaumer, N. (1993). Hypochondriacal attitudes, pain sensitivity, and attentional bias. *Journal of Psychosomatic Research, 37,* 745–752.

Peal, R. L., Handal, P. J., & Gilner, F. H. (1985). A group desensitization procedure for the reduction of death anxiety. In R. A. Kalish (Ed.), *The final transition* (pp. 331–339). New York: Baywood.

Penfield, W., & Faulk, M. E. (1955). The insula: Further observations on its function. *Brain, 78,* 445–470.

Penfield, W., & Jasper, H. (1954). *Epilepsy and the functional anatomy of the human brain.* Boston: Little, Brown.

Pennebaker, J. W. (1980). Perceptual and environmental determinants of coughing. *Basic and Applied Social Psychology, 1,* 83–91.

Pennebaker, J. W. (1982). *The psychology of physical symptoms.* New York: Springer.

Pennebaker, J. W. (2000). Psychological factors influencing the reporting of physical symptoms. In A. A. Stone, J. S. Turkkan, C. A. Bachrach, J. B. Jobe, H. S. Kurtzman, & V. S. Cain (Eds.), *The science of self-report: Implications for research and practice* (pp. 299–315). Mahwah, NJ: Erlbaum.

Pennebaker, J. W., & Skelton, J. A. (1978). Psychological parameters of physical symptoms. *Personality and Social Psychology Bulletin, 4,* 524–530.

Peters, S., Stanley, I., Rose, M., & Salmon, P. (1998). Patients with medically unexplained symptoms: Sources of patients' authority and implications for demands on medical care. *Social Science and Medicine, 46,* 559–565.

Phillips, K. A. (1991). Pimozide in clinical psychiatry. *Journal of Clinical Psychiatry, 52,* 514–515.

Pickering, G. (1974). *Creative malady.* New York: Oxford University Press.

Pilowsky, I. (1967). Dimensions of hypochondriasis. *British Journal of Psychiatry, 113,* 89–93.

Pilowsky, I. (1968). The response to treatment in hypochondriacal disorders. *Australian and New Zealand Journal of Psychiatry, 2,* 88–94.

Pilowsky, I. (1997). *Abnormal illness behaviour.* New York: Wiley.

Pilowsky, I., Chapman, R. C., & Bonica, J. J. (1977). Depression, illness behaviour and pain. *Pain, 4,* 183–192.

Pilowsky, I., Murrell, T. G. C., & Gordon, A. (1979). The development of a screening method for abnormal illness behaviour. *Journal of Psychosomatic Research, 23,* 203–207.

Pilowsky, I., & Spence, N. D. (1994). *Manual for the Illness Behavior Questionnaire (3rd ed.)*. Unpublished manual, University of Adelaide, Department of Psychiatry, Adelaide, Australia.

Pylko, T., & Sicignan, J. (1985). Nortriptyline in the treatment of a mono-symptomatic delusion. *American Journal of Psychiatry, 142*, 1223.

Quality Assurance Project. (1985). Treatment outlines for the management of the somatoform disorders. *Australian and New Zealand Journal of Psychiatry, 19*, 397–407.

Rahe, R. H., & Arthur, R. J. (1978). Life change and illness studies: Past history and future directions. *Journal of Human Stress, 4*, 3–15.

Raven, J. C. (1998). *Raven's standard progressive matrices*. San Antonio, TX: Psychological Corporation.

Resnicow, K., Jackson, A., Wang, T., de Anindya, K., McCarty, F., Dudley, W. N., & Baranowski, T. (2001). A motivational interviewing intervention to increase fruit and vegetable intake through black churches: Results of the Eat for Life trial. *American Journal of Public Health, 91*, 1686–1693.

Rief, W., Hiller, W., & Margraf, J. (1998). Cognitive aspects of hypochondriasis and the somatization syndrome. *Journal of Abnormal Psychology, 107*, 587–595.

Rifkin, B. G. (1968). The treatment of cardiac neurosis using systematic desensitization. *Behaviour Research and Therapy, 6*, 239–240.

Robbins, J. M., & Kirmayer, L. J. (1996). Transient and persistent hypochondriacal worry in primary care. *Psychological Medicine, 26*, 575–589.

Roberts, J., & Roberts, R. (1977). Delusions of parasitosis. *British Medical Journal, 1*, 1219.

Romanik, R. L., & Kellner, R. (1985). Case study: Treatment of herpes genitalis phobia and agoraphobia with panic attacks. *Psychotherapy, 22*, 542–546.

Ross, C. A., Siddiqui, A. R., & Matas, M. (1987). DSM-III: Problems in diagnosis of paranoia and obsessive–compulsive disorder. *Canadian Journal of Psychiatry, 32*, 146–148.

Rowe, M. K., & Craske, M. G. (1998). Effects of an expanding-spaced vs. massed exposure schedule on fear reduction and return of fear. *Behaviour Research and Therapy, 36*, 701–717.

Safer, D. L., Wenegrat, B., & Roth, W. T. (1997). Risperidone in the treatment of delusional parasitosis: A case report. *Journal of Clinical Psychopharmacology, 17*, 131–132.

Salkovskis, P. M. (1989). Somatic problems. In K. Hawton, P. M. Salkovskis, J. Kirk, & D. M. Clark (Eds.), *Cognitive behaviour therapy for psychiatric problems: A practical guide* (pp. 235–276). Oxford, UK: Oxford University Press.

Salkovskis, P. M., & Warwick, H. M. (1986). Morbid preoccupations, health anxiety and reassurance: A cognitive-behavioural approach to hypochondriasis. *Behaviour Research and Therapy, 24*, 597–602.

Salkovskis, P. M., & Warwick, H. M. (2000). Making sense of hypochondriasis: A cognitive theory of health anxiety. In G. J. G. Asmundson, S. Taylor, & B. J. Cox (Eds.), *Health anxiety: Clinical and research perspectives on hypochondriasis and related conditions* (pp. 46–64). New York: Wiley.

Salkovskis, P. M., & Warwick, H. M. (2001). Meaning, misinterpretations, and medicine: A cognitive-behavioral approach to understanding health anxiety and hypochondriasis. In V. Starcevic & D. R. Lipsitt (Eds.), *Hypochondriasis: Modern perspectives on an ancient malady* (pp. 202–222). New York: Oxford University Press.

Sato, T., Takeichi, M., Shirahama, M., Fukui T., & Gude, J. K. (1995). Doctor shopping patients and users of alternative medicine among Japanese primary care patients. *General Hospital Psychiatry, 17*, 115–125.

Sayar, K., Ebrinc, S., & Ak, I. (2001). Alexithymia in patients with antisocial personality disorder in a military hospital setting. *Israel Journal of Psychiatry and Related Sciences, 38*, 81–87.

Scarone, S., & Gambini, O. (1991). Delusional hypochondriasis: Nosographic evaluation, clinical course and therapeutic outcome of 5 cases. *Psychopathology, 24*, 179–184.

Schatz, I. J. (1986). *Orthostatic hypotension.* Philadelphia: Davis.

Schmidt, A. J. M. (1994). Bottlenecks in the diagnosis of hypochondriasis. *Comprehensive Psychiatry, 35*, 306–315.

Schmidt, A. J. M., Wolfs-Takens, D. J., Oosterlaan, J., & van den Hout, M. A. (1994). Psychological mechanisms in hypochondriasis: Attention-induced physical symptoms without sensory stimulation. *Psychotherapy and Psychosomatics, 61*, 117–120.

Schwartz, S. M., Gramling, S. E., & Mancini, T. (1994). The influence of life stress, personality, and learning history on illness behavior. *Journal of Behavior Therapy and Experimental Psychiatry, 25*, 135–142.

Scrignar, C. B. (1974). Exposure time as the main hierarchy variable. *Journal of Behavior Therapy and Experimental Psychiatry, 5*, 153–155.

Seaward, B. L. (1997). *Managing stress: Principles and strategies for health and wellbeing* (2nd ed.). Boston: Jones & Bartlett.

Sharpe, M., & Bass, C. (1992). Pathophysiological mechanisms in somatization. *International Review of Psychiatry, 4*, 81–97.

Sharpe, M., Bass, C., & Mayou, R. (1995). An overview of the treatment of functional somatic symptoms. In R. Mayou, C. Bass, & M. Sharpe (Eds.), *Treatment of functional somatic symptoms* (pp. 66–86). Oxford, UK: Oxford University Press.

Shear, M. K., Kligfield, P., Harshfield, G., Devereux, R. B., Polan, J. J., Mann, J. J., Pickering, T., & Frances, A. J. (1987). Cardiac rate and rhythm in panic patients. *American Journal of Psychiatry, 144*, 633–637.

Sheppard, N. P., O'Loughlin, S., & Malone, J. P. (1986). Psychogenic skin disease: A review of 35 cases. *British Journal of Psychiatry, 149*, 636–643.

Sifneos, P. E. (1972). *Short-term psychotherapy and emotional crisis.* Cambridge, MA: Harvard University Press.

Simons, A. D., Garfield, S. L., & Murphy, G. E. (1984). The process of change in cognitive therapy and pharmacotherapy for depression: Changes in mood and cognition. *Archives of General Psychiatry, 41*, 45–51.

Slavney, P. R. (1987). The hypochondriacal patient and Murphy's "law." *General Hospital Psychiatry, 9*, 302–303.

Smeets, G., de Jong, P. J., & Mayer, B. (2000). If you suffer from a headache, then you have a brain tumour: Domain-specific reasoning "bias" and hypochondriasis. *Behaviour Research and Therapy, 38*, 763–776.

Smith, R. C. (1985). A clinical approach to the somatizing patient. *Journal of Family Practice, 21*, 294–301.

Smith, T. W., Snyder, C. R., & Perkins, S. C. (1983). The self-serving function of hypochondriacal complaints: Physical symptoms as self-handicapping strategies. *Journal of Personality and Social Psychology, 44*, 787–797.

Snyder, A. G., & Stanley, M. A. (2001). Hypochondriasis and health anxiety in the elderly. In G. J. G. Asmundson, S. Taylor, & B. J. Cox (Eds.), *Health anxiety: Clinical and research perspectives on hypochondriasis and related conditions* (pp. 246–274). New York: Wiley.

Songer, D. A, & Roman, B. (1996). Treatment of somatic delusional disorder with atypical antipsychotic agents. *American Journal of Psychiatry, 153*, 578–579.

Speckens, A. E. M. (2001). Assessment of hypochondriasis. In V. Starcevic & D. R. Lipsitt (Eds.), *Hypochondriasis: Modern perspectives on an ancient malady* (pp. 61–88). New York: Oxford University Press.

Speckens, A. E. M., Spinhoven, P., Sloekers, P. P. A., Bolk, J. H., & van Hemert, A. M. (1996). A validation study of the Whiteley Index, the Illness Attitudes Scales, and the Somatosensory Amplification Scale in general medical and general practice patients. *Journal of Psychosomatic Research, 40*, 95–104.

Speckens, A. E. M., Spinhoven, P., van Hemert, A. M., & Bolk, J. H. (2000). The Reassurance Questionnaire (RQ): Psychometric properties of a self-report questionnaire. *Psychological Medicine, 30*, 841–847.

Speckens, A. E. M., Spinhoven, P., van Hemert, A. M., Bolk, J. H., & Hawton, K. E. (1997). Cognitive behavioural therapy for unexplained physical symptoms: Process and prognostic factors. *Behavioural and Cognitive Psychotherapy, 25*, 291–294.

Speckens, A. E. M., van Hemert, A. M., Spinhoven, P., Hawton, K., Bolk, J. H., & Rooijmans, H. G. M. (1995). Cognitive behavioural therapy for medically unexplained physical symptoms: A randomized controlled trial. *British Medical Journal, 311*, 1328–1332.

Starcevic, V., & Lipsitt, D. R. (2001). *Hypochondriasis: Modern perspectives on an ancient malady.* New York: Oxford University Press.

Stefanek, M., Hartmann, L., & Nelson, W. (2001). Risk-reduction mastectomy: Clinical issues and research. *Journal of the National Cancer Institute, 93*, 1297–1306.

Stein, D. J. (2000). Neurobiology of the obsessive–compulsive spectrum disorders. *Biological Psychiatry, 47*, 296–304.

Steptoe, A., & Noll, A. (1997). The perception of bodily sensations, with special reference to hypochondriasis. *Behaviour Research and Therapy, 35*, 901–910.

Stern, R., & Fernandez, M. (1991). Group cognitive and behavioural treatment for hypochondriasis. *British Medical Journal, 303*, 1229–1231.

Stern, R., & Marks, I. (1973). Brief and prolonged flooding: A comparison in agoraphobic patients. *Archives of General Psychiatry, 28*, 270–276.

Stewart, S. H., & Watt, M. C. (2000). Illness Attitude Scale dimensions and their association with anxiety-related constructs in a non-clinical sample. *Behaviour Research and Therapy, 38*, 83–99.

Stewart, S. H., & Watt, M. C. (2001). Assessment of health anxiety. In G. J. G. Asmundson, S. Taylor, & B. J. Cox (Eds.), *Health anxiety: Clinical and research perspectives on hypochondriasis and related conditions* (pp. 95–131). New York: Wiley.

Stone, A. A., & Neale, J. M. (1981). Hypochondriasis and tendency to adopt the sick role as moderators of the relationship between life-events and somatic symptomatology. *British Journal of Medical Psychology, 54*, 75–81.

Stone, A. B. (1993). Treatment of hypochondriasis with clomipramine. *Journal of Clinical Psychiatry, 54*, 200–201.

Sureda, B., Valdes, M., Jodar, I., & de Pablo, J. (1999). Alexithymia, Type A behaviour and bulimia nervosa. *European Eating Disorders Review, 7*, 286–292.

Taylor, G. J. (2000). Recent developments in alexithymia theory and research. *Canadian Journal of Psychiatry, 45*, 134–142.

Taylor, S. (1995). Assessment of obsessions and compulsions: Reliability, validity, and sensitivity to treatment effects. *Clinical Psychology Review, 15*, 261–296.

Taylor, S. (1996). Meta-analysis of cognitive-behavioral treatments for social phobia. *Journal of Behavior Therapy and Experimental Psychiatry, 27*, 1–9.

Taylor, S. (1999). *Anxiety sensitivity.* Mahwah, NJ: Erlbaum.

Taylor, S. (2000). *Understanding and treating panic disorder.* New York: Wiley.

Taylor, S. (2001). Invited article: Breathing retraining in the treatment of panic disorder: Efficacy, caveats, and indications. *Scandinavian Journal of Behaviour Therapy, 30*, 1–8.

Taylor, S. (2004). Understanding and treating health anxiety: A cognitive-behavioural approach. *Cognitive and Behavioral Practice, 11.*

Taylor, S. E. (1999). *Health psychology* (4th ed.). Boston: McGraw-Hill.

Taylor, S. E., & Brown, J. D. (1988). Illusion and well-being: A social psychological perspective on mental health. *Psychological Bulletin, 103*, 193–210.

Tearnan, B. H., Goetsch, V., & Adams, H. E. (1985). Modification of disease phobia using a multifaceted exposure program. *Journal of Behavior Therapy and Experimental Psychiatry, 16*, 57–61.

Thompson, W. G. (1984). The irritable bowel. *Gut, 25*, 305–320.

Thompson, W. G. (1989). *Gut reactions: Understanding symptoms of the digestive tract.* New York: Plenum Press.

Torgersen, S. (1986). Genetics of somatoform disorders. *Archives of General Psychiatry, 43*, 502–505.

Trabert, W. (1995). 100 years of delusional parasitosis: Meta-analysis of 1,223 case reports. *Psychopathology, 28*, 238–246.

Tsao, J. C. I., & Craske, M. G. (2000). Timing of treatment and return of fear: Effects of massed, uniform-, and expanding-spaced exposure schedules. *Behavior Therapy, 31*, 479–497.

Tyrer, P., Lee, I., & Alexander, J. (1980). Awareness of cardiac function in anxious, phobic and hypochondriacal patients. *Psychological Medicine, 10*, 171–174.

Tyrer, P., Seivewright, N., & Behr, G. (1999). A specific treatment for hypochondriasis? *Lancet, 353*, 672–673.

Ungvari, G., & Vladar, K. (1986). Pimozide treatment for delusion of infestation. *Activitas Nervosa Superior, 28*, 103–107.

Vaillant, G. (1984). The disadvantages of the DSM-III outweigh its advantages. *American Journal of Psychiatry, 141,* 542–545.

van Etten, M., & Taylor, S. (1998). Comparative efficacy of treatments for post-traumatic stress disorder: A meta-analysis. *Clinical Psychology and Psychotherapy, 5,* 126–145.

Vervaeke, G. A. C., Bouman, T. K., & Valmaggia, L. R. (1999). Attentional correlates of illness anxiety in a non-clinical sample. *Psychotherapy and Psychosomatics, 68,* 22–25.

Visser, S., & Bouman, T. K. (1992). Cognitive-behavioural approaches in the treatment of hypochondriasis: Six single case cross-over studies. *Behaviour Research and Therapy, 30,* 301–306.

Visser, S., & Bouman, T. K. (2001). The treatment of hypochondriasis: Exposure plus response prevention vs. cognitive therapy. *Behaviour Research and Therapy, 39,* 423–442.

Viswanathan, R., & Paradis, C. (1991). Treatment of cancer phobia with fluoxetine. *American Journal of Psychiatry, 148,* 1090.

Walitzer, K. S., Dermen, K. H., & Connors, G. J. (1999). Strategies for preparing clients for treatment. *Behavior Modification, 23,* 129–151.

Walker, J., Vincent, N., Furer, P., Cox, B., & Kjernisted, K. (1999). Treatment preference in hypochondriasis. *Journal of Behavior Therapy and Experimental Psychiatry, 30,* 251–258.

Walter, G. (1991). An unusual monosymptomatic hypochondriacal delusion presenting as self-insertion of a foreign body into the urethra. *British Journal of Psychiatry, 159,* 283–284.

Warwick, H. (1992). Provision of appropriate and effective reassurance. *International Review of Psychiatry, 4,* 76–80.

Warwick, H. M. C. (1995). Treatment of hypochondriasis. In R. Mayou, C. Bass, & M. Sharpe (Eds.), *Treatment of functional somatic symptoms* (pp. 163–174). Oxford, UK: Oxford University Press.

Warwick, H. M., Clark, D. M., Cobb, A. M., & Salkovskis, P. M. (1996). A controlled trial of cognitive-behavioural treatment of hypochondriasis. *British Journal of Psychiatry, 169,* 189–195.

Warwick, H. M., & Marks, I. M. (1988). Behavioural treatment of illness phobia and hypochondriasis: A pilot study of 17 cases. *British Journal of Psychiatry, 152,* 239–241.

Warwick, H. M., & Salkovskis, P. M. (1985). Reassurance. *British Medical Journal, 290,* 1028.

Warwick, H. M., & Salkovskis, P. M. (1989). Cognitive and behavioural characteristics of primary hypochondriasis. *Scandinavian Journal of Behaviour Therapy, 18,* 85–92.

Warwick, H. M., & Salkovskis, P. M. (1990). Hypochondriasis. *Behaviour Research and Therapy, 28,* 105–117.

Warwick, H. M. C., & Salkovskis, P. M. (2001). Cognitive-behavioral treatment of hypochondriasis. In V. Starcevic & D. R. Lipsitt (Eds.), *Hypochondriasis: Modern perspectives on an ancient malady* (pp. 314–328). New York: Oxford University Press.

Watt, M. C., & Stewart, S. H. (2000). Anxiety sensitivity mediates the relationships between childhood learning experiences and elevated hypochondriacal concerns in young adulthood. *Journal of Psychosomatic Research, 49,* 107–118.

Weinstein, M. C., Berwick, D. M., Goldman, P. A., Murphy, J. M., & Barsky, A. J. (1989). A comparison of three psychiatric screening tests using receiver operating characteristic (ROC) analysis. *Medical Care, 27,* 593–607.

Weintraub, E., & Robinson, C. (2000). A case of monsymptomic hypochondriacal psychosis treated with olanzapine. *Annals of Clinical Psychiatry, 1,* 247–249.

Wells, A. (1997). *Cognitive therapy of anxiety disorders.* New York: Wiley.

Wells, A. (2000). *Emotional disorders and metacognition.* New York: Wiley.

Wells, A., & Hackmann, A. (1993). Imagery and core beliefs in health anxiety: Contents and origins. *Behavioural and Cognitive Psychotherapy, 21,* 265–273.

Wesner, R. B., & Noyes, R. (1991). Imipramine: An effective treatment for illness phobia. *Journal of Affective Disorders, 22,* 43–48.

Wessely, S. (2000). Responding to mass psychogenic illness. *New England Journal of Medicine, 342,* 129–130.

Wetchler, J. L. (1994). Brief strategic treatment of a male with HIV hypochondria. *Journal of Family Psychotherapy, 5,* 1–9.

White, K. L., Williams, T. F., & Greenberg, B. G. (1961). The ecology of medical care. *New England Journal of Medicine, 265,* 885–892.

Whitehead, W. E., Busch, C. M., Heller, B. R., & Costa, P. T. (1986). Social learning influences on menstrual symptoms and illness behavior. *Health Psychology, 5,* 13–23.

Whitehead, W. E., Crowell, M. D., Heller, B. R., Robinson, J. C., Schuster, M. M., & Horn, S. (1994). Modeling and reinforcement of the sick role during childhood predicts adult illness behavior. *Psychosomatic Medicine, 56,* 541–550.

Whitehead, W. E., Winget, C., Fedoravicius, A. S., Wooley, S., & Blackwell, B. (1981). Learned illness behavior in patients with irritable bowel syndrome and peptic ulcer. *Digestive Diseases and Sciences, 27,* 202–208.

Williams, J. B. W., Gibbon, M., First, M. B., Spitzer, R. L., Davis, M., Borus, J., Howes, M. J., Kane, J., Pope, H. G., Rounsaville, B., & Wittchen, H.-U. (1992). The Structured Clinical Interview for DSM-III-R (SCID): II. Multisite test–retest reliability. *Archives of General Psychiatry, 49,* 630–636.

Williamson, P. N. (1984). An intervention for hypochondriacal complaints. *Clinical Gerontologist, 3,* 64–68.

Wilson, A., Hickie, I., Lloyd, A., Hadzi-Pavlovic, D., Boughton, C., Dwyer, J., & Wakefield, D. (1994). Longitudinal study of outcome of chronic fatigue syndrome. *British Medical Journal, 308,* 756–759.

Wise, T. N., Mann, L. S., Hryvniak, M., Mitchell, J. D., & Hill, B. (1990). The relationship between alexithymia and abnormal illness behavior. *Psychotherapy and Psychosomatics, 54,* 18–25.

Wittchen, H.-U. (1996). Critical issues in the evaluation of comorbidity of psychiatric disorders. *British Journal of Psychiatry, 168 (Suppl.),* 9–16.

Woods, S. M., Natterson, J., & Silverman, J. (1966). Medical students' disease: Hypochondriasis in medical education. *Journal of Medical Education, 41,* 785–790.

Wooley, S. C., Blackwell, B., & Winget, C. (1978). A learning theory model of chronic illness behavior: Theory, treatment, and research. *Psychosomatic Medicine,* *40,* 379–401.

Yaryura-Tobias, J. A., & Neziroglu, F. A. (1997). *Obsessive–compulsive disorder spectrum.* Washington, DC: American Psychiatric Press.

Yehuda, R., Steiner, A., Kahana, B., Binder-Byrnes, K., Southwick, S. M., Zemelman, S., & Giller, E. L. (1997). Alexithymia in Holocaust survivors with and without PTSD. *Journal of Traumatic Stress, 10,* 93–100.

Yorston, G. (1997). Treatment of delusional parasitosis with sertindole. *Journal of Geriatric Psychiatry, 12,* 1127–1128.

Zalaquett, C. P., & Wood, R. J. (1997). *Evaluating stress: A book of resources.* Landham, MD: Scarecrow Press.

Zlotnick, C., Mattia, J. I., & Zimmerman, M. (2001). The relationship between posttraumatic stress disorder, childhood trauma and alexithymia in an outpatient sample. *Journal of Traumatic Stress, 14,* 177–188.

Zomer, S. F., de Wit, R. F. E., van Bronswijk, J. E. H. M., Nabarro, G., & van Vloten, W. A. (1998). Delusions of parasitosis: A psychiatric disorder to be treated by dermatologists?: An analysis of 33 patients. *British Journal of Dermatology, 138,* 1030–1032.

Zonderman, A. B., Heft, M. W., & Costa, P. T. (1985). Does the Illness Behavior Questionnaire measure abnormal illness behavior? *Health Psychology, 4,* 425–436.

Index

t indicated material in a table, *f* indicated material in a figure